PIONEERS

In

Surgical
Gastroenterology

Edited by

Walford Gillison & Henry Buchwald

tfm Publishing Limited
Castle Hill Barns
Harley
Shrewsbury
SY5 6LX, UK

Tel: +44 (0)1952 510061
Fax: +44 (0)1952 510192
E-mail: nikki@tfmpublishing.com
Web site: www.tfmpublishing.com

Design: Nikki Bramhill, tfm publishing Ltd.
Typesetting: Nikki Bramhill, tfm publishing Ltd.

Cover images:
Top row (from left to right): Theodor Billroth (1829-1894). Reproduced with permission from Elsevier. Rutledge RH. In commemoration of Theodor Billroth on the 150th anniversary of his birth. *Surgery* 1979; 86: 688; John Hunter (1728-1793). Reproduced with permission from the Royal College of Surgeons of England; Andreas Vesalius (1514-1564). Reproduced with permission from BIUM/Service Comptabilite, MME Martin, 12 rue de l'Ecole de Médecine, 75270 Paris CEDEX 06; Ambroise Paré (1510-1590). Reproduced with permission from the Académie de Médecine, Paris, France.
Bottom row (from left to right): Theodor Kocher (1841-1917). Reproduced with permission from the National Library of Medicine, Bethesda, Maryland, USA; Louis Pasteur (1822-1895). Reproduced with permission from the Académie de Médecine, Paris, France; Owen H Wangensteen (1898-1981). Reproduced with permission from the National Library of Medicine, Bethesda, Maryland, USA; Joseph Lister (1827-1912). Reproduced with permission from the Wellcome Library, London.
Background image of Vesalius' drawing. Reproduced with permission from the Classics of Surgery Library (Gyphon Editions), New York, USA.

First Edition   © 2007

ISBN 1 903378 35 4

Printed by Gutenberg Press Ltd., Gudja Road, Tarxien, PLA 19, Malta.
Tel: +356 21897037; Fax: +356 21800069.

Contents

Contributors

Paul Benfredj MD Médecin adjoint de l'hôpital Bellan, Paris, France, Praticien attaché du Centre Hospitalier de Versailles, France

Henry Buchwald MD PhD FACS Professor of Surgery and Biomedical Engineering, Owen H. and Sarah Davidson Wangensteen Chair in Experimental Surgery Emeritus, University of Minnesota, Minnesota, USA

Robert E Bulander MD Surgical Resident, Department of Surgery, University of Minnesota School of Medicine, Minneapolis, USA

Dick C Busman MD PhD Emeritus Consultant Surgeon, Leeuwarden, The Netherlands

Michael KH Crumplin FRCS Honorary Curator and Archivist at the Royal College of Surgeons of England and Honorary Consultant Surgeon, Wrexham Maelor Hospital, Wrexham, UK

James B Elder MD FRCS Ed Eng & Glasgow Emeritus Professor and Consultant Surgeon, North Staffordshire Hospitals, Stoke-on-Trent, University of Keele, Staffordshire, UK

Walford Gillison FRCS Ed FRCS Emeritus Consultant Surgeon, Kidderminster General Hospital, Kidderminster, UK and Honorary Consultant Surgeon, City Hospital, Birmingham, UK

Jay L Grosfeld MD Emeritus Lafayette Page Professor of Surgery, Indiana University School of Medicine, Indianapolis, USA

Glyn G Jamieson MD FRCSA FRCS Dorothy Morlock Professor of Surgery, University of Adelaide, Australia

John R Kirkup MD FRCS Emeritus Consultant Orthopaedic Surgeon, Royal United Hospital, Bath, Somerset, UK and Honorary Curator, Historical Instrument Collection, Royal College of Surgeons of England, London, UK

Bernard Launois MD FACS FRCST (Hon) Emeritus Professor of Surgery, Department of Surgery, University of Rennes, France and University of Adelaide, Australia

Anders F Mellgren MD PhD Adjunct Associate Professor, Department of Surgery, University of Minnesota School of Medicine, Minneapolis, USA

Abdool R Moossa MD FRCS (Eng & Edin) FACS Professor of Surgery and Emeritus Chairman, Associate Dean and Special Counsel to the Vice Chancellor for Health Sciences, Director of Tertiary and Quarternary Referral Services, UCSD Thornton Hospital, San Diego, California, USA

John F Murray DA FRCA Emeritus Consultant Anaesthetist, Kidderminster General Hospital, Kidderminster, UK

John Nicholls MD FRCS EBSQ (Coloproctology) St. Mark's Hospital, Harrow, UK

Johan F Nordenstam MD Post Doctoral Associate, Department of Surgery, University of Minnesota School of Medicine, Minneapolis, USA

David A Rothenberger MD Professor and Interim Chair, Department of Surgery, University of Minnesota School of Medicine, Minneapolis, USA

Luis Ruso MD Professor of Surgery, Department of Surgery, Hospital Maciel, University of Montevideo, Uruguay

Felicien M Steichen MD FACS Professor of Surgery, New York Medical College, New York, USA

Jackie Y Tracey MD Postdoctoral Fellow in Surgery, UCSD Thornton Hospital, San Diego, California, USA

David FL Watkin MChir FRCS Emeritus Consultant Surgeon, Leicester Royal Infirmary, Leicester, UK

Foreword

Sir Isaac Newton said: "If I have seen further it is by standing on the shoulders of giants."[1] True, but giants have not been right all the time. This book aims to illustrate where the giants have gone wrong, and how subsequent pioneers have got back on the right track to make modern surgery what it is today. For example, the surgical giant Mikulicz was a very astute clinician, a real pioneer in oesophagoscopy and oesophageal cancer, but for many years misled the medical world by labelling achalasia as 'cardiospasm'.

The book's title was chosen with great care; a comprehensive book on the history of surgical gastroenterology would have to be in several volumes, be beyond the pockets of the people we wanted to reach, and run the risk of gathering dust in large university or hospital shelves. While most of the historical events have been gleaned from books written in the English language and journals, we are obliged to our authors fluent in other languages who have helped with the necessary translations to broaden the scope to discoveries in the rest of the world.

By choosing *Pioneers in Surgical Gastroenterology*, we have unashamedly chosen the pioneers we wanted to include, and regretfully excluded many others. We wanted to recount memorable anecdotes whenever possible, to illustrate surgical principles, and have as many 'aides de mémoire' for the students and trainees of the future. Our definition of a pioneer did not include that person having to be a practising surgeon, not did he or she have to be deceased. Furthermore, we wanted to produce a strong reference section for each chapter, to help researchers as well as medical historians.

Teamwork in a multiple author book is essential. As practising surgeons, it has been a bonus to have made new friendships among our chapter authors, whose expertise has been appreciated in putting this book together. Their input on their own and on other chapters has been invaluable; furthermore, this whole team has contributed to the final chapter, which we believe will be a useful 'ready reckoner' for checking up on these remarkable pioneers.

The target readership

◆ The surgical trainee with sufficient fire in his or her belly who might want to know how surgical gastroenterology arrived, and who needs to know what has been tried before to avoid repetition.

◆ The professor, consultant, or senior surgeon who wants to put memorable flesh on the bare bones of a lecture, tutorial or ward round.

◆ The scientific surgeon needing a starting point in any major gastroenterological research. Our illustrations may well provide the first two or three slides for a thesis or presentation. What better start to a presentation on gastric cancer than a portrait of Theodor Billroth?

◆ The medical student or trainee who appreciates a good story and requires an inkling of which career direction to choose. For example, a firm grasp of our chapter on "The Challenge of Intestinal Obstruction" would enable a basic knowledge of what is in debate in a modern Intensive Care Unit.

◆ Finally anyone, medical or non-medical, with an enquiring mind on what problems our pioneers faced, given the facilities of their time, and how they tried to alleviate and sometimes cure their patients of some desperate conditions.

Our own discoveries on writing this book

In Chapter 1, we discovered that contrary to the commonly held belief, the Roman Catholic Church was not guilty of forbidding dissection in halls of learning throughout the centuries after Galen's death about 200 AD. It was the sensible practice of boiling the deceased down to bare bones after wars that was prohibited. We were surprised to learn that Vesalius during his lifetime would have regarded himself as a 'Galenist', despite being the very person who destroyed Galen's alleged infallibility.

In Chapter 2, we realised that although nitrous oxide was processed commercially by the eminent Humphrey Davy in 1880, it took about 40 years until some dentists realised the clinical importance of a popular fairground recreational drug. Despite the lack of fast communications to spread the news, once the public demonstration in Boston had taken place in October 1846, a surgeon across the Atlantic painlessly amputated a limb in a matter of seconds, using this means of pain relief only two months later. This historic moment was witnessed by a medical student called Joseph Lister who was to become the father of antiseptic surgery.

In Chapter 3, we learned that others had carried out aseptic surgery long before Lister, but they could not have appreciated the full significance of their results. Had they done so they could have saved hundreds of lives in their time. The attacks against Lister and the neglect of his message in his own country were no surprise. True it is indeed that "a prophet is not without honour save in his own country" [2].

In Chapter 4, it was unbelievable to us that Chevalier Jackson had to fight for 20 years in America before commercial caustics and other noxious substances were required to be properly labelled to avoid severe damage to the oesophagus and stomach.

Chapter 5 deals with the management of morbid obesity, which many would think was not history but modern contemporary surgery. Procedures carried out a few years ago are indeed history. Morbid obesity is now known as a serious global gastroenterological problem and bariatric surgery is today the only effective therapy available for this disease.

Most students at all levels may have heard of Theodor Billroth and the first surviving gastrectomy. Digging deep into the accounts of these events, Chapter 6 reveals how the impact of this success at the time was sensational, and thus began the reluctant relinquishing of many gastrointestinal disorders from physicians to surgeons. It is no surprise now that the tables have been turned since the discovery and treatment of the *Helicobacter* organism.

In Chapter 7, we found English language books should never have summarised Courvoisier's findings as 'Courvoisier's Law'. It should now, as stated in Chapters 7 and 8, be referred to as the 'Courvoisier-Terrier guide or rule'. We realise, since asking Professor Launois to write the chapter, that would-be liver surgeons must be thoroughly familiar with the distribution of the eight segments of the portal vein, hepatic artery and bile duct derivatives to best manage liver trauma efficiently and relieve obstructive jaundice from whatever cause, to offer the chance of cure.

In Chapters 9 and 10, we came to realise how patients with intestinal obstruction, from whatever cause, were killed in large numbers not because of their surgeons' technical failures, but because of ignorance of the all important physiological fluid and electrolyte imbalances. We learned that the belief in nebulous 'toxins' were to contribute to this ignorance for some time.

In Chapter 11, we are told the fascinating story of the origins of stapling in surgery. It was a surprise to learn that during the unsuccessful quest for a revolutionary method of saving and storing blood in the Soviet Union, came the discovery of stapling devices. One stapler, encountered as a paperweight in a patent office, led to the development of a universal instrument for dividing, sealing or anastomosing parts of the alimentary tract with user-friendly disposable cartridges. Now that minimally invasive surgery has come to stay, stapling devices are now able to pass through cannulas to provide safe, quick and less painful gastrointestinal manouevres. As the great American scientist and politician Benjamin Franklin said in 1748: "Remember that time is money!" [3].

In Chapter 12, we learned that while Littré can be fairly remembered for the hernia containing Meckel's diverticulum, the more common right inguinal hernia containing an appendix should be remembered as 'Amyand's hernia', as it was he who succeeded in the first recorded appendicectomy. The laparoscopic removal of an appendix once scorned as an expensive way of emulating the routine open operation, can now be realised as a significant way of reducing the unnecessary removal of normal appendices. Unlike the surgeon doing a standard appendicectomy, the laparoscopist is not obliged to remove a normal appendix. This surely must be good news for health economists.

Chapter 14 on colorectal cancer describes the questioning of a number of old wives' tales, such as the 5cm rule for rectal cancer, and the reduction of time-consuming staged bowel resections including emergencies. This has resulted in modern surgeons providing a shorter hospital stay and better survival and quality of life.

Chapter 15 on peri-anal disease includes a host of abnormal functional problems, which if it were not for sound physiological investigations, might well have left the patients and proctologists in the Middle Ages. For example, the revelation that various military battles in history may have had different durations and outcomes because of acutely thrombosed piles during various heat of the moment episodes was indeed an eye-opener!

Where one individual made the outstanding contribution, authors were encouraged to include an extended biography.

Synchronous advances

We found that advances in the past have often been duplicated or reciprocated, not because of plagiarism, but because the technological advances of that particular period of time allowed certain procedures to become feasible. Despite the increasing exchange of ideas globally, some pioneers, unaware of another's existence, coincided with the same procedure or philosophy.

As discussed in Chapter 6, Walther Heinecke devised his simple pyloroplasty in 1886 and Johann von Mikulicz independently the year after. To keep the proverbial peace between these surgical giants, the pyloroplasty was hyphenated to the Heinecke-Mikulicz pyloroplasty.

In 1889, Terrier found his landmark physical sign of an easily palpable gallbladder in obstructive jaundice was usually associated with malignant disease at or near the ampulla. When Ludwig Courvoisier published the same message the next year, again, it was decided diplomatically in France that the rule or guideline should be named the 'Courvoisier-Terrier rule'.

Following the very public appendix abscess operation on royalty in 1902, the floodgates opened around the world for appendicectomies here, there and everywhere, several times with a fatal outcome. In 1902, Albert Ochsner realised many subsiding appendix masses could be allowed to settle and have a safe appendicectomy perhaps after three months; so too, James Sherren realised and published this wise regime three years later, and so this was since called the 'Ochsner-Sherren regime'.

Finally, in recent years, François Dubois in 1989 had published a successful series of laparoscopic cholecystectomies, and in the very same year, a not too far distance away, his compatriot Jacques Perissat demonstrated a visual recording of a very similar procedure at an international meeting across the Atlantic Ocean.

Serendipidity

Good luck has played a part in science as every schoolboy and schoolgirl knows. In 1911, Conrad Ramstedt was operating on an infant with pyloric stenosis who had an oedematous hypertrophied pyloric muscle. Ramstedt wanted to perform the then established operation of extramucosal pyloroplasty, but his sutures kept cutting out. As Professor Grosfeld described in Chapter 16, Ramstedt was forced to leave the myotomy alone, only to find the child not only survived but subsequently thrived.

Likewise, Ernst Heller was trying to do what we now know was the wrong drainage procedure for achalasia, which would have later caused severe reflux oesophagitis. For technical reasons he performed a myotomy as a temporising measure, which to his surprise produced an excellent result. Our staples chapter author, Felicien Steichen, while a junior, was able to see the same patient many years later and confirm the result to be long lasting.

The future

Our authors needed little persuasion to collaborate in this undertaking because they felt as we did, that both the distant and recent past are known to provide crucial aids to learning at all levels of education. We hope this book will allow students of surgical gastroenterology to expand their understanding of the past by associating contributions to the field with the people who made them - a process both pleasant and rewarding.

Walford Gillison
Henry Buchwald

References

1.   Newton Isaac (1642-1727). Letter to Robert Hooke February 5th 1676. In: *Correspondence of Isaac Newton.* HW Turnbull. 1659; 1: 416.
2.   New Testament. Matthew 5: verse 57.
3.   Benjamin Franklin (1706-1790). *Advice to a young salesman,* 1748.

The editors

The editors of this book are surgeons from the UK and USA, and the chapter authors are from Europe, North and South America, and Australia.

Walford Gillison FRCS Ed FRCS

Walford Gillison graduated from the London Hospital (now The Royal London Hospital) in 1959, and after ten years of clinical surgery experience in the UK, spent a year in research with Dr. Lloyd Nyhus at the University of Illinois in Chicago. His research work, on both sides of the Atlantic, has been focused on gastroenterology, in particular in gastro-oesophageal reflux disease (GORD), duodenogastric reflux as a component of GORD, and oesophageal cancer. He demonstrated increased oesophagitis when the GORD refluxate contained duodenal contents. He detailed the changes in oesophageal cancer in a selected UK population of five million. A Fellow of both the Royal College of Surgeons of England and Edinburgh, he has served as the President of the West Midlands Surgical Association (2000-2001), and he is an Honorary Consultant to the City Hospital of Birmingham. Medical history is a life-long, cherished avocation of Mr. Gillison.

Henry Buchwald MD PhD

Henry Buchwald attended Columbia College (valedictorian, 1954) and Columbia University College of Physicians and Surgeons. He studied under Wangensteen and Varco at the University of Minnesota, where he is Professor of Surgery and Biomedical Engineering, and was the first Owen H. and Sarah Davidson Wangensteen Chair of Experimental Surgery. He has served as President of the International Study Group for Implantable Insulin Delivery Devices, Central Surgical Association, American Society for Bariatric Surgery, and the International Federation for the Surgery of Obesity. Dr. Buchwald is best known for being the Principal Investigator of the Program on the Surgical Control of the Hyperlipidemias, the first randomised clinical trial of the lipid hypothesis to demonstrate that cholesterol lowering resulted in reductions in the comorbidities of atherosclerosis and extension of life expectancy. He is also known for being the inventor and operating surgeon for the first implantable infusion pump, and a pioneer of bariatric surgery, having performed about 4,000 cases.

Acknowledgements

A work of this magnitude has deserved our gratitude to many other people, for whom we do not have the space to acknowledge.

To start with we are indebted to Professor Dorothea Liebermann-Meffert from Munchen (Munich), Germany, who not only procured a fine portrait of Rudolf Nissen, but also details of Nissen's remarkable life described in Chapter 4. Wendy Husser of the American College of Surgeons spent time with us to advise on the size of the task and pitfalls of writing a book of this nature.

We visited several libraries besides the British and Wellcome libraries in London and the National Library of Medicine in North America. Tina Craig, Assistant Librarian at the Royal College of Surgeons of England, was a mine of information on what was, or was not, possible to achieve. Suzanne Ostini, of the Institut d'Histoire de la Médecine et de la Santé in Lausanne, Switzerland, permitted access to detailed files on César Roux. In the Netherlands, Miriam Wetzels and her staff of the Atrium Medical Centre in Heerlen, were invaluable to Dick Busman (Chapter 6). Paul Benfredj wished to thank Bibliothèque Inter-Universitaire de Médecine (History of Medicine section) in Paris for the competence and dedication of the librarians and quality of their web site. Also in Paris, Laurence Camous and Sylvie Morant at the Académie de Médecine, kindly allowed access to precious original works and provided many useful images seen in the book. Thanks too to librarian Jez Conolly at Bristol University for tidying up incomplete references at the eleventh hour.

As regards the detective work of finding manuscripts around the world and getting photocopies sent by post, we will forever be obliged to Sue McEnroe, Annette Giles, Carol Anne Regan, and David Chambers of the Medical Library at the Musgrove Park Hospital in Taunton, UK, who made the task so much easier.

John Murray (Chapters 1 and 2) is obliged to Dr. David Zuck from Chase Farm Hospital London, for advice on the history of anaesthesia. Dick Busman also wanted to thank Professor Suy from Leuven (Louvain) in Belgium who allowed him to use several fine illustrations, especially the 60 pfennig Austrian postage stamp, seen at the end of Theodor Billroth's biography.

Mick Crumplin (Chapter 12) wanted to express his thanks to the Secretary of the New Club, Edinburgh, for help, especially for the portrait of King Edward VII in that chapter. In addition, Professor Martin Kemp from Oxford corrected some minor historical errors and told us where to find the best likeness of Leonardo da Vinci by his pupil, Francesco Melzi.

We wanted to add our thanks to Bobbie Randolph, Secretary to Professor David Rothenberger, who communicated quickly at all times, organised no less than four co-authors to work together so effectively to complete Chapter 14, and achieved permission for all their images without mishap. We are everlastingly grateful to Dr. Buchwald's Secretary, Danette Oien, for her organisational skills and for maintaining a fluid flow of the information necessary to complete this task.

Ceri Keene's computer-graphic skills were highly valued for the tidying up and making presentable several of the images, especially the older ones, suitable for reproduction.

Last and by no means least, both editors are very grateful to Nikki Bramhill of tfm publishing, who added considerable editing chores to her high standards of proof reading. We believe this resulted in the book coming out many months earlier than otherwise.

Walford Gillison
Henry Buchwald
October 2006

Dedication

This book is dedicated to our wives

Susan Gillison and Emilie Buchwald

who have supported us throughout our

entire professional lifetimes and

always with great forbearance.

Chapter 1

Early origins of anatomy and surgery

John F Murray DA FRCA
Emeritus Consultant Anaesthetist, Kidderminster General Hospital, Kidderminster, UK
Walford Gillison FRCS Ed FRCS
Emeritus Consultant Surgeon, Kidderminster General Hospital, Kidderminster, UK and
Honorary Consultant Surgeon, City Hospital, Birmingham, UK

Introduction

Surgical gastroenterology has changed and is perpetually changing; like so many other branches of medicine, it owes much to the early clinicians who tended the sick. The word 'surgery' is derived from the Greek 'cheirourgia' (Cheir = hand, urgos or ergos = work). In the Oxford Dictionary a surgeon is someone who treats injury or disease by manual means. The accumulated knowledge from professional historians comes from records written or carved over 3000 years, and from archaeologists who have taken us back even further in time.

We can only speculate on the practice of medicine and surgery before records of written communication. Certainly our ancestors tripped and broke an ankle, strained a back or groin, got crushed by falling rocks or trees, or were bitten by predators exactly as can be experienced today. A foreign body in the eye or a thorn in a foot was a potential emergency. At times the patient had to act the part of the surgeon in a harshly competitive hunter-gatherer community; he or she would be left for dead if unable to keep up. There are many examples even today of climbers, drivers, fishermen and others trapped by a limb when working alone, having to perform their own amputation or perish. Although a patient may be forced to act

surgically, clearly it was better to have someone in the family or tribe with skill and experience to help, so early 'surgeons' appeared. There must have been gifted people who could promptly squeeze out splinters, straighten fractures, remove grit from eyes etc., for the survival of the human race.

Gross wrote as late as 1866 [1]: "If it were not for the frightful hemorrhage (sic) which so frequently attends them, operations would be robbed of nearly all their terror, and few men would shrink from their performance." Arrest of haemorrhage by mechanical means was slow to develop and often frustrated by infection. The means to achieve the arrest included digital pressure, limb elevation, bandages, tourniquets, cautery using hot irons, boiling oil or electrical diathermy, long and short ligatures, as well as other methods learned over several centuries.

Written evidence of disease and injury is found in the earliest human records. The many histories of medicine and surgery list the evidence that man has been mostly prepared to infringe the body's external barriers with good rather than evil intent. Evidence of trepanation of some Neolithic skulls has been noticed near fractures, with evidence of healing to prove many of the subjects survived even when several cranial holes had been made. There is a fine example of trepanation in the Jordanian National Museum in Amman.

The paths of surgery including surgical gastroenterology have followed a long, tortuous, and contentious route, fraught with wrong turnings, confrontations against local and national laws and religious institutions, as well as naked ignorance.

Stages in evolution

Attempts to relate clinical features with illness

Since the development of writing and keeping of records in Mesopotamia, payments or punishments of the priest-physicians usually depended on their successes or failures. From earliest times empirical treatments were based on observation combined with philosophical or religious concepts which inhibited proper understanding.

Hippocrates (ca 460-377 BC) was one of the first to relate symptoms and signs to all known disease. His beliefs have been quoted in several of the chapters in this book. Celsus, who lived in the 1st century AD, described many things in his writing, including rhinoplasty and the treatment of hernias, which were as advanced as any authority of the 16th century [2].

Medicine and surgery really developed from the Renaissance when the old rules in science and philosophy became challenged. At the same time widespread literacy produced a ferment of intellectual activity, which led to the development of our modern world. The acceptance, without question, of the ancient teachings of Galen (Figure 1), Hippocrates, Avicenna (Figure 8, Chapter 15) and others, gave way to critical scrutiny and the beginning of experimental method. Paracelsus (1493-1541), a shrewd clinician, and very much aware of blind repetition of past heresies, even burnt the works of the ancient authorities in public to show his contempt for them.

The importance of anatomy

It took several centuries for the enlightened to realise that to operate on the human body without an accurate knowledge of anatomy was like taking a journey into the unknown without a map. A simple example of this is described in Chapter 12; as far as it is possible to learn, no illustration of the humble human appendix had been drawn until Leonardo drew it about 1515 AD, and confirmed by Vesalius shortly after in 1543. Thus, many young people, and some of our own pioneers, such as Ernst von Bergmann and Ryerson Fowler, died from complications when this organ became inflamed, because the medical profession did not realise it was there.

The ban on dissection of the human body by the Egyptian, Greek and Roman cultures inhibited progress. Fortunately there were some exceptions. The Hindu, Sushruta, was allowed to dissect the bodies of children under the age of two [3], and around 300 BC, Herophilus of Calcedon, from the famous centre of learning at Alexandria, was permitted to dissect living criminals.

In China the phrase for surgery was 'Wai Ke' meaning science of the exterior, as distinct from 'Nei Ke' (medicine) meaning science of the interior. According to Yap and Cotterell [4], Hua T'o was a physician and surgeon about the same time as Galen. He developed massage, physiotherapy, and practised dissection in spite of the local authorities who were against it. It is uncertain as to whether his knowledge of primitive anaesthetics and surgery survived his death.

Later these authors found that the medical profession was recognised during the Tang Dynasty between 619 and 629 AD. An Imperial Medical College was set up in Ch' Ang (now Sian) with satellite institutions in the provincial towns around. About 1111 AD, 12 eminent doctors compiled the Imperial Medical Encyclopaedia as part of a movement to code medical disorders, symptoms, diagnoses and treatment. Anatomy was reintroduced allowing dissection using the bodies of rebel soldiers! Their classifications held for a long time until replaced by translated Western Medical Works several centuries later.

Galen (130-200 AD), also educated in Alexandria, gained all his anatomical knowledge from the dissection of animals including apes.

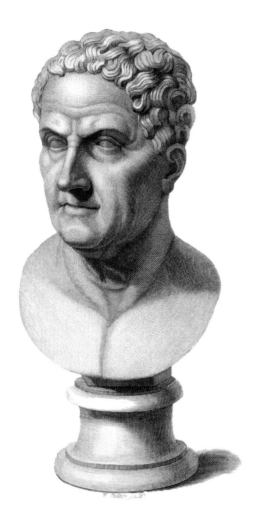

Figure 1. Claudius Galenicus (Galen) (130-200 AD). *Reproduced with permission from Argosy Books, New York, USA.*

His works remained unchallenged as a source of anatomical facts for many centuries until the Renaissance.

The Christian church, according to many histories of medicine, was said to have banned dissection, but this was a misinterpretation of the Bull *De Sepulturis* promulgated by Pope Boniface VIII in 1300 [5]. The translated text is as follows: "Persons cutting up the bodies of the dead, barbarously cooking them in order that the bones being separated from the flesh to be carried for burial in their own country, are by that very act excommunicated." Until this edict, the packaging of the dried bones had been an economic and compact way of returning warriors to their homelands from remote fields of battle. The sending of the deceased by long sea voyages was otherwise repulsive unless funds were available for them to be sent home in a barrel of wine or spirits, like Horatio Nelson who died during the battle of Trafalgar in 1805. Islam, which came to North Africa in the 7th century, also forbade dissection.

Even though dissection had been widely practised for many years, Galen's errors were rarely questioned. Mondino di Luzzi, Professor at Bologna in 1315, wrote a new compendium of anatomy which still contained many of Galen's inaccuracies. Public dissections at universities, though practised once or twice a year, failed to improve anatomical knowledge.

Whereas the Arab conquerors of North Africa inherited their learning from Alexandria, the turmoil of the 'Dark Ages' in Europe saw the disappearance of Romano-Greek traditions. When more peaceful times returned, nuns and monks cared for the sick, and controlled the universities. The lay School of Salerno, established in the 9th century, introduced Greek learning to Europe. For centuries the teaching of medicine and surgery was initially confined to the writings of the ancients whose work was accepted without question.

The Council of Tours in 1163 declared that monks should not shed blood ("Ecclesia abhorret sanguine") [6]. In consequence when they ceased the practice of surgery, uneducated barbers with no knowledge of Latin filled the vacuum. As these barbers were excluded from the universities, they were forced to acquire their knowledge by apprenticeship and experience. Doctors, who were more academically trained, continued to rely on ancient lore and ancient dogma.

Italy led Europe at the start in acquiring human anatomical knowledge. Antonio Bienvieni studied pathology and Alessandro Benedetti gave public demonstrations of dissection in Verona and Venice.

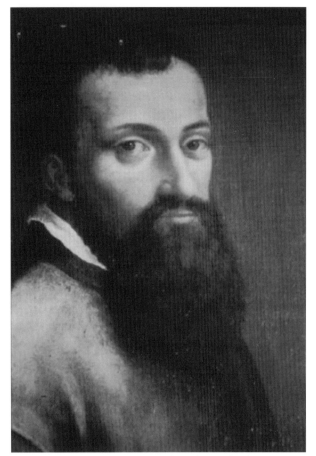

Figure 2. Andreas Vesalius (1514-1564). *Reproduced with permission from the Musée de L'histoire de la Médecine, Paris, France.*

Andreas Vesalius (Figure 2), a Fleming, who studied in Louvain, Paris, Padua, and finally Spain, was rightly named the 'father of anatomy'. He dissected extensively, having to steal parts from criminal gallows, or purchasing bodies from cut-throats or grave robbers at great risk to his life and reputation. As a result he denounced the many errors in the ancient accounts. This brought him many enemies including renowned anatomists such as Silviuc of Pario and Euctachiuc of Padua.

His great work *De Humani Corporis Fabrica Libri Septem* was first published in Basle in 1543 and later editions were enhanced by engravings in wood by Titian's pupil, Calcar. For uncertain reasons he relinquished his academic life and became a physician to Charles Vth of Spain. An ill-founded story was told about performing an autopsy on a living patient, but it is not believed by the majority of scholars today [7].

More biographical details of Vesalius are described at the end of the chapter.

William Harvey [8] was an Englishman who trained in Padua, kept animals for vivisection and lectured on surgery, but did not practise the craft. He is known for demonstrating the circulation of blood in the 17th century.

Schools of Anatomy appeared all over Europe in the 18th century. John Hunter (Figure 3), after a very rudimentary medical education, lectured in surgery and anatomy, first employed by his brother William, but later formed his own private anatomy school near Leicester Square in London.

Dissection schools were busy in the winter because in the summer heat, cadavers deteriorated too quickly without preservatives such as formalin. Before his appointment to St. George's Hospital in London, Hunter, like so many others without private means, had to obtain clinical and operative surgical

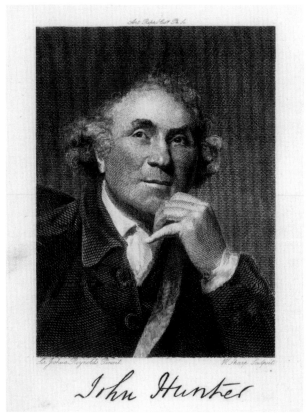

John Hunter

Figure 3. John Hunter (1728-1793). *Reproduced with permission from The Royal College of Surgeons of England.*

experience in the armed forces in order to earn a living until the 'dissecting season' came around again. To obtain the required large numbers of fresh cadavers for dissection he too had to adopt Vesalius' methods of procurement. Why did he consort with grave robbers and other characters that disobeyed the law? The first reason was because the Company of Surgeons (later the College of Surgeons) decreed that only six public dissections were permitted per year. The second reason was because Hunter was aware that the human anatomy was full of variations and anomalies in its structure, and he was also aware of the limited time available to map these structures before cadavers became repugnant.

As 'father of British surgery' and at his own private anatomy school, Hunter attracted many students from other countries, and was eventually appointed to the teaching staff of St. George's Medical School in London against fierce opposition by jealous contemporaries. Two fine student examples were Samuel Physick who later founded the early medical school in Philadelphia in the US, and the bright Astley Cooper (Figure 3, Chapter 9) who himself formed an anatomy school when appointed to Guy's Hospital in London. By the time of Hunter's death, his private human and animal anatomical and pathological collections were of such quality that they were purchased by the government and presented to the College of Surgeons. He had invested so much of his income into his famous collection, leaving few resources to provide for his widow, who was forced to earn her living as a paid companion [9].

Surgical college pioneers

Ambroise Paré (Figure 4) is given the credit of doing for surgery what Vesalius had done for anatomy. He had no knowledge of Latin, so he wrote up all his notes in French. It was a happy chance during a campaign battle in Italy that his supply of boiling tar was exhausted, so he was forced to ligature bleeding vessels and apply simple clean linen, rose-water dressings to amputation stumps. After a sleepless night he found the latter group of patients had less pain and were not inevitably subject to infection.

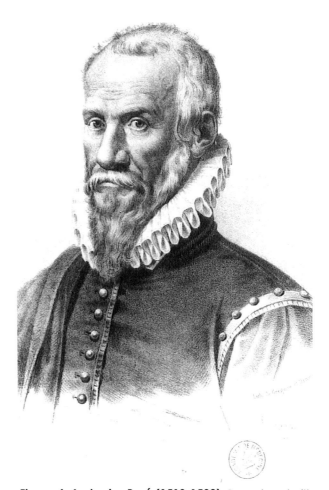

Figure 4. Ambroise Paré (1510-1590). *Reproduced with permission from the Académie de Médecine, Paris, France.*

He was renowned for his kindness and his modesty. His motto was "Je le Pansay et Dieu le guarist" ("I treated but God healed him").

Colleges of Surgeons were set up in France as early as the 14th century. Lanfranc trained at Verona, and fortunately obtained the support of King Louis IX to found the College of St. Côme in Paris. The Medical Faculty, jealous of the éclat of Paré and others, obtained the removal of surgeons from the university, not only because they had no Latin, but also because of their association with the barbers. Consequently, surgeons, barbers and bonesetters, were less given to high-flown theorising than contemporary physicians.

Bleeding, cupping and crude cautery were in use until the early 19th century. Nancy Mitford who wrote *The Sun King* (p 151) [10] said: "The surgeons did a better job than the physicians. They tied the patient to a board with linen bands and paid no attention to his screams; but they honestly tried to hurt as little as possible, and seem to have undertaken quite major procedures such as lithotomy via the perineum with some survivors." Physicians at one stage were blamed for the deaths of most of Louis XIVth's progeny because of their regimes of weekly cupping and purging of previously healthy children.

A company of barber surgeons was recognised by Edward IV of England in 1461. Barbers were prevented from operating, except for blood-letting and the pulling of teeth, following an ordinance of Henry VIII in 1540. The King also decreed that apprenticed surgeons be called 'Master', which has evolved into 'Mister', the title still given to surgeons in the UK and the Commonwealth today [11]. Richard Wiseman, who published two volumes in surgery in 1676, set up the first School of Surgery in England. Surgeons later separated from the barbers in the Company of Surgeons in 1745. The College became the Royal College by a charter granted by Queen Victoria in 1800 [12].

In Scotland [13], the City of Edinburgh granted a charter (Seal of Cause) to both barbers and surgeons in 1505. This was ratified by James IV of Scotland in 1506, in a writ which incorporated teaching responsibilities as well. King George III of the UK granted the Edinburgh College a Royal Charter in 1778. In Glasgow a unique and surviving institution was created in 1599 uniting the Colleges of Physicians and Surgeons together.

In Germany, four prestigious pioneers founded the German Surgical Society in 1872: Bernhard von Langenbeck, Friedrich von Eomarch, Theodor Billroth and Ernst von Bergmann. The journal, founded in 1860, was von Langenbeck's *Archiv fur Klinische Chirurgie*. This changed to *Langenbeck's Archives of Surgery* in 1998. In the same year the German Society of Visceral Surgery (Gastroenterological Surgery) was founded by Messrs Beger, Siewert, Bauer, Kremer and Enke [14].

According to de Moulin [15], the barbers and surgeons in the Netherlands separated in the second half of the 16th century. Their roles were strictly regulated from 1552 onwards. Barbers were not allowed to operate but surgeons retained the right to cut hair as this practice was so profitable! Philip II, who ruled Spain as well as the Netherlands, granted the right to surgeons to continue dissection of cadavers. Leyden was the first city to acquire an anatomy theatre (1595) used for both teaching and entertainment.

The story of the American College of Surgeons is that of the development and progress of surgery in America [16]. No other medical organisation, voluntarily entered into by its Fellows, has exerted such a profound influence on the discipline and art of surgery in the US. The founder was Franklin Martin, a gynaecologist, from Wisconsin, practising in Chicago, who established the journal *Surgery, Gynecology & Obstetrics* in 1905. Subsequent national clinical congresses were so popular that Martin proposed and promulgated the American College of Surgeons in 1912 during a meeting in New York City. Prestigious presidents were appointed and the future of the College became secure. Membership in 2005 reached 67,550.

The Polish Association of Surgeons had a much harder time to maintain a distinct identity because it was surrounded by political turmoil. Much credit is due to the energy, the status and determination of Ludwig Rydygier (Figure 5) [17].

He was schooled in Chelmo, and had to go to Greifswald in Germany for his medical education. As a student he was a co-founder of the Polish Student Union called 'Polonia', but he himself went to Berlin and Strasbourg to complete his studies before graduating at Greifswald in 1873. His MD thesis the next year was on the benefits and dangers of carbolic acid in surgery and obstetrics. After this he visited contemporaries in Warsaw and particularly Billroth in Vienna. His next appointments were in Chelmo and later, Krakow, where he was appointed Professor in the Jagiellian University. It was while he was there that he founded the Polish Association of Surgeons in 1889, in spite of Poland losing its nationality when annexed by the three

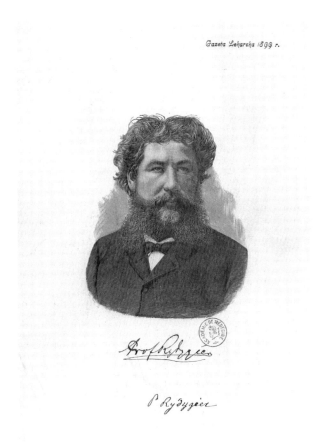

Gazeta Lekarska 1899 r.

Figure 5. Ludwig Rydygier (1850-1920). *Reproduced with permission from the Académie de Médecine, Paris, France.*

surrounding empires of Prussia, Austria and Russia. The current borders of Poland were not actually restored until 1945, following the negotiations by Stalin, Roosevelt and Churchill at Yalta.

Separation into surgical gastroenterology

Surgical gastroenterology was born as a result of the following historic events:

- availability of general and local anaesthesia from 1846 (Chapter 2);
- the increased survival following antiseptic and aseptic surgery (Chapter 3), as well as the expanding knowledge of the infective organisms and how they may be treated;

- the dramatic ripple effect following Billroth's successful resection of the distal stomach (Chapter 6). As Busman implied, most gastrointestinal conditions were managed, sometimes jealously by physicians, until this event. As a consequence, more and more patients with disorders of the alimentary tract were referred to surgeons after 1881, not only those with life-threatening alimentary conditions, but also those with less pressing problems;
- the gradual awareness of the need for proper resuscitation and better nutrition (Chapters 2 and 9), to survive major operations;
- surgeons all over the globe eventually realised that in operations from the oesophagus to the anal margin, anastomoses required a good blood supply, perfect apposition of the resection margins without tension, and finally, no distal obstruction in a reasonably nourished patient. These criteria are well described in Chapters 10 and 11;
- curative cancer surgery in gastroenterology no longer meant simple extirpation of the tumour. For patients to experience hope after an operation, it required the search for early diagnosis, preferably at the pre-malignant stage. Curative surgery required adequate clearance both proximally and distally from the tumour, and crucially, clearance of the whole regional lymphatic field.

Though many thousands of years have gone by, some things have not changed. All surgical contemporaries can remember during student days, during training, or when established, that some individual surgeons were especially gifted with an innate manual dexterity. They were swift without appearing to hurry, and at the same time gentle when handling tissues. Should these elite operators possess shrewd clinical judgement and organising ability, they became surgical 'giants'. On the subject of giants, Isaac Newton confirmed what we have since learned, when he quoted Bernard of Chartres who lived about 1130 AD: "We are like dwarfs standing on the shoulders of giants, so that we can see more than they, and things at a greater distance." [18]

Surgical gastroenterology developed in fits and starts in varying ways across the world. The colleges and legal protection societies had variable powers to maintain standards. Earlier diagnoses by endoscopists and improved radiological techniques increased both the survival and the expectations following treatment, which meant huge training implications everywhere. Some of the burden of this work has returned to the physicians who also dilate or intubate strictures safely, inject sclerosants into varices as well as bleeding peptic ulcers, and conduct screening and surveillance programmes where economically justified.

Theodor Kocher (Figure 14, Chapter 12) a surgical giant and Nobel Prize winner once said: "A good surgeon is a doctor who can operate and who knows when not to operate." It was true in his lifetime, and it is just as true for surgeons today.

Biographical footnote on Andreas Vesalius

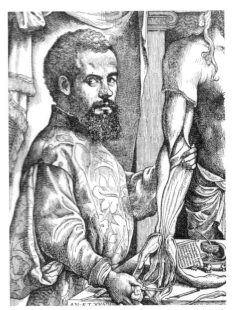

Figure 6. Andreas Vesalius (1514-1564) frontispiece. *Reproduced with permission from the Classics of Surgery Library (Gryphon Editions), New York, USA.*

This remarkable scientific and scholastic pioneer came from a distinguished medical family, a member of a fifth generation of doctors. One of his ancestors had written about Avicenna, and another was an expert of the works of both Rhazes and Hippocrates. His father was physician to Emperor Charles V of the Hapsburg dynasty for several years [19].

1514-1533

Vesalius was born in Brussels on New Year's Eve but his family moved to Nijmegen soon after, which he always regarded as home. At school he was an avid reader of the classics, and a fluent Latin scholar. He intended to study Greek and Hebrew at the University of Louvain, but he soon changed to Medicine having been fascinated with animal dissection since school [19].

1533-1537

Thanks to family influence Vesalius was able to transfer to the University of Paris which had a fine reputation, but he was disappointed to discover very few anatomical demonstrations in the basement of the Hotel Dieu Hospital. The Professor of Anatomy, Johann Guinther, who had recently translated Galen's works, was too proud to dirty his hands in the dissecting room. The disappointed Vesalius said: "I would not mind as many cuts inflicted on me as I have seen him make on man or brute, except at the banqueting table!" Another celebrated teacher was Jacques du Bois (Latinised to Sylvius) who owed fanatical allegiance to the teachings of Galen. If any human structure differed from Galen's text, Sylvius declared it was due to "the decadence and degeneration of mankind!" [19]

In fairness even Vesalius respected the works of Galen. He tried to modify Galen's writings when he encountered differences, and discreetly tried to 'update' them. Frustrated by ubiquitous ignorance, he frequented the Hill of Montfaucon at night which then was outside Paris, featuring several gallows for criminals before their incineration in a local charnel house. Fresh corpses provided him with a huge knowledge of anatomy, and bones from the 'Cemetery of the Innocents', where plague victims had been buried, provided him with knowledge of the human skeleton.

1537-1542

He had to leave Paris without graduation because of the outbreak of war, as he was technically an enemy citizen. He returned briefly to Louvain, and presented an old school friend an intact articulated skeleton purloined from a roadside gallows near his home! The authorities unofficially encouraged this practice because of the gathering prestige of his public dissections for both education and entertainment.

He left Louvain after disputes with the hierarchy about the practice of blood-letting and eventually enrolled at the prestigious University of Padua. On the way he stayed in Basle where he befriended Robert Winter, a printer, who published Vesalius' Baccalaureate. From Padua he visited Venice and met compatriot Jan van Kalkar, a member of the Titian School of Art.

In Padua he was conferred with his doctorate on one day, and appointed Professor of Surgery the next, at the age of 23! Unlike his predecessors he rolled up his sleeves and started public anatomical demonstrations at once. His rough drawings were seized upon by students, so he needed to get them drawn accurately and published properly to avoid errors and plagiarism.

Though there is much debate on who did what, it is believed as he was no mean artist, he drew most of the vascular drawings himself. Although reluctant to give credit elsewhere, he did concede that Jan Kalkar was responsible for most of the drawings of the human skeleton, which art experts subsequently recognised from Kalkar's other work. A hundred years later experts wondered if Titian himself had contributed, because several artists had been employed by Vesalius. At that time Vesalius was honoured by being asked to contribute to a modernised translation of Galen's works in Venice called *Opera Galeni*.

1543

His own work *De Humani Corporis Fabrica* and its companion to *Epitome* which shook the Renaissance world were published from Basle by his friend Oporinus, who had once been tutored by Paracelsus. However, the latter's tantrums had driven Oporinus away from medicine to work for a famous printing company called Froben. The quality of the woodcuts and of the copper plates was of the highest quality thanks to Oporinus' meticulous work. The venous drawings were most popular because of the widespread blood-letting (phlebotomy) practices by physicians and 'quacks' at that time. Another teaching aid was the use of paper 'cut-outs', as in children's books, to teach internal anatomy. The Latin text was very elaborate according to scholars but the illustrations spoke eloquently for themselves.

Once the seven books were published and he seemed established, he looked for experience in clinical surgery. He had prudently dedicated *Fabrica* to Charles V, so it was no surprise when he resigned his chair in Padua that he became Physician to the Emperor in the same year. One can easily suspect his successor in Padua, Realdus Columbus (Columbo), criticised his work out of jealousy or pique; added to that Sylvius from Paris publicly demanded Vesalius to recant!

1544-1562

During a Franco-Imperial conflict at Saint-Dizier, it transpired that Vesalius attended wounded Imperial troops on one side, while Ambroise Paré attended the enemy wounded on the other!

Vesalius was accused of a fiery temper, perhaps because he suffered fools badly. He certainly made enemies yet he also made a lot of friends. His surgical exploits were quite impressive; he was the first to drain osteomyelitis from a soldier's femur, he re-introduced the Hippocratic method of draining empyema in the chest and successfully drained a previously neglected extradural abscess from the son of Philip II who succeeded Charles V.

1562-1564

The reason for leaving Spain is subject for debate. There was much jealousy in the Spanish court and certainly he was not appreciated by Emperor Phillip. His enemies alleged he performed an autopsy on a subject while the heart was still beating. Against that rumour, Paré, who was in Spain at the time and had met Vesalius, said this had happened to another surgeon [19]. Whatever the reason, Vesalius made a journey (possibly a pilgrimage) to Jerusalem, but tragically died near the Island of Zante on the way back to resume work in Padua.

He was directly the father of anatomy, indirectly a father of surgery, and an honest perpetual seeker of truth.

References

1. Gross SD. *A System of Surgery.* 4th edition. Philadelphia: Henry Lea, 1866; Volume 1: 635.
2. Celsus A. *De Medicina.* Leipzig: Daremberg, 1859.
3. Garrison FH. *History of Medicine. The Sushruta.* WB Saunders Company, 1924: 63.
4. Yap Y, Cotterell A. *The Early Civilisation of China.* London: Weidenfeld and Nicholson, 1975: 117 and 207.
5. Pope Boniface VIII. New Advent Encyclopaedia, Volume II: 1-19.
6. Dingwall HM. *A Famous and Flourishing Society. The History of the Royal College of Surgeons of Edinburgh, 1505-2005.* Edinburgh University Press, 2005: 12.
7. BBC.co.uk. 4th November 2005. BBC-History - Andreas Vesalius (1514-1564).
8. Harvey W. *De Motu Cordis.* (The Circulation of the blood and other writings). Everyman Library. London: JM Dent and Sons, 1963.
9. Moore W. *The Knife Man.* Bantam Press, 2003: 396.
10. Mitford N. *The Sun King.* Hamish Hamilton, 1966: 151.
11. Eibel P. *Doctor or Mister.* (The Correct Appellation of British Surgeons). *Can J Surg* 1988; 31(6): 452-3.
12. Blandy JP, Lumley JSP. *The Royal College of Surgeons of England. 200 years of History at the Millennium.* The Royal College of Surgeons of England. Oxford: Blackwell Science Ltd., 2000: 18.
13. Dingwall HM. *A Famous and Flourishing Society. The History of the Royal College so Surgeons of Edinburgh, 1505-2005.* Edinburgh University Press, 2005: 25.
14. Beger H. Personal Communication.
15. De Moulin D. *A History of Surgery.* Dordrecht: Martinus Nijhoff publishers, 1988.
16. Husser W. Personal Communication. Executive editor; *Journal of the American College of Surgeons.*
17. Rudowski W. *Surgery of the Esophagus, Stomach and Small Intestine,* Fifth Edition. Nyhus LM, Wastell C, Donahue P. 1995: 382-5.
18. Letter to Robert Hooke. February 5th 1676. In: *Correspondence of Isaac Newton.* Turnbull HW, Ed. 1959; 1: 416.
19. De CM, Saunders JB, O'Malley CD. *The Illustrations from the works of Andreas Vesalius of Brussels.* New York, USA: The Classics of Surgery Library, 1993.

Chapter 2

The battles against pain and the inception of resuscitation

John F Murray DA FRCA

Emeritus Consultant Anaesthetist, Kidderminster General Hospital, Kidderminster, UK

Introduction

In the new age of experimentation, huge advances were made in physics, chemistry, mathematics and all branches of science. Isaac Newton (1642-1727) characterised gravity and laid the ground rules of mechanics and calculus. Robert Boyle (1627-1691) showed the relationship between the volume and pressure of gases and Jacques Charles (1746-1823) showed the effect of temperature on gases in 1788. In 1774, Priestley discovered oxygen which he called dephlogisticated air because he was working from the erroneous phlogiston theory. Lavoisier, a year later, showed the gas in question was present in air and called it oxygen from the Greek 'oxus' (acid) and 'gennao' (I produce) thinking it was present in all acids. He realised its connections with combustion, respiration and metabolism. By the turn of the 19th century, nitrous oxide and carbon dioxide had been isolated. Numerous chemical substances were synthesised or extracted from natural products and some of these were used subsequently in anaesthesia.

Dalton produced his law of partial pressures of gases, very relevant to anaesthesia in 1801 and subsequently, his atomic theory in 1803. The latter stated that matter is made of indivisible particles, all those of one element being alike and of the same weight. When they combine to form molecules, they do so in simple proportions. This theory opened a new chapter in our understanding of chemistry.

The relief of pain; evolution of anaesthesia

Until inhalation anaesthesia was developed in the 19th century, the pain of surgery had to be borne by the majority unless they fainted. Death from vaso-vagal shock was not unknown.

Opium and its derivatives such as laudanum had been available for centuries. Twenty minims of opium tincture (solution) was described as having been given before suturing a severe laceration of the scalp in 1829. Many other substances were administered, such as an extract of mandrake, a relative of deadly nightshade, whose value was uncertain, and hemp, as used in Chinese acupuncture. Alcohol was also used, notably in the Navy, to relieve the pain of war surgery. Hypnosis (mesmerism) had been tried with mixed success but fell into disrepute because of trickery. Baron Larrey, surgeon to Napoleon's Imperial Guard, noted that frozen limbs could be amputated painlessly, and others tried nerve compression by external clamps with mixed success.

The advent of inhalation anaesthesia

In 1800, Humphrey Davy [1], who noticed the analgesic qualities of nitrous oxide, was able to manufacture it in significantly large quantities. He is said to have used it as a recreational drug for many years, but that did not prevent him from being a brilliant President of the Royal Society for some time. He suggested its use in surgery, but he was ignored. Henry Hill Hickman of Ludlow, UK, anaesthetised animals with carbon dioxide and even appealed to the King of France for the recognition which he did not receive in his own country [2]. Baron Larrey, Napoleon's favourite Marshal, was interested but did not enquire further.

Eventually it was the widespread use of nitrous oxide and ether for amusement in 'laughing gas' and 'ether frolics' that led to their use in surgery. Gardner Quincy Colton gave lectures in chemistry to the public, which included the effects of nitrous oxide inhalation. One day on December 11th 1844, he visited Hartford in Connecticut. Horace Wells, a local dentist, noticed that a young man under the influence of nitrous oxide felt no pain on banging his shin. Wells, suffering from toothache at the time, persuaded Colton to give him the nitrous oxide so that his dental colleague John Riggs could remove the tooth without pain. This worked, and after performing several painless extractions, Wells enlisted the help of a former partner to arrange a dental demonstration before a distinguished surgeon, Dr. John Collins Warren, at the Harvard Medical School. Unfortunately, as can happen with nitrous oxide, the dose of anaesthetic agent was inadequate, the patient complained bitterly of pain throughout, and poor Wells was hissed out of the theatre [3]. His subsequent career deteriorated, culminating in suicide at the age of 33 by cutting his femoral artery [4].

It is clear from contemporary accounts that most patients suffered agonies during operations. This would explain the rapid and widespread use of inhalation anaesthesia after the first successful public demonstration of ether by William Morton at the Massachusetts General Hospital in Boston on October 16th 1846 (Figure 1). Morton had wisely

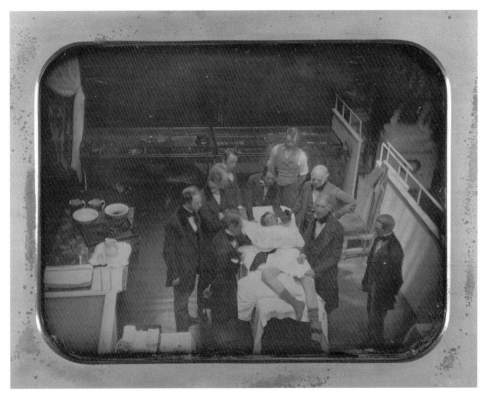

Figure 1. Re-enactment of Morton's anaesthetic. *Reproduced with permission from The J. Paul Getty Museum, Los Angeles, USA. Southworth & Hawes. Early Operation Using Ether for Anesthesia. Late Spring 1847. Daguerreotype.*

given a number of anaesthetics before the planned demonstration. Using equipment modified at the last moment, Morton gave ether to a young man for the removal of a vascular tumour below the mandible. The result greatly impressed Warren who remarked: "Gentlemen, this is no humbug." Morton's attempts to keep the recipe a secret caused uproar in the medical fraternity; in addition he spent much time and money unsuccessfully defending his right of copyright of the discovery [5]. Crawford Long, a General Practitioner from Jefferson, Georgia, claimed to have used ether for the painless removal of a tumour of the neck in 1842, but did not publish that experience until 1849. Thus, disputes about the discovery took place against William Morton for many years afterwards.

Within two months the news reached the UK in a letter from Jacob Bigelow, who had witnessed Morton's success, to Francis Boott, a General Practitioner in London. Boott's dentist friend, James Robinson, gave ether for a dental extraction on December 19th. Just two days later, Robert Liston performed an above knee amputation for osteomyelitis at University College Hospital, the anaesthetic being given by a 21-year-old medical student, William Squire [6]. The limb was in the sawdust in 28 seconds, and the patient was returned to bed in five minutes! Liston's reputed comment was "This Yankee dodge, Gentlemen, beats Mesmerism hollow!"

By January 12th 1847, Malgaigne reported five operations under ether to the Académie de Médecine in Paris [7] and by 1st June, ether had been successfully used at St. John's Hospital in Launceston, Tasmania. The report in that journal of three anaesthetics having been given prompted a rather over-cautious editor to describe the practice as a "dangerous ephemeral fad"!

Widespread experimentation with other agents and methods of administration followed. John Snow (1813-1858) used amylene extensively until two deaths occurred [8].

Chloroform was shown to have anaesthetic properties by Fluorens (as was ethyl chloride) in 1847 [9]. Sir James Young Simpson (Figure 2) pioneered its

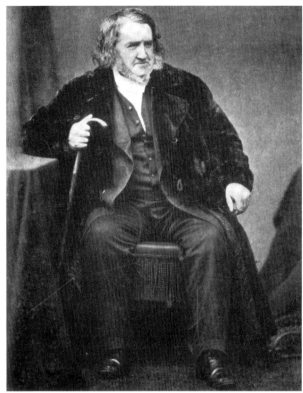

Figure 2. Sir James Young Simpson (1811-1870). *Reproduced with permission from The Royal Society of Medicine, London, UK.*

clinical use and declared it superior to ether. It became widely used in the UK, particularly after Queen Victoria received it as an analgesic for labour pain during two deliveries.

The first anaesthetic death recorded in England in 1848 was attributed to chloroform. The patient, a healthy 15-year-old girl called Hannah Greener, had undergone an uneventful ether anaesthetic two weeks previously. Chloroform was easier to administer, non-flammable, but more dangerous. Fatal cardiac arrhythmias could occur during induction, the blood pressure could fall steadily during anaesthesia and liver damage was reported in the 1890s. Snow recognised these problems and took safety precautions [8]. Nonetheless, chloroform was the most widely used anaesthetic agent in Britain and Europe for many years, and in Scotland, it was used up to the 1970s. In the US, ether was more widely used in the Northern states, perhaps due to the residual influence of the Boston School, except during the Civil War when the convenience of chloroform outweighed the risks. The Southern armies mainly used chloroform because they were influenced by Parisian practice emanating from New Orleans [3].

Morton's apparatus required the patient to breathe through a tube between his lips, his nostrils being pinched closed by an assistant. By 1848, a number of masks covering the nose and mouth had appeared; Snow's modification of Sibson's inhaler in 1847 is seen below (Figure 3).

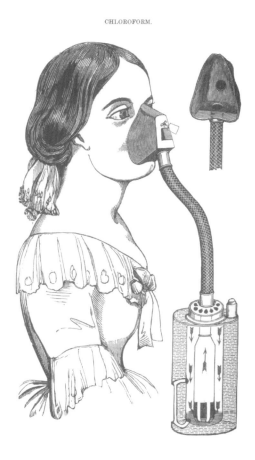

Figure 3. Snow's modification of Sibson's inhaler. *Reproduced from Snow J. On chloroform and other anaesthetics, 1858.*

The scientific investigation of anaesthesia

John Snow was a farmer's son born in 1813 (Figure 4), who received his medical education in Newcastle and London. He held a number of posts including a lectureship in forensic medicine, before

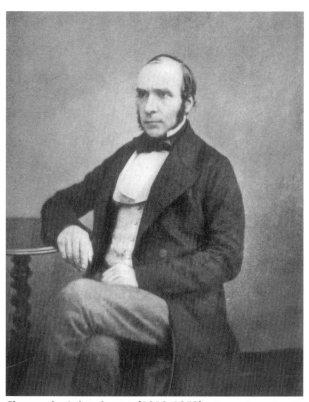

Figure 4. John Snow (1813-1858). *Reproduced with permission from The Royal Society of Medicine, London, UK.*

becoming the first full-time anaesthetist in the UK. His exploits regarding cholera are mentioned in the Appendix.

The principal problem facing early anaesthetists was giving the right amount of anaesthetic agent. John Snow and others determined the effect of different concentrations of most agents on animals. Once the importance of the concentration of inhaled vapour had been established (as opposed to the amount used), quite sophisticated attempts were made to provide a known percentage. Snow [8] ascertained that a 4% chloroform vapour would induce anaesthesia and that higher concentrations were dangerous. He used a metal chloroform inhaler adapted from a design of

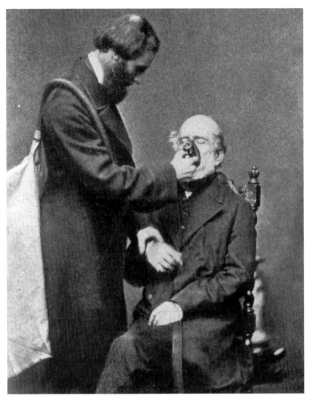

Figure 5. Joseph Clover's apparatus for chloroform. Note finger on pulse! *Reproduced with permission from The Royal Society of Medicine, London, UK.*

Sibson. The inner vaporising chamber was surrounded by a water-filled container to reduce the cooling effect of chloroform evaporation. He published a series of 4000 successful chloroform anaesthetics but, tragically, one death occurred soon after this series.

After Snow's early death in 1858, Joseph Clover, who like Snow, suffered from chronic poor health, became the leading British anaesthetist. To prevent the prolonged inhalation of more than 4% chloroform, he devised a large bag filled with 4.5% chloroform in air working from Avogadro's hypothesis. This sufficed for induction, after which more air was allowed into the inspiratory tube to dilute the mixture (Figure 5).

Despite the existence of numerous devices that gave a reasonably precise inhaled concentration of anaesthetic, the crude method of dropping of an anaesthetic liquid onto a cloth, pad or open mask was still widely used, and aptly described as 'flying by the seat of the pants'. This method may have been used because of the costs of the more sophisticated devices.

By the late 1860s, nitrous oxide was available in cylinders and was becoming widely used in dentistry. Andrews of Chicago mixed it with 20% oxygen, thereby obviating asphyxia, but many years were to elapse before nitrous oxide and oxygen were combined with a volatile agent. Clover developed a nitrous oxide/ether device. The French physiologist, Paul Bert, having noted that the partial pressure of the inhaled agent determined its effect, developed a mobile barometric chamber for giving nitrous oxide and air at two atmospheres (Figure 6). Whilst the apparatus seemed to work, the problems of operating in a confined space, fully clothed, under high pressure, and in increasing heat, proved intolerable.

As already stated, Clover and others had investigated the scientific basis of anaesthesia and

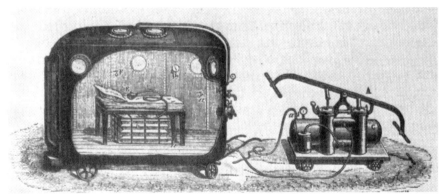

Figure 6. Paul Bert's anaesthetic 'car'. *Reproduced with permission from The Royal Society of Medicine, London, UK.*

had developed sophisticated devices to provide precise concentrations of the agents. Despite their efforts, their progress did not compare with the speed of progress in surgery, largely due to Lister's measures to prevent sepsis based on the fundamental work of Pasteur.

Maintenance of a clear airway during anaesthesia was crucial. Sir William Macewen, after huge experience treating diphtheria in Glasgow, preserved airways by intubating conscious patients before each operation [10]. Friederich Trendelenburg's [11] precaution was to perform a preliminary tracheotomy. Many anaesthetists were part-time or inexperienced, so that endotracheal intubation remained a minority skill until the arrival of muscle relaxants in the 1940s.

While nurse-anaesthetists, working under the direction of a surgeon were common in some countries, anaesthesia was only given as now by doctors and dentists in Britain. The average abdominal surgeon of the era needed to be swift and robust, since muscle relaxation of the abdominal wall was often minimal. There are still accounts of operations being performed without anaesthesia in European centres up to the 1880s.

It took some time before the use of nitrous oxide and oxygen as carrier gases for volatile agents became possible, with the introduction of pressurised cylinders and better drying of the gases within them.

Local anaesthesia

Cocaine was introduced into medical practice in 1884 by Koller [12] who demonstrated its effectiveness in ophthalmic surgery. In the same year Halsted (Figure 6, Chapter 10) and Hall in New York carried out mandibular nerve blocks on each other. Their experiments resulted, alas, in cocaine addiction for both men. Hans Finisterer, one of many surgeons, was famous for his skill not only for hundreds of gastric operations, but also for the technique of infiltrating diluted local anaesthetic solutions.

Credit for the first planned spinal anaesthetic in man was given to Auguste Bier [13] in 1898, but the toxicity of cocaine limited its use. Both Sicard and

Cathelin performed caudal epidural injections in 1901, but only in the 1920s were lumbar epidural injections performed by Pages of Madrid. Although synthetic agents, such as stovaine (Amylocaine) and procaine were introduced in the early 1900s, these ester-based local anaesthetics were short-acting and liable to produce allergic and other reactions. The first long-acting amide agent, cinchocaine, was developed in 1927, and a series of safer amide agents commenced with lignocaine in 1943. All the agents now in use are non-irritant amides, chemically stable and heat-resistant, with little allergic potential. Useful drugs amongst these are prilocaine, which has a high therapeutic ratio, and ropivacaine, which has a long duration of action.

The techniques for blocking elements of the nervous system were remarkably advanced by the 1920s, as can be seen in Labat's *Regional Anaesthesia*, published in 1922. Prolonged anaesthesia could only be achieved by repeated blocks. Edwards and Hingson, in 1943 [14], produced an in-dwelling malleable needle for caudal analgesia, but progress was not really made until plastics replaced larger cumbersome rubber tubes. Tuohy's needle, now used for epidural cannulation, had originally been designed for sub-arachnoid puncture and cannulation. One can assume that a high proportion of post-spinal headaches resulted from the large dural punctures! The introduction of fine nylon catheters and bacterial filters in the 1960s, together with better agents, made the provision of operative and postoperative abdominal, trunk, limb and obstetric analgesia, simpler and safer.

The 20th century, the arrival of anaesthesia as a specialty

James Tayloe Gwathmey [15] produced an anaesthetic apparatus in 1912 which combined oxygen and nitrous oxide cylinders with a vaporiser for ether. The basic principle has continued to this day. Henry Gaskin Boyle's machine (Figure 7) was really a modification of Gwathmey's apparatus. Boyle's arrangement had one oxygen and four nitrous oxide cylinders equipped with reducing valves, carried on a trolley with spirit lamps to prevent moisture in the gases from freezing. The gases passed through water

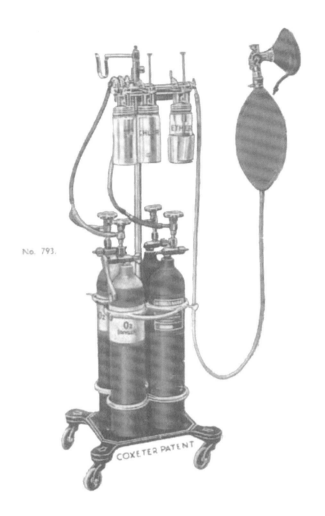

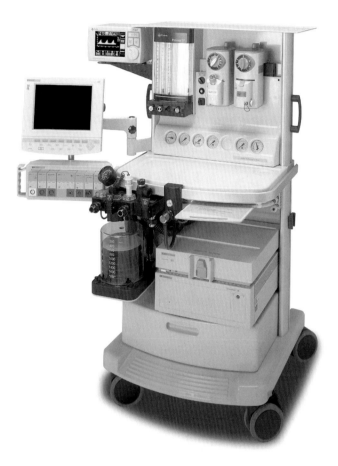

Figure 7. Early Boyle's machine. *Reproduced with permission from British Oxygen, UK.*

Figure 8. A more modern Boyle's machine. *Reproduced with permission from Penlon Ltd., Abingdon, UK.*

sight meters, which were vertical tubes with multiple perforations submerged in water. Bubbles emerged further down, as pressure and flow increased. In addition, there was a simple ether vaporiser from which the mixed gases passed through a bag and thence to the patient.

Later, flow meters, working on the decline in pressure across an orifice, were designed by Foregger and Connell. 'Rotameters' which originated from the chemical industries were introduced in the 1930s.

Major wars are said to produce major advances. The First World War in 1914-1918 was no exception. The huge numbers of major casualties in that war accelerated change. For the first time anaesthetists undertook transfusions, mostly infusing saline, to prevent surgical shock, as well as provide analgesia in the pre- and postoperative period. Furthermore, a portable form of Boyle's machine, made available to the British Army, became very popular. Modern anaesthetic machines today embody the same principles but carry a variety of monitors, warning devices, and lung ventilators (Figure 8).

Intravenous agents

Glass and metal syringes, such as Luer (Paris) and Rekord (Berlin), developed around the end of the 19th century, were to have an important effect later, when better agents were developed. Chloral hydrate by intravenous injection was introduced in France in 1872 and paraldehyde in Britain in 1912. At times both were found to be dangerous. Similar results were obtained with intravenous ether. Barbituric acid had been synthesised in 1864, but the first of the barbiturates to be used clinically was diethyl barbituric acid (Veronal) in 1912. Hexabarbitone, the first acceptable intravenous barbiturate anaesthetic, was introduced into medicine by Weese of Düsseldorf [16] in 1932. Thiopentone replaced it within a few years and remained the standard induction agent until the early 1980s. Thiopentone's main drawbacks were depression of the cardiovascular system, which could be fatal in compromised patients, and also a relatively slow recovery time. Repeated injections or prolonged infusion could therefore be dangerous. Another barbiturate, methohexitone, introduced in the US in 1957, allowed a more rapid recovery than thiopentone; it also showed long-term accumulation.

Alternatives were sought which could be rapidly broken down in the body after injection. Althesin, a mixture of two steroids, was popular in the early 1970s, but a high incidence of hypotension and anaphylactoid reactions led to its withdrawal. Cremophor EL, an emulsifying agent used to dissolve the steroids, was the suspected culprit. Etomidate, introduced in 1973, initially seemed the ideal agent because it was short-acting and had minimal effects on the cardiovascular system. Its use was limited to induction because cardiovascular instability from adrenocortical suppression occurred after prolonged administration.

Ketamine, introduced in 1965, differed from other anaesthetics in that it produced dissociative anaesthesia. Respiration and blood pressure were well maintained but the latter was sometimes elevated. Analgesia was obtained at sub-anaesthetic concentrations and could be used via both epidural and spinal routes. Disadvantages were excessive salivation and unpleasant vivid psychic phenomena. The salivation was often controlled by a phenothiazine and the psychic phenomena by diazepam.

Propofol, introduced by ICI in 1977, is a polyphenol [17], known in some quarters as 'instant amnesia'. It was originally dissolved with cremophor EL, but later with soya oil and other agents. The combination of rapid recovery, even after prolonged infusion, seldom accompanied by nausea, led to a major change in anaesthetic practice. Total intravenous anaesthesia (TIVA) using computerised pumps for propofol and other agents, such as rapid acting analgesics, provided an alternative to inhalational anaesthesia. Prolonged administration in the Intensive Care Unit has shown little evidence of cumulation. The use of propofol for this purpose is contraindicated in children and adolescents because of possible heart and liver damage.

As said at the beginning of the chapter, morphine and its analogues were given by injection or by mouth before inhalation anaesthesia. However, its use has continued as an adjunct or as pre-medication. A series of powerful agents, developed from pethidine, such as fentanil and sufentanil, were found to cause less cardiovascular depression when used with propofol.

The excessive salivation after ether led to prescription of anticholinergics, such as hyoscine, to dry up secretions. Excessive quantities sometimes produced a central anti-cholinergic syndrome. Fortunately, glycopyrollate, introduced in 1971, was found not to cross the blood brain barrier and therefore caused less tachycardia than the older anticholinergics.

Muscle relaxants

Modern anaesthesia for major surgery would be impossible without the use of muscle relaxants. Curare, the first agent to be used, was extracted from *Chondrodendron tomentosum*, and used by the Amazonian Indians as an arrow poison. Small quantities were brought to Europe by explorers. Von Humboldt and his companion, Bonpland [18], noted that the man preparing the poison tasted the mixture from time to time and correctly concluded that for paralysis to occur the substance had to be injected. In 1814, Charles Waterston (the explorer who had brought back a native form of curare called 'Wourali'), with Sir

Benjamin Brodie and Sewell, paralysed an ass with curare and kept it alive by artificial respiration, employing bellows via a tracheotomy for two hours until it recovered [19]. Claude Bernard (Figure 8, Chapter 7) noted in 1850 that although curare paralysed a frog, the muscles responded to direct stimulation [20]. He concluded that the block was between the nerve and muscle. His then assistant, Kukne, subsequently demonstrated the site of action to be the neuromuscular junction.

Extracts of curare were used in a number of conditions, such as the management of tetanus, particularly in the 1930s, but its introduction into anaesthetic practice is attributed to Griffith and Johnson of Montreal in 1942 [21]. Tubocurarine, the first commercial product, produced occasional untoward reactions such as bronchospasm, hypotension and sensitivity phenomena which could be life-threatening and a substitute was sought from the outset. Decamethonium and suxamethonium, both depolarising relaxants, unlike curare, were introduced in 1948 and 1949 respectively and the latter is still used for rapid paralysis for intubation of the trachea. Occasional side effects include muscle pain.

Alcuronium derived from *Strychnos toxifera* was introduced in 1958 to be followed by synthetic agents like the steroid Pancuronium. Other 'designer' drugs followed as a consequence of the revolution in biochemistry. Vecuronium (1979), derived from Pancuronium, is broken down by the liver, and Atracurium (1980) undergoes initial Hoffman degradation. These agents assured complete and safe recovery from paralysis and, unlike curare, were unaffected by renal function. Mivacurium, a short-acting non-depolarising agent with an onset nearly as rapid as suxamethonium, was introduced in 1993. Like suxamethonium, it is broken down by the plasma enzyme, pseudo-cholinesterase. Both can cause prolonged paralysis if there is an abnormality of that enzyme. Rocuronium, which combines a rapid onset with a longer duration of action and minimal untoward effects, appeared in 1994.

Control of the airway

Airway obstruction tends to occur under anaesthesia for a number of reasons; for example, a reduction of tone in the pharyngeal muscles. Assorted oro- and nasopharyngeal airways were used until the Guedel airway became popular. Surgical access to the head and neck was a major problem for surgeons, which pioneers such as McEwen, who intubated patients while awake using his fingers, and Trendelenburg, who performed a pre-operative tracheotomy, resolved. Faced with large numbers of injured servicemen after the First World War, Magill and Rowbotham developed 'blind' intubation of the trachea with rubber tubes passed through the nose. The technique was difficult, but once mastered, was found to be safe and allowed rapid deepening of anaesthesia without coughing. When muscle relaxants were introduced, endotracheal tubes became indispensable and were easier to insert. A laryngoscope developed by Sir Robert Macintosh [22] in 1943, specifically for intubation was, and is, even today, used most frequently. The original tubes were simple red rubber pipes to which inflatable cuffs were added over time. Low allergy vinyl has now replaced the original rubber.

The pioneers of thoracic surgery were faced with the problem of lung collapse on opening the pleura. As early as 1891, Tuffier [23] of Paris performed a partial lung resection and he and his colleague, Hallion, used an endotracheal intubation technique and subsequently, tracheal insufflation. Sauerbruch [24] initially tried operating in a low pressure chamber with the patient's head outside, but subsequently, he followed others and placed the patient's head and the anaesthetist in a positive pressure environment. Neither was satisfactory, and like Bert's car, Sauerbruch's chamber was an uncomfortable place to work. Matas [25] of New Orleans used a Fell-O'Dwyer resuscitation system with bellows and an endotracheal tube in the late 1880s. Once the advantages of positive pressure ventilation had been established, isolation of diseased segments to prevent the spread of infection was achieved by bronchial tampons and inflatable bronchial blockers. Bronchoscopy was required to ensure proper placement of these devices, which could easily become displaced. The isolation of one lung by an endobronchial tube was described by Gale and Waters in 1932. With the appearance of the Carlens [26] double-lumen tube for broncho-spirometry in 1946, several variants more suited to anaesthetic use were developed, such as those of Bryce-Smith, Pallister and Robertshaw and similar available designs in polyvinyl chloride.

It is worth noting that thoracic surgery was performed in Eastern Europe up to the 1960s using local anaesthesia alone. Patients could talk whilst the thorax was open and most survived these procedures [27]. Open thoracotomies under acupuncture in conscious patients have been filmed in China during the 20th century; it is uncertain for how long thoracotomy using acupuncture has taken place.

In the early 1980s, Brain developed the laryngeal mask, which has been an enormous boon to anaesthetists [28]. It covered the larynx, although it was not guaranteed to prevent contamination of the trachea, and was well tolerated at light levels of anaesthesia, particularly after propofol induction. Apart from its use in routine anaesthesia, it is invaluable after failed intubation, because artificial ventilation of the lungs can be satisfactorily maintained.

New inhalational agents

It is surprising that no new satisfactory agent had appeared to replace ether and chloroform until after the end of the Second World War. Many anaesthetists knew chloroform was potentially dangerous but easier to use than ether. Cyclopropane, introduced in 1933, was not only an explosive and expensive gas, which had to be used in a closed circuit for safety reasons and to avoid waste, but could be a profound depressant of respiration. Artificial ventilation solved the problem of respiratory depression, but the cost and inflammability led to its replacement by newer agents such as halothane.

Employees using trichlorethylene in dry cleaning establishments discovered it could relieve pain. Although potentially toxic and a poor muscle relaxant, it was widely used for pain relief after 1939. Nerve damage was reported when used in closed circuit anaesthesia. For a while temperature-compensated

inhalers (e.g. TECOTA) were used in domiciliary midwifery, but they are no longer available in the Western hemisphere.

Halothane, a fluorinated hydrocarbon, which was developed from a series of substances used as engine coolants during World War II, was introduced in 1952. It was a pleasant smelling non-irritant liquid which vaporised easily. It was potent, enabling easy induction in children. When it was first introduced it was used, as ether had been, in a vaporiser within a closed circuit. Its greater potency and volatility led to dangerous concentrations, especially if the patient's ventilation was manually assisted. Once the danger was recognised two steps were taken to prevent overdose: the first was to remove the vaporiser from within the closed circuit; and the second, was the introduction of vaporisers, such as the Fluotec in 1957, which gave a constant concentration over a range of temperature and flow (Figure 9).

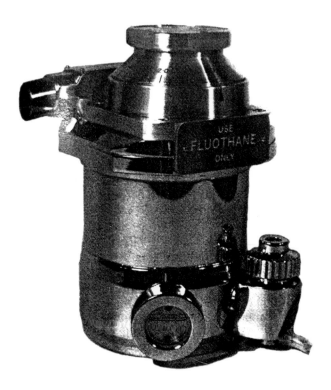

Figure 9. Fluotec vaporiser. *Reproduced with permission from British Oxygen, UK.*

Unexplained jaundice after halothane administration, especially if repeated, had been noted from its introduction. The phenomenon was eventually traced to breakdown products, which combined with body proteins, resulted in an autoimmune reaction. This spurred the introduction of a series of halogenated ethers, which were less subject to chemical breakdown in the body.

Unfortunately, one of the early varieties called methoxyflurane was shown to break down to such an extent that the excess free fluoride ions caused renal damage. Safer versions, such as enflurane and isoflurane synthesised by Ross Terrell in the US, were introduced into clinical practice in 1966 and 1971 respectively. These and newer halogenated ethers were safer, although less pleasant to inhale than halothane. However, improvements in intravenous anaesthesia have significantly reduced the importance of inhalation anaesthesia over the past ten years.

Transfusion and intravenous fluids

In 1832, Thomas Aitcheson Latta of Edinburgh who had noted the work of O'Shaughnessy on the blood of cholera victims, transfused a mixed solution of half normal saline and bicarbonate with some benefit [29]. On one occasion he gave 33oz or one litre over 12 hours in three sessions, using a Reads pump via a silver tube inserted into a vein; the fluid was filtered through a 'shammoy leather', producing doubts about sterility. The technique, which must have been difficult, was used only rarely for the remainder of the century (even during a cholera epidemic in London in the 1850s). Saline and related infusions were used extensively during World War I (1914-1918) when blood was less available.

Colloidal substitutes were tried as an alternative to blood. Gum acacia as an early example, introduced in 1919, was effective but fatal allergic reactions occurred. Other agents, including modified gelatins, dextrans, and etherified starch, have been widely used for blood volume replacement to treat surgical shock. Albumin, a component of blood, was extensively used in burns resuscitation in some centres and to raise serum albumin levels in other conditions. Recent changes in the understanding of fluid and solute movement in and out of capillaries have reduced its use.

The transfusion of blood from animal to animal as a means of treatment of illness, rather than for resuscitation, was performed by Richard Lower in 1666 and Sir Christopher Wren [30], perhaps as an experimental exercise. Jean Denis, at the University of Montpellier, transfused animal blood to man in 1667 [31]. He claimed his first two patients survived, but the remaining two died, which led to a charge of murder and a ban on the procedure. Human-to-human transfusion was performed by the obstetrician Blundell, who designed his own pump and syringe [32] in 1818. The first patient died, but a second one survived. He later showed that interspecies transfusions were dangerous. Aveling, in 1864, and Halsted, in 1880, succeeded using vein-to-vein transfusion. On one occasion, Halsted was himself the donor for his sister, after post-partum haemorrhage.

Regarding the storage of blood, Braxton Hicks succeeded in preservation with sodium phosphate in 1881, but this agent proved to be too toxic. Sodium citrate introduced by Richard Lewishon in 1915 was a more satisfactory replacement. Cadaver blood, having no fibrinogen, therefore needing no anticoagulant, was alleged to be available in Russia throughout the 1930s. The true story of this is described in Chapter 11, which destroyed the myth, but by sheer chance led to the discovery of the use of staples in surgery of the bronchus and gastrointestinal tract in the Soviet Union, and subsequent revolution of the use of staples in the whole surgical world.

Autotransfusion was described in 1874 and widely used between the two World Wars. It required the discovery of the ABO agglutinogens in 1901 by Landsteiner of Vienna [33] (Figure 10), and glucose to prolong red cell life in 1916 for blood transfusion to become a more routine procedure. Archibald [34] installed blood transfusion services at forward military casualty stations during the First World War in 1916, and by the 1930s, blood banks had been developed in several centres. The Barcelona Blood Bank in the Spanish Civil War used only Group O blood, which was then called 'universal donor' blood. The existence of the Rhesus factors was not known until they were discovered by Landsteiner and Weiner [35] in 1940.

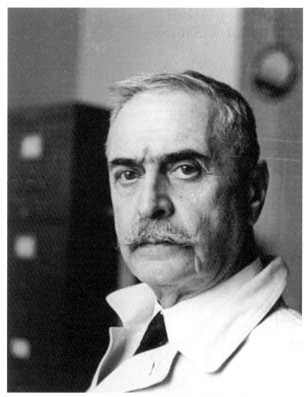

Figure 10. Karl Landsteiner (1868-1943). *Reproduced from www.peoples.ru/medicine/immunologist/landsteiner/.*

Roscoe Clark at the Birmingham Accident Hospital emphasised the need for adequate blood transfusion in trauma, particularly major bone trauma, and so he trained all staff, including ambulance staff, to assess blood loss more accurately. Concern over viral and sub-viral infections has brought about a more stringent approach to transfusion over the past few years.

The administration of all intravenous fluids became easier in the 1960s with the arrival of single-use sterile sets and plastic intravenous cannulas with steel trocars. The former were a major advance on the re-usable rubber and glass kits previously provided by transfusion services, which often accumulated deposits however sterile from previous use. The new cannulas were easy to insert, did not cut out, and caused less irritation and infection than the previous steel needles. They were followed by special cannulas for insertion into arteries, central veins, and in the pulmonary arterial tree for pressure measurement. The direct measurement of arterial pressure and central venous pressure became routine for major operations. Developments in physics and electronics led to the production of minute pressure sensors, gas-sensitive electrodes for measuring partial pressures of gases and vapours in the airway, and refined electrocardiography. Cardiac output and associated variables, such as left ventricular filling pressure, could be measured on a minute-to-minute basis using in-dwelling pulmonary catheters and the appropriate drugs subsequently titrated against results.

In Chapter 9, the sequence of events is described of the large volumes of fluid required for resuscitation and management of intestinal obstruction, and the value of the more sensitive central venous pressure measurement to manage intestinal obstruction and many other major gastrointestinal conditions.

Conclusions

Anaesthesia in the 21st century may have become more complicated, but it has also become much safer and more pleasant for patients than a hundred years ago. Evaluation of the performance of surgeons and anaesthetists by bodies such as the Confidential Enquiry into Perioperative Deaths (CEPOD) in the UK and the Patient Safety Association in the US have clarified errors and increased safety especially during emergency conditions [36].

Those who have attempted induction with ether in the past appreciate the ease with which patients lose consciousness nowadays with modern intravenous agents. Nausea and pain after operations have been greatly diminished and patients are often able to return home within hours of their operations.

Intensive Care Units (ICUs) in which highly skilled staff and advanced equipment enhance the chances of a patient's recovery are an essential component of care for major surgery and patients with pre-existing illnesses. The development of ICUs had been impelled initially by events, such as epidemics of poliomyelitis and the realisation that the support of functions such as respiration and of the heart and circulation for a short period could result in full recovery.

The use of advanced methods of pain relief, such as continuous epidural infusion, patient-controlled analgesic pumps and other interventions led to the development of pain clinics for the relief of chronic pain in which anaesthetists have played a major role. As a consequence, the role of the anaesthetist has changed enormously through the 20th century. The anaesthetist is no longer a 'gasman' charged with keeping the patient quiet (while remaining awake!) during an operation; the role has changed to becoming a specialist in resuscitation, intravenous therapy, postoperative pain relief, and respiratory support. Active participation by anaesthetists in peri-operative management has been shown to improve outcomes in patients with all surgical problems. Management is enormously helped by the availability of electrolyte and blood gas analysis, as well as acid / base measurement at the bedside. Despite the availability of so much monitoring equipment, the clinical skill and judgement of the anaesthetist remains as essential today as it did a century ago.

References

1. Davy H. *Researches, Chemical and Philosophical; Chiefly Concerning Nitrous Oxide.* Johnson London facsimile. London: Butterworths, 1972.
2. Hickman H. A letter on suspended animation containing experiments showing that it may be safely employed during operations on animals with a view to ascertaining its probable utility in the human subject. *Survey of Anaesthesiology Classical file* 1966; 10: 91-6.
3. Duncum BM. *The Development of Inhalation Anaesthesia. (1846-1900).* London: Wellcome Historical Medical Museum, 1946.
4. Rushman GB, Davies NJ, Atkinson RS. *Wells' Life. A Short History of Anaesthesia.* Butterworth Heinmann, 1996.
5. Rutkow IM. *Surgery. An Illustrated History.* St. Louis, USA: Mosby, 1993: 335.
6. Zuck D. Dr. Nooth and his apparatus. The role of carbon dioxide in medicine in the 18th century. *Br J Anaes* 1978; 50: 393-405.
7. Neveu R. The introduction of surgical anaesthesia in France. *J Hist Med Allied Sci* 1946; 1: 607-10.
8. Snow J. *On Chloroform and Other Anaesthetics.* Classics of Surgery Library, New York, 1992.
9. Fluorens PJ, Hebd CR. Seances. *Acad Sci Paris* 1847; 24: 161, 253 and 340.
10. Macewen W. Clinical Observations. *Survey of Anaesthesiology* 1969; 13: 105-20.
11. Trendelenburg F. Beitragen zu den Operationen den Luffwwegen. *Arch Clin Chir* 1871; 12: 112-4.
12. Koller C. Preliminary report on local anaesthesia of the eye. *Archives of Ophthalmology* 1934; 12: 473-4.
13. Bier A. Classical file: experiments regarding the cocainisation of the spinal cord. *Surv Anaesthiol* 1962; 6: 352-8. Reprint from *Zeitschrift fur Chirurgie* 1899; 51: 361-9.
14. Edwards RA, Hingson WB. Continuous caudal anaesthesia in obstetrics. *Am J Surg* 1942; 57: 459-64. Repr. Classical File. *Surv Anaesthiol* 1980; 24: 275-80.
15. Gwathmey JT. *Anaesthesia.* New York: Appleton, 1914: 174.
16. Jarman R, Abel LA. Intravenous anaesthesia with pentothal sodium. *Lancet* 1936; 1: 422-5.
17. Rogers KM, Dewar KMS, McCubbin TD. Preliminary experience with ICI 35868 as an IV induction agent; comparison with Althesin. *Br J Anaes* 1980; 52: 807-10.
18. Humboldt FHA von. *Voyages aux regions equinoxiale du nouveau continent 1859-1860.* Hauf, Ed. JG Cotta. Stuttgart.
19. Irwin RA. Letters of Charles Waterston, London. Cited by Maltby JR. In: *Anaesthesia Essays on its History.* Rupreht J, *et al,* Eds. Springer Verlag, 1985.
20. Bernard C. Analyse physiologique des systemes musculaire et nerveux au moyen du curare. *Comptes Rendu Acad Sci* (Paris). 1856; 43: 825-9.
21. Griffith HR, Johnson E. Anaesthesiology 1942. Classical File. *Surv Anaesthesiol* 1985; 29: 358-68.
22. Macintosh RR, Leatherdale RAC. Bronchus tube and bronchus blocker. *Br J Anaes* 1955; 27: 556-7.
23. Tuffier T, Hallion J. Operation intrathoracique avec respiration artificial par insufflation. *Compte Rendu Soc de Biol* 1896; 48: 951-1026.
24. Sauerbruch F. Uber die Ausschaltung der schadlichen Wirkung des Pneumothorax bei intrathorakalen Operationen. *Zbl Chur* 1904; 31: 146-9.
25. Matas R. On the treatment of traumatic pneumothorax. *Ann Surg* 1899; 29: 951.
26. Carlens EJ. A new flexible double lumen catheter for bronchospirometry. *J Thorac Surg* 1949; 18: 742-6.
27. Vidra G. Personal communication.
28. Brain AIJ. The laryngeal mask - a new concept in airway management. *Br J Anaes* 1983; 55: 801-5.
29. Masson AHB. Latta - pioneer in saline infusion *Br J Anaes* 1971; 43: 681-6.
30. Lower R. *Tractatus de Corde.* London: Jacobi Allestry, 1669.
31. Denis JB. *Transactions giving some account of the present undertakings, studies, and labours of the ingenious in considerable parts of the world.* London: John Martyn, 1667.
32. Blundell J. Observations on the transfusion of blood, with a description of his Gravitator. *Lancet* 1928; 2: 321-4. Reprint. *Surv Anaesthesiol* 1986; 30: 103-6.
33. Landsteiner K. 1901 reprint & trans. *Haematology landmark papers of the twentieth century.* Lichtman, *et al.* London: Academic Press, 2000.
34. Archibald E. A note upon the employment of blood transfusion in war surgery. *J R Army Med Corps* 1916; 27: 636-44.
35. Landsteiner K, Weiner AS. An agglutinable factor in human blood recognised by immune sera for human blood. *Proceedings for the Society for Experimental Biology and Medicine* 1940; 43: 223-4.
36. Buck N, Devlin HB, Lunn JN, Eds. The Report of the Confidential Enquiry into Perioperative Deaths. London: The Nuffield Provincial Hospitals Trust and King's Fund, 1987.

Chapter 3

The battle against infection

John R Kirkup MD FRCS

Emeritus Consultant Orthopaedic Surgeon, Royal United Hospital, Bath, Somerset, UK

Honorary Curator, Historical Instrument Collection, Royal College of Surgeons of England, London, UK

"For it is not necessary ... that pus should be generated in wounds. No error can be greater than this." [1]

Early responses to wound infection

Until the 19th century, wound infection was viewed as a mysterious and inevitable complication, even applauded by some as necessary to healing and recovery; hence the expression 'laudable pus' [2]. This notion was not universally adopted, as the above quotation indicates, and empirical applications of water, wine, spirits, turpentine and other substances to cleanse fresh wounds against putrefaction have a long history. Although Leeuwenhoek of Leiden visualised protozoa and bacteria before 1693 [3] and Spallanzani of Modena disputed the doctrine of spontaneous generation in 1776 by boiling liquids in flasks, which he then closed to exclude the entry of air, demonstrating no subsequent formation of organisms [4], their work had no effect on wound management. Statistical evidence of wound care is sparse before 1782 when Alanson of Liverpool reported 35 consecutive major amputations without a death in a city hospital, normally a source of high mortality. He fashioned flaps carefully, ligated vessels, and permitted wound drainage using adhesive strips only; importantly, he

isolated his surgical cases, instituted frequent changes of bed-linen and clean clothing for patients, refused admission for ulcerated cases, isolated gangrenous patients, and oven-baked clothing and linen of all infected cases [5]. Unfortunately, few surgeons were capable of repeating his results. In 1802, Crowther of Halifax, UK, reported the successful healing of 28 consecutive compound fracture wounds treated with a dressing of wood tar, later shown to contain phenol. Wood tar was a Crowther family remedy employed for several generations. Most of these fractures were due to industrial accidents in mines and quarries which, formerly, were submitted to immediate amputations to avoid death from wound suppuration and gangrene [6]. Unhappily, Crowther's evidence did not influence established surgical management.

Earlier, in 1760, Pouteau of Lyons recognised a similarity between puerperal fever and surgical wound infections, and in 1773, White of Manchester stressed cleanliness and the isolation of patients with puerperal fever, as did Clarke of Dublin in 1790 [7]. Meanwhile, in 1795, Gordon of Aberdeen and in 1843, Holmes of Boston advocated rigorous hand washing to prevent the spread of puerperal fever in maternity wards [8]. This was proven statistically by Semmelweiss of Vienna (Figure 1) in 1847 when he

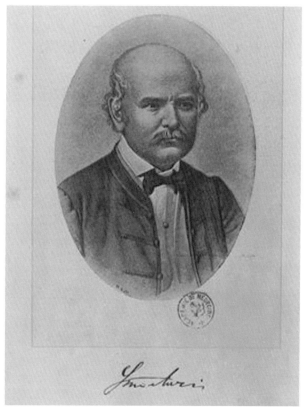

Figure 1. Ignaz Phillipp Semmelweiss (1818-1865). *Reproduced with permission from the Bibliothèque Académie Nationale de Médecine, Paris, France.*

instituted hand scrubbing with soap followed by chorine water for all participants involved in a delivery, and similar disinfection of obstetric instruments, to reduce parturient mortality from 10% to 1% [9]. Once again, compelling evidence was ignored and, unjustly, Semmelweiss was dismissed for arousing his seniors' jealousy.

Prophylactic wound antisepsis by chemical sterilisation

Runge of Leipzig isolated phenol, that is carbolic acid, in 1834, and this was employed sporadically in the dissecting room and to sweeten wounds; after systematic research Lemaire of Paris published a comprehensive analysis of its antiseptic effects on contaminated wounds in 1865 [10]. Significantly, Lemaire, Calvert of Manchester, Declat of Paris,

Bottini of Milan [11] and others who demonstrated that phenol promoted the healing of infected wounds, sinuses and ulcers, failed to establish its prophylactic role in preventing the contamination of clean wounds. In 1864, Wells of London drew attention to the work of Pasteur (Figure 2) in Paris on spontaneous generation, fermentation and putrefaction and its significance to surgical practice [12].

Whether Lister (Figure 3) in Glasgow was aware of Wells' paper is uncertain for Godlee maintained it was his colleague, Anderson, a chemist, who alerted him to Pasteur's work, that contact with the air rendered sterile fluids cloudy, and how micro-organisms contributed to fermentation [13]. This suggested to Lister that particles in the air caused wound infection and treatment should be directed towards their exclusion before suppuration ensued, especially for compound fractures usually subjected to immediate

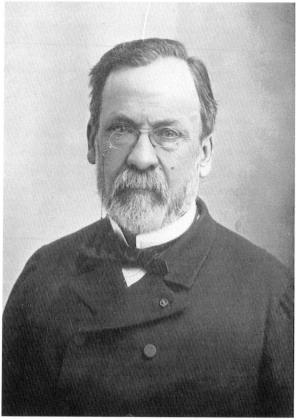

Figure 2. Louis Pasteur (1822-1895). *Reproduced with permission from the Bibliothèque Académie Nationale de Médecine, Paris, France.*

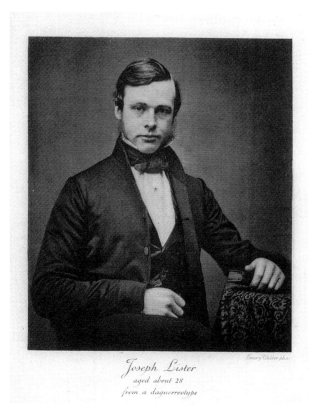

Figure 3. Joseph Lister (1827-1912) aged about 28 years. *Reproduced from a daguerreotype. In: Godlee RJ. Lord Lister. London: Macmillan, 1917: facing page 42.*

amputation, with a mortality of 45% in the Royal Infirmary, Glasgow.

Aware of the efficient use of phenol to treat sewage in the town of Carlisle, he applied undiluted antiseptic to his hands and patients' wounds in 1865; although effective he realised pure phenol was strongly irritant to intact skin. By 1867 he reported a significant reduction in sepsis and of the need to amputate in his wards [14]. Finding 5% phenol satisfactory, his system evolved, and Lister began to perform elective surgery soaking his hands, instruments and dressings in antiseptic and saturating the air surrounding the wound by a phenol spray, achieving primary healing. Nevertheless, he had many critics who claimed failure to repeat Lister's results, almost certainly because they did not follow his exacting instructions; however, he recognised that the spray was unnecessary in 1887. Fortunately, his pupils, house surgeons and many impartial visitors including Saxtorph of Copenhagen,

Lucas-Championnière of Paris, von Volkmann of Halle and Nussbaum of Munich disseminated the true practice of his antiseptic system [15]. It is said that Lister rejected thermal sterilisation but in fact he retired in 1893 when practical aseptic techniques had barely been published in the surgical literature.

Ovariotomy and abdominal surgery

During the establishment of antiseptic surgery and emergence of aseptic techniques, Wells of London, Keith of Edinburgh and Tait of Birmingham (Figure 6, Chapter 12) developed safe ovariotomy following the pioneer work by McDowell of Kentucky, Clay of Manchester and others [16]. They also performed uterine fibroid excision, hysterectomy, splenectomy and, in the case of Tait, cholecystostomy in 1879 and appendicectomy in 1880 [17]. Whilst repudiating Listerian antisepsis, they observed scrupulous cleanliness using soap and water, employed nickel-plated and phenolised instruments, antiseptic dressings, boiled sponges and silk sutures, applied cautery and lavaged the peritoneal cavity with large volumes of clean but unsterile water. In reality they had adopted certain antiseptic procedures and Pasteur's advice on heat. Lister himself had warned that the phenol would damage the peritoneum which he considered had particular vital power against infection [18].

Prophylactic wound asepsis by heat sterilisation

Pasteur stated in 1874: "If I had the honour of being a surgeon, I would never introduce into a human body an instrument that had not been passed through boiling water and better yet a flame, just before an operation, and rapidly cooled." [19] He amplified this in 1878, recommending careful hand washing and flaming, the use of dressings subjected to heating at 130-150°C, and water to 110-120°C. Regrettably, surgeons were slow to seize on these revolutionary instructions, although one of Lister's pupils, Macewen, is reported to have commenced boiling instruments, ligature and gauze in a fish-kettle during the late 1870s [20].

a   b

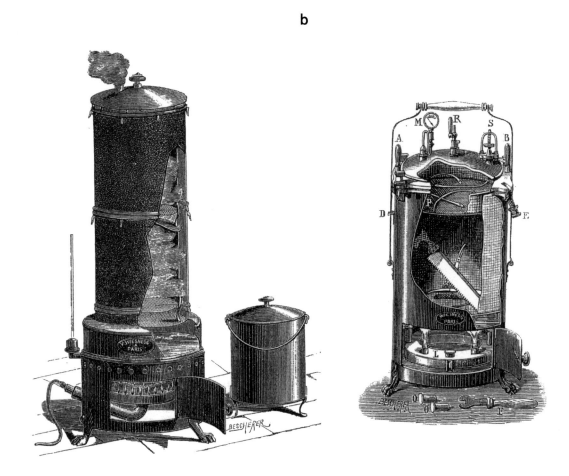

Figure 4. a) Koch's laboratory autoclave (1881); b) Redard's surgical autoclave (1888). *Reproduced from Vinay C. Manuel d'Asepsie. Paris: J-B Bailliere, 1890: figures 28 & 29.*

By 1881, Pasteur with Chamberland in Paris and Koch in Berlin had developed steam autoclaves to sterilise culture media and laboratory equipment (Figure 4). They showed that moist steam under pressure was best at killing organisms and spores and by 1883, the autoclave was available in many laboratories [21]. Finally, a few surgeons began to transfer laboratory practice to the operating theatre.

Primed with the science of bacteriology, several contributors increasingly introduced heat sterilisation for surgery in France and Germany. In 1883, Tripier of Lyons boiled instruments in oil but this blunted blades and damaged organic instrument handles [22]. In the same year Neuber of Kiel autoclaved operative gowns and in 1886 he advocated sterile caps and rubber

shoes whilst continuing to use antiseptics [23]. Redard of Paris commenced autoclaving instruments in 1888 (Figure 4) [24] and in 1890, von Bergmann (Figure 5) claimed that for two years he had operated aseptically, autoclaving linen, swabs and silk sutures; instruments were boiled in 10% soda, and the operative site and his hands were cleaned with antiseptics in which he also preserved catgut [25].

At last this resembled the basis of modern practice, much clarified by von Bergmann's assistant Schimmelbusch in 1892, who described boilers for instruments, steam sterilisers of metal drums containing operative clothing, linen, dressings and suture, and also novel glass and metal theatre furniture (Figure 6) [26]. Gloves and masks were to come later.

Aseptic heat sterilisation techniques raised important financial issues for hospitals who were faced with costly redesigns of operating theatres, necessitating totally new furniture and equipment. For example, required instruments handled in ebony, ivory and tortoiseshell, destroyed by heat, demanded instant replacement in crucible steel protected by nickel plate, proving a major challenge for instrument manufacturers. Those hospitals reluctant to change, could not ignore for long a revolution which ensured safe exploration of all body cavities and joints. In effect, aseptic practice combined with antiseptic procedures transformed surgery's progress, triggering a unique expansion in operative techniques, surgical literature and instrument makers' catalogues.

Twentieth century developments

Serious wound infections, due to tetanus and gas gangrene organisms are now avoided by immunisation or treated by antibodies or antibiotics. Streptococcal infections had proved sensitive to sulphonamides and

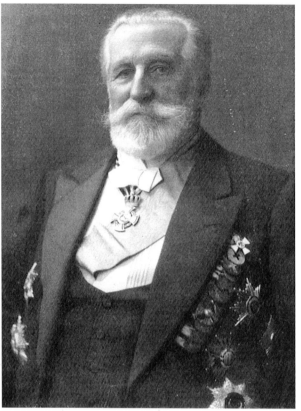

Figure 5. Ernst von Bergmann (1837-1907). *Reproduced with permission from the Bibliothèque Académie Nationale de Médecine, Paris, France.*

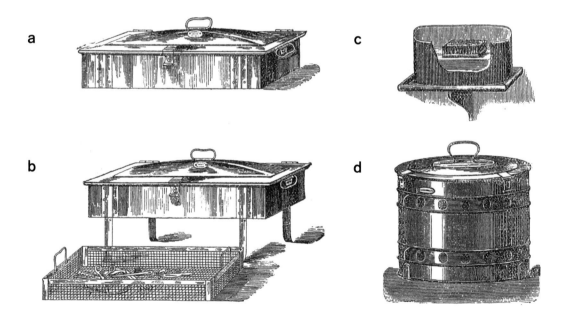

Figure 6. Examples of Schimmelbusch's aseptic equipment, c. 1892. a) Portable instrument steriliser ready for transport. b) The same opened to show legs, permitting use of a spirit lamp and the removable tray for instruments. c) Sterilised nail brush in sublimate solution. d) Sterilising drum for use with a steam autoclave. *Reproduced from Schimmelbusch C. The Aseptic Treatment of Wounds. Translated by AT Rake from 2nd German edn. London: Lewis, 1894: figures 3, 5, 6 & 16.*

staphylococcal infections to penicillin, although the emergence of resistant strains is now a worrying issue, especially as discoveries of new antibiotics diminish. Persistent infections of bones and joint prostheses have diminished by operating in 'clean-air' theatres, confirming Lister's suspicions about organisms floating in air. For infections related to gastroenterology it became apparent in the mid-1970s that *Bacteroides* species were not uncommon in post-appendicectomy wound infections [27], and a dramatic reduction in wound sepsis was achieved (0% against 19%) when placebo was compared with prophylactic intrarectal metronidazole [28].

Conclusions

Lucas-Championnière said in 1878: "There are only two periods in surgery, that before Lister, and that since Lister". [29] Others who celebrate asepsis deny Lister a place in the development of safe surgery, forgetting that the patient's skin, the surgeon's hands and many instruments, such as endoscopes, cannot be submitted to heat sterilisation, whilst the scandal over MRSA (methicillin-resistant *Staphylococcus aureus*) at the beginning of the 21st century reflects neglect of simple Listerian prophylaxis. In reality, operative surgery's battle against infection is linked inescapably to both aseptic and antiseptic practices.

Biographical footnote on Joseph Lister

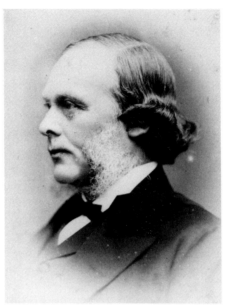

Figure 7. Joseph Lister (1827-1912) aged about 58 years. *Reproduced with permission from the Wellcome Library, London.*

Joseph Lister, the founder of safe surgery, was born in Upton, Essex, the son of Joseph Jackson Lister FRS, a Quaker, wine merchant and dedicated amateur scientist, who perfected the microscope by inventing achromatic lenses, a factor of importance to his son's research. After attending the Quaker School in Tottenham, he entered University College, London in 1844 to study for a BA in arts and in December 1846, witnessed Robert Liston perform the first major operation under general anaesthesia in Britain. He transferred to medical studies in 1847, also at University College, and was among the first British surgeons not to be traditionally apprenticed, graduating MB (London) and FRCS (England) in 1852, appointed house physician to Dr. W.H. Walshe, and house surgeon to Mr. John Erichsen at University College Hospital. Meanwhile, he undertook experimental work on smooth muscle function of the iris and hair follicles, being much influenced by William Sharpey, Professor of Physiology who, noting Lister's interest in surgery, introduced him in 1853 to James Syme, Professor of Clinical Surgery in Edinburgh [30].

Intending to stay for a month, he impressed Syme greatly and was made his supernumerary clerk before being promoted resident house surgeon. After the 60 surgical beds at University College Hospital, Lister was amazed to find 200 at the Edinburgh Royal Infirmary, offering wide experience both to him and his 12 surgical dressers. At the same time he started experiments on inflammation, stimulating a frog's web observed under a microscope. His rapport with Syme flourished and at Syme's house he met many important colleagues, foreign visitors and Syme's eldest daughter Agnes, who he married in 1856. Soon he was appointed Assistant Surgeon and became fully occupied with clinical responsibilities, teaching and research into coagulation of the blood.

In 1860, he took up the Chair of Surgery in Glasgow which stimulated one of the most vital stages of his career. Initially, he had no beds at the Glasgow Royal Infirmary, permitting him to concentrate on teaching and to invent a number of surgical instruments, including a sinus dressing forceps and an ear hook for foreign bodies; his screw tourniquet for the abdominal aorta to promote hip disarticulation was eventually abandoned as too dangerous [31].

Once in the wards he pioneered wrist joint excision for tuberculosis, thus avoiding hand amputation, and noted the Infirmary's high rate of operative wound infections. Pondering a mortality of some 45% for major amputations, Lister's attention was drawn to Pasteur's work on the fermentation of wine and the action of yeasts, which made him suspect it was not the air, but something in the air which fermented wine and putrefied wounds. Searching for an antidote to combat infection, he introduced carbolic acid wound dressings applied immediately after surgery or wounding, as a prophylactic agent in 1865. By 1867, he reported a reduction in amputation mortality to 15%. If others claimed priority in treating wounds with carbolic acid, they only applied it for established infection or gangrene. Lister's antiseptic principle for clean wound management aroused widespread discussion, many in London claiming it was unnecessary, too complicated and it was better to rely on improved hospital hygiene, disbelieving evidence of a germ theory [32].

In the US, Watson noted: "The great objections come not from those who have tried 'Listerism', but from those who are willing to raise their hands and thank God that they have neither witnessed its application nor used it." [33] Fortunately, Lister's surgical assistants and students, and impartial visitors from Europe promulgated his methods, which underwent gradual modification with experience.

In 1860, Lister returned to Edinburgh as Professor of Clinical Surgery, to replace Syme who had become ill and retired, where he had an enthusiastic student following. In addition to employing carbolic acid solutions for sterilising instruments, for cleaning surgeon's hands and patient's skin and to impregnate dressings, Lister now introduced a carbolic spray to saturate the operative field and also medicated gauze dressings. Meanwhile he investigated the souring of

milk to produce a pure culture of *Bacillus lactis* by ultra-dilution in 1877; this first isolation of a pure bacterial culture preceded Koch's isolation on solid media in 1881. He also noted the common presence of *Penicillium glaucum* as a contaminant. Lister was not only an innovative surgeon but a pioneer bacteriologist, a competent physiologist, a botanist and chemist.

When an additional Chair of Clinical Surgery was created at King's College, London, in 1877, he agreed to accept considering it his duty to persuade a largely sceptical metropolis to adopt antiseptic surgery, although very reluctant to leave Edinburgh. Fortified by four members of his Edinburgh team, he slowly won over students and younger surgeons, and in the process introduced better methods of surgical teaching. At this time he pioneered the open reduction of displaced fractures of the patella and olecranon, internally fixing them with silver wire successfully, and he continued research on ligature materials. Eminent internationally, fluent in French and German, he was acclaimed at conferences in Europe and the US, meeting Pasteur, Koch and many leading surgeons who had adopted 'Listerism'.

Lister retired from active practice in 1893, declining the Presidency of the Royal College of Surgeons of England to become President of the Royal Society in 1895; he was created Lord Lister in 1898. Throughout his active surgical career until late in retirement, he investigated chemical methods of hardening catgut to prolong its ligature-holding power, giving his last paper on this subject in 1908. This and much of his experimental work is recorded in four massive volumes, written mostly in the hand of his wife, often noting experiments which began late at night [34]. Agnes Lister was an intelligent and dedicated partner, grievously missed by Lister when she died of pneumonia in 1893, during a holiday in Italy. His *Collected Papers* in two volumes were published in 1909; he died aged 84 at Walmer, Kent in 1912.

If heat sterilisation, introduced after Lister's retirement, proved an essential key to successful gastroenterological surgery, all operative procedures continued to embrace indispensable chemical sterilisation techniques pioneered by Lister's scientific sagacity and relentless endeavour.

References

1. Campbell E, Colton J, Eds. *The Surgery of Theodoric ca. 1267.* New York: Appleton-Century-Crofts, 1955-60; 2: ch.27.

2. Garrison FH. *An Introduction to the History of Medicine*, 4th ed. Commentary on Galen's concept of laudable pus. Philadelphia: Saunders, 1929: 144.

3. Morton LT. *A Medical Bibliography* (noting Antonj Leeuwenhoek's contributions 1693-1718). London: Deutch, 1970; item 67.

4. Spallanzani L. *Saggio di osservazioni microscopiche relative al sistema della generazione.* Modena, 1767.

5. Alanson E. *Practical Observations on Amputation, and the After-treatment.* London: Johnson, 1782: 87-103.

6. Crowther J. A successful mode of preventing gangrene in compound fractures. *Med & Phys J* 1802; 7: 307-10.

7. Wangensteen OH, Wangensteen SD. *The Rise of Surgery.* Folkestone: Dawson, 1978: 410-1.

8. Ibid, 689-90.

9. Semmelweis IP. *Die Aetiologie, der Begriff und die Prophylaxis des Kindbettfiebers.* Budapest: Hartleben, 1861.

10. Lemaire FJ. *Du Coaltar Saponiné, Désinfectant Énergetique.* Paris: Germer-Ballière, 1865.

11. Wangensteen OH, Wangensteen SD. *The Rise of Surgery.* Folkestone: Dawson, 1978: 321.

12. Wells TS. Some causes of excessive mortality after surgical operations. *Br Med J* 1864; ii: 384-8.

13. Godlee RJ. *Lord Lister.* London: Macmillan, 1917: 162-3.

14. Lister J. On a new method of treating compound fractures, abcess, etc with observations on the conditions of suppuration. *Lancet* 1867; i: 326-9, 357-9, 387-9, 507-9; ii: 95-6. On the antiseptic principle in the practice of surgery. *Br Med J* 1867; ii: 246.

15. Godlee RJ. *Lord Lister.* London: Macmillan, 1917: 336-56.

16. Shepherd JA. *Lawson Tait the Rebellious Surgeon (1845-1899).* Lawrence, Kansas: Coronado, 1980: 36-54, 108.

17. Ibid, 90.

18. Lister J. An address on the treatment of wounds. *Lancet* 1881; ii: 369.

19. Pasteur L. A l'occasion de la note de MM Gosselin et A Robin. *Compt Rend Acad D Sc* 1874; 78: 46.

20. Bowman AK. *The life and teaching of Sir William Macewen.* London: Hodge, 1942: 63-5.

21. Wangensteen OH, Wangensteen SD. *The Rise of Surgery.* Folkestone: Dawson, 1978: 491.

22. Tripier L. Du chauffage des instruments en chirurgie. *Lyon Méd* 1883; 2: 551.

23. Neuber G. *Die aseptische Wundbehandlung in meinen chirurgischen Privat-Hospitalern.* Keil, 1886.

24. Redard P. De la désinfection des instruments chirugicaux et des objets de pansements. *Rev D Chir* 1888; 8: 509.

25. Bergmann E von. Méthode aseptique suivie à la clinique de Berlin. *Rev D Chir* 1890; 10: 844-5.

26. Schimmelbusch C. *The Aseptic Treatment of Wounds.* Translated by AT Rake from 2nd German edn. London: Lewis, 1894.

27. Leigh DA, Simmons K, Norman E. Bacterial flora of the appendix fossa in appendicitis and postoperative wound infection. *J Clin Path* 1974; 27: 997-1000.

28. Willis AT, Ferguson IR, Jones PF, *et al.* Metronidazole in prevention and treatment of *Bacteroides* infections after appendicectomy. *Brit Med J* 1976; 1: (3) 18-20.

29. Cameron HC. *On the Evolution of Wound-Treatment During the Last Forty Years.* Glasgow: MacLehose, 1907: 4.

30. Godlee RJ. *Lord Lister.* London: Macmillan, 1917.

31. Cheyne WM, Watson. *Lister and his achievement.* London: Longmans, 1925.

32. Lister J. *Collected papers.* Oxford: Clarendon, 1909.

33. Watson BA. Lister's system of aseptic wound treatment versus its modifications. *Trans Am Surg Assoc* 1882; 1: 205-23.

34. Archives of The Royal College of Surgeons of England.

Chapter 4

The changing tides in oesophageal surgery

Walford Gillison FRCS Ed FRCS

Emeritus Consultant Surgeon, Kidderminster General Hospital, Kidderminster, UK and
Honorary Consultant Surgeon, City Hospital, Birmingham, UK

James B Elder MD FRCS Ed Eng & Glasgow

Emeritus Professor and Consultant Surgeon, North Staffordshire Hospitals, Stoke-on-Trent,
University of Keele, Staffordshire, UK

Introduction

"The oesophagus is a difficult surgical field .... for its inaccessibility, its lack of serous coat, and its enclosure in structures where infection is especially dangerous and rapid." (Ivor Lewis) [1].

Most of the oesophagus is situated behind the heart, between the lungs, in a fairly rigid bony cage. Instrumentation and surgical procedures on the oesophagus are relatively recent events compared with other parts of the body. Many patients are frail. Such frailty and absence of modern peri-operative support was the cause of so little progress taking place until half way through the 20th century.

With the benefit of hindsight the evolution of oesophageal surgery is made easier by looking at four important milestones or time-zones.

Milestones in oesophageal surgery

First milestone: before general anaesthesia in 1846

Earliest endeavours before 'Ether Day' in 1846 were mainly on the cervical oesophagus. The situations were desperate: one can imagine the fear, the pain and the fortitude required of the patients at that time, despite the help of liberal doses of laudanum and alcohol. Frequently the patient was held down, possibly strapped to a hard operating table, with the single-minded surgeons of the day gritting their teeth to achieve the goal as quickly as possible. It is no wonder the operating theatres were placed as far from the wards as practicable. As Nuland [2] wrote: "It took a particular kind of man to do this work...... he is not the kind of man or woman who would be a surgeon of this century."

Surgery in that time was limited to instrumental pushing or pulling foreign bodies, dilating both benign and malignant strictures, or opening the oesophagus through the neck.

Second milestone: 1846 to the advent of thoracotomy until 1913

Before thoracotomy, access to the oesophagus from above or below the mediastinum was limited. Theodor Billroth, the father of gastrointestinal surgery, at one stage said: "Surgery should halt at the pleura!"

Ingenious reconstructions were tried, using rubber tubes, skin tubes, skin grafts, or later, lengths of large or small intestine illustrated later.

Johann von Mikulicz-Radecki (Figure 1), referred to as von Mikulicz, was determined to solve the problem of fatal pneumothorax when the chest cavity was opened, deliberately or otherwise.

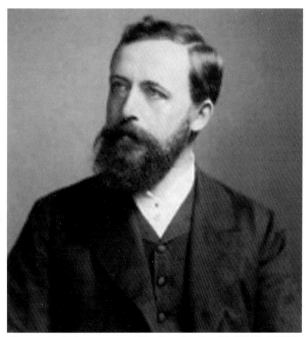

Figure 1. Johann von Mikulicz-Radecki (1850-1905). *Reproduced with permission from the Académie de Médecine, Paris, France.*

He appointed his pupil Ferdinand Sauerbruch to research in the laboratory a means of avoiding it. Sauerbruch realised that if the relatively negative pressure in the pleural cavity could be reproduced outside the chest, surgical intervention should be possible. After several trials and tribulations, he succeeded during a public demonstration in 1904 [3].

The chambers were difficult to seal against leakage, the costs were high and the working environment uncomfortable. Fortunately, following the pioneer work of Brauer and Petersen [4] and others, positive pressure endotracheal ventilation provided an alternative and safer method of providing anaesthesia. Sauerbruch was not amused and advised against positive pressure endotracheal anaesthesia! It took a very short time before he lost that argument.

The third milestone: advent of thoracotomy

In 1913, Torek [5] performed the first successful transthoracic resection with the intention of restoring swallowing outside the chest at a later date. Others attempted to emulate him with varying success.

Later, Rowbotham and Magill's [6] endotracheal tube devised in 1921 permitted access to the chest interior. Surgeons were gradually entering the chest cavity, opening or repairing the oesophagus, but after resection the majority restored continuity outside the rib cage.

The fourth milestone: after 1938

In 1938, Marshall's successful transthoracic resection [7] combined with immediate anastomosis, changed oesophageal surgery forever. When muscle relaxants, blood transfusion and antibiotics arrived in the 1940s, the oesophagus could more safely be resected and restored in this manner. The Copenhagen polio epidemic [8] in 1952 stimulated development of long-term ventilation which further involved anaesthetists, as well as intensive and critical care units. Endotracheal tubes permitted 'one-lung anaesthesia' allowing one lung to collapse on the operated side while the other lung continued to absorb the anaesthetic gases. Plastic cannulas transformed intravenous therapy, and the explosion of laparoscopic and endoscopic surgery in the last 25 years has made a huge surgical impact.

Common oesophageal disorders

Foreign body impaction

Conservative treatment

In 1889 the *Journal of Medical Progress* quoted the "Potato Cure" by a Dr. Cameron at a meeting of the Imperial Society of Physicians in Vienna. He cited several patients with impacted foreign bodies, who were fed by mashed potato, in order to propel the bolus into the stomach.

Hochenegg and Billroth at the same meeting agreed. This might be questioned, as this method would only work in mild obstructions, and in the event of failure would only complicate the solution.

Blind extraction

Johannes Arculanus in 1493 [9], designed a flexible multi-perforated leaden tube for extraction of impacted foreign bodies which might be caught in its perforations. About the same time, Ambroise Paré devised leather tubes, osiers (willow wands) and swans' quills to dispel boluses. After these, flexible lead or silver probes and whalebone probes were used. They were understandably called 'sounds' especially if the foreign body was metallic.

About a century later, Guilemus Fabricius Hildanus designed a perforated silver tube, about 75cm in length with a small sponge at its tip, for retrieving or pushing objects through to the stomach. Hieronymus Fabricius from Aquapendente (Wilhelm Fabry) confirmed that if an impacted object in the oesophagus could not be extracted up through the mouth, it was reasonable to push it distally into the stomach. Furthermore, he once covered a similar tube with sheep intestine to reduce friction to be retained *in situ* for feeding purposes. He also used thin waxed tapers, hence 'bougies' (French for waxed candle) to push obstructing objects into the stomach.

Open operation

According to Meade [10], Habicot in 1620 saved a young boy from death by asphyxiation, who had swallowed a bag of coins which impacted in the upper oesophagus. He first performed an emergency tracheotomy; later, an assistant passed a sound by mouth to the obstruction. Habicot squeezed the bag of coins safely into the stomach without opening the oesophagus. Over a century later, Guttani, according to Goursault from Limoges, removed an impacted bone from the cervical oesophagus in 1738. He wisely laid the wound open to allow delayed healing. Therefore, in the 16th and 17th centuries, some surgeons were conscious of the risks of infection, and that fistulas would close in the absence of distal obstruction.

Cheever [11], in 1867, was the first American to perform a successful oesophagotomy for impacted foreign body. He noted seven oesophagotomies had been reported in France, five in England, and one each in Belgium, Italy and India. Cheever's foreign body was an impacted fish-bone in the oesophagus which had stuck below the cricoid cartilage for three days despite repeated attempts to remove it endoscopically.

It was hoped a posterolateral extrapleural route for surgical access to the thoracic oesophagus would reduce the risk of empyema. In 1924, Enderlen [12] of Heidelberg did succeed in such an attempt; however, most contemporaries thought it too dangerous.

Visual extraction

Successful treatment was related to the advances in endoscopy and instruments of retrieval. The reader is recommended to an excellent detailed review by Edmondson [13] for the broader picture. Endoscopic removal replaced most operative measures because general and topical anaesthesia gradually became safer and more comfortable.

Upper gastrointestinal endoscopy is conveniently divided into three eras: the rigid, semi-flexible and fiberoptic eras.

The rigid endoscope era (1805-1932)
Adolf Kussmaul, father-in-law to Vincenz Czerny, was driven by the discovery that emptying of the stomach in pyloric stenosis produced excellent but temporary relief. He realised that seeing the interior of the oesophagus and stomach was crucial. He extended the advances by Bozzini's lichtleiter and Desormeux' cystoscopes, which were mainly of benefit for seeing the pharynx, vagina or bladder, to looking further. In 1868 [13], he got a glimpse of the oesophagus but was hindered by poor light and no suction. He once saw a tumour of the oesophagus at the level of the tracheal bifurcation with an instrument similar to that shown in Figure 2.

He established, thanks to a co-operative sword swallower, the important principle that both the oesophagus and part of the stomach could be examined with a straight instrument.

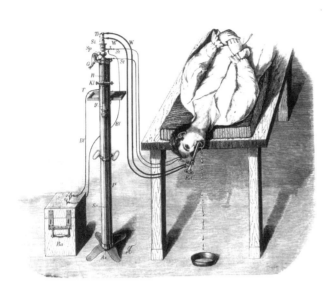

Figure 2. First oesophagoscopic examination. *Reproduced from Phillipp Bozzini and Endoscopy in the 19th century. By H.J. and M.A. Reuter, with collaboration by D. Loenicker. Max Nitze Museum, Stuttgart, 1988.*

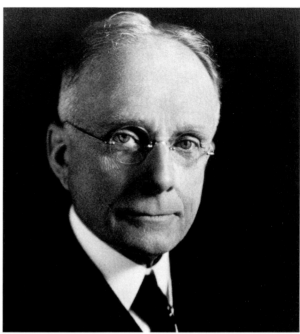

Figure 3. Chevalier Jackson (1865-1958). *Reproduced with permission from the Wellcome Library, London.*

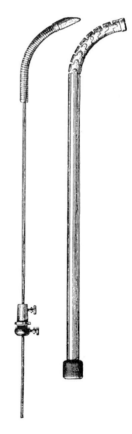

Progress continued when Leiter, a technician, collaborated with Mikulicz using electric light sources and straight tubular endoscopes.

Von Hacker [14] first successfully removed a foreign body through an oesophagoscope in 1898. As oesophagoscopes were being developed globally, increasing patient comfort and safety, adequate light, adequate suction and clear views made oesophagotomy less necessary.

Doyens such as Chevalier Jackson (Figure 3) perfected examination and retrieval of foreign objects, performing biopsies and occasionally, he saw part of the stomach using straight instruments. An accolade to Jackson was made by Edmondson [13] who said no contemporary was able to see as much, nor perform endoscopy so safely. Rigid oesophagoscopes are occasionally required to retrieve foreign bodies today.

The semi-flexible (Schindler) era (1932-1957)

Schindler, an expert with rigid equipment, devised with Wolf an endoscope which was able to visualise most of the stomach as well as the oesophagus after several attempts (Figure 4). Such instruments were

Figure 4. Schindler semi-flexible endoscope (Down Bros. London). *Reproduced with permission from B. Braun Medical Ltd.*

easier to introduce, safer to use and could have camera attachment. After setting up teaching centres around Munich in Germany, he was seized during a Nazi purge in Munich because he was Jewish, but thanks to his non-Jewish wife and his American colleagues, he was released to perform a lecture tour on endoscopy in America, and wisely decided to remain.

The fiberoptic era (since 1957)

Basil Hirschowitz utilised advances in the physics of light-bending glass fibres until he could examine his own gastric interior. Now the proximal duodenum and the whole stomach could be seen, and side-viewing equipment allowed the duodenum and biliary tree to be inspected and cannulated. Fiberoptic colonoscopy followed soon after.

Perforation and rupture

Instrumental damage is still the commonest cause of oesophageal rupture today. Management and survival depend on the speed of diagnosis and the extent of the damage. Spontaneous rupture is more rare an event.

No surgical intervention was possible when the famous Dutch physician Hermann Boerhaave (Figure 5) attended the gourmand, the Grand Admiral of Holland, Baron de Wassenaer in 1723.

A fine account has been given by Liebermann-Meffert and colleagues [15]: "Three days earlier the patient had taken part in what he called a light meal from the following menu:

Veal Soup with herbs.
Boiled lamb with cabbage.
Fried sweetbread (pancreas) and spinach.
Duck.
Two larks.
Compôte of apples.
Dessert.
Pears, Grapes, Sweetmeats.
Beer and Moselle.

He went out riding after this repast, but at 10.30pm he suffered intense pains in the stomach. Despite several doses of his favourite emetic, vomiting produced no relief. Desperately he tickled his throat with a feather which caused even greater pain which spread round his left chest.

After careful examination of both patient and his urine, Boerhaave believed the patient was dehydrated despite the huge fluid intake; so poultices, blood letting, oral sweet almond oil and enemata were tried with no relief before the patient died.

Autopsy showed surgical emphysema all over his torso, his intestines were full of air, despite an empty stomach and the left chest full of fluid smelling of roast duck. Both the patient's emetic solution and Boerhaave's almond oil were floating on the surface. Above the hiatus was a ragged tear in the left wall of the pleura communicating with a cavity between two completely disrupted ends of the previously healthy oesophagus."

Norman Barrett [16] performed the first successful operative repair in 1947. Menguy in 1971 repaired a huge tear in the thoracic oesophagus and protected his suture line with a loop cervical oesophagostomy

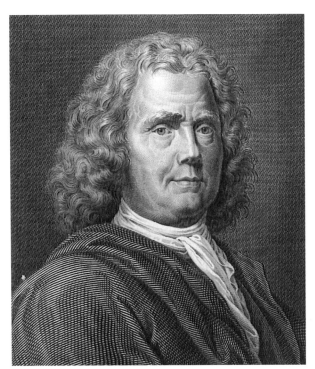

Figure 5. Hermann Boerhaave (1668-1738). *Reproduced with permission from the Académie de Médecine, Paris, France.*

above and fed the patient by gastrostomy until the oesophagus was proved to have healed later [17].

Wise surgeons soon learned to look for other injuries: blunt injuries to the thoracic oesophagus were often too ragged to suture, so T-tubes used by Abbott and colleagues [18], with temporising cervical oesophagostomies were used, or restoration using the stomach or colon later. For distal obstruction or tumour, the case for immediate oesophagectomy was justified by Seybold, Johnson and Leary [19] in 1950, and Blalock [20] in 1957.

Damage by noxious acids and caustics

Postlethwait found in nearly 4000 poison ingestions that only 5.7% developed permanent stenoses. Most accidental strictures occur in children. About 60% in his study were due to lye (sodium hydroxide) ingestion [21]. Some medications, such as potassium chloride, caused localised stricture especially in motility disorders. Ingestion of caustics left in wine bottles by retreating troops in battle proved devastating weapons.

Acute stages

The knowledge of the site and extent of the stricture was crucial in order to save some of these desperate cases. Prompt skilled endoscopy was often paramount; likewise, care for respiratory complications, relief of pain, and rehydration were critical. If surgical intervention was not indicated, Constanzo and colleagues [22] splinted the lumen with a nasogastric tube to feed the patient and prevent complete fibrosis.

The treatment options with acute necrosis were:

- transhiatal oesophagectomy [23] (vide infra) if the stomach were spared;
- diversion by cervical oesophagostomy, with washing and drainage of the contaminated mediastinum and peritoneum;
- replacement with pedicled colon if stomach was unavailable. Yudin [24] published a most remarkable series reported in 1944 of 88 resections followed by colonic substitution with only two deaths;

- pedicled or free jejunal graft [25], if localised to the neck or lowermost oesophagus, described in the cancer section below.

Late stages

The clinician had to look out for, anticipate and treat if necessary:

- reflux oesophagitis from shortening of the longitudinal muscle pulling the cardia through the hiatus;
- hard, resistant, fibrotic strictures. Tucker [26], in 1924, employed string dilatations threaded from mouth to preliminary gastrostomy, until most fibrotic narrowing ceased. Tucker realised that retrograde dilatation by the gastrostomy was often safer in tough late strictures;
- occasionally strictures resistant to dilatations had to be resected, as described later in this chapter;
- malignant (usually squamous) change occurring approximately 24 years later. Kiviranta [27] found increased frequency of dilatations an ominous sign.

Chevalier Jackson, who had a huge reputation for dilating oesophageal strictures, fought for 20 years to get caustics clearly labelled and out of reach of children [28]. It eventually became law by statute in the US in 1927.

Damage by reflux of noxious digestive juices (gastro-oesophageal reflux)

Hiatal hernia and gastro-oesophageal reflux

Diaphragmatic hernias

Ambroise Paré [29] in the 16th century, described autopsy findings of two patients with traumatic diaphragmatic hernia in his book *Oeuvres complètes*. Bright [30] from Guy's Hospital in London reported the phenomenon in 1836. Bowditch [31], 17 years later, suggested that it should be corrected or repaired. In 1912, Scudder [32] from Boston reported on 53 surgical attempts at reduction and repair of all types of hiatal hernia. He recorded a survival of seven in 11 thoracic repairs, but only seven survived out of 42 abdominal repairs! There was no mention of associated abdominal disease.

Sliding hiatal hernias

Everything changed when Allison [33] drew attention in 1951 to reflux symptoms being different from other abdominal conditions. Without the aid of manometry, Allison believed simple anatomical repair alone was sufficient to cure reflux; he deserves credit for admitting it was insufficient later. Before laparoscopic surgery, surgeons had heated arguments for and against abdominal or thoracic access. The advantages of the abdominal approach included:

- treatment of coexisting peptic ulcer or gallbladder disease;
- alleged fewer disturbances of the left lung;
- a potentially painless scar.

Advantages of the thoracic approach included:

- direct access to a badly inflamed lower oesophagus;
- better access in obese patients;
- incarcerated herniated stomach reduction.

The principles, whatever the route, included restoration of original anatomy, a thorough cleaning of the hiatal area, with preservation of the vagus nerves and spleen.

Some of the commoner anti-reflux operations are described below.

Classical Nissen fundoplication

Rudolf Nissen (Figure 20) discovered an anti-reflux procedure by chance, following a resection of the cardia for oesophageal ulcer in 1936, which he described in 1937 [34]. He fashioned the oesophagus into the fundus of the stomach, similar to the valve of a Witzel gastrostomy (Figure 3, Chapter 6). To his delight, he found this patient had no reflux symptoms after 16 years. Other patients without this valve developed oesophagitis.

Initially, he added a gastropexy, but discarded it later. However, after the 1937 experience, he

recreated a new valve by wrapping a tongue of intact stomach near the cardia, which he called a 'fundoplication'. The stages are shown in Figure 6.

The principles of Nissen's anti-reflux operation were:

- sub-costal incision, though most surgeons used an upper midline incision;
- division of the short gastric vessels, but his assistant Rossetti tried to avoid it. The spleen was preserved if possible;
- thorough clearance behind the restored abdominal oesophagus;
- three or four non-absorbable sutures inserted transversely from the fundus on the left to the plicated fundus on the right of the oesophagus. These included the anterior wall of the lower oesophagus to prevent the oesophagus retracting upward from the plication. His unit later reduced the number of sutures to one or two;
- Nissen seldom repaired the hiatus as he believed that the bulk of the plication was too large to enter the chest. He declared that should this postoperative event take place, the 'wrap' would still act as a reflux barrier even in the chest.

However, Mansour and colleagues [35] found some prolapsed plications through the hiatus developed gastric ulceration above the diaphragm. Many agreed with Polk and Zeppa [36] in 1969 who routinely repaired the diaphragm.

There is no doubt that the Nissen fundoplication or 'wrap' has been a very successful anti-reflux barrier. It has been too successful in some patients, causing occasional dysphagia and 'gas-bloat'. The latter could cause inability to belch or vomit, and socially embarrassing flatulence. It is because the principle of Nissen's fundoplication is applicable to laparoscopic surgery that many surgeons have modified the 'wrap' to reduce the chances of gas bloat. These modifications include that of Donahue [37] who devised a 'floppy' 360° fundoplication, and DeMeester's [38] shortened version. The Lind [39] and Toupet [40] partial fundoplications are very similar. Watson's [41] fundoplication of only 120° was even less of a wrap.

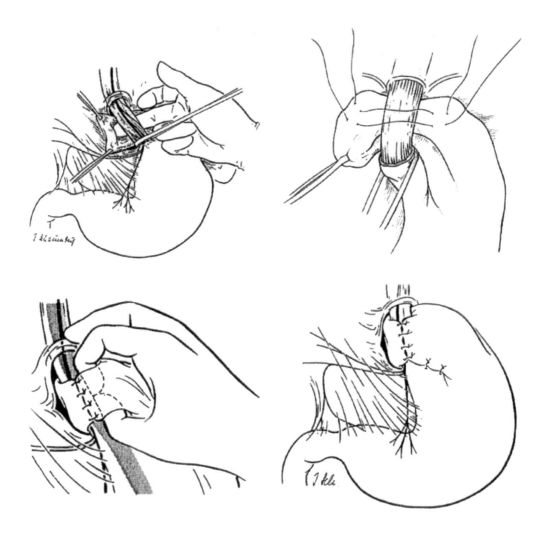

Figure 6. Classical Nissen fundoplication by his first assistant Mario Rossetti. *Reproduced with permission from Elsevier Science Inc. Surgery of the Oesophagus. Jamieson GG, Ed. Churchill Livingstone, 1988: 250-1.*

DeMeester's total fundoplication was short, all short gastric vessels were divided, and the 2cm wrap placed between the oesophagus and the posterior vagal trunk. Like Donahue's wrap, there was space between it and the oesophagus, which incorporated a # 60 bougie during plication. If the cardia could not be brought into the abdomen, he would open the chest to gain more oesophageal length, or change to a Collis-Nissen anti-reflux operation described below.

Tom DeMeester

During the US-Vietnam War, DeMeester was conscripted into the American armed forces. In charge of healthy troops he had time on his hands. Acid reflux measured by pH recordings above the cardia encountered by people such as Spencer [42] was recent news. How much and how often was reflux abnormal? DeMeester was able to test symptomatic and asymptomatic volunteers over 24 hours. The response of the airmen for the reward of an extra week's annual leave by swallowing a pH probe for 24 hours resulted in a deluge of volunteers! He found asymptomatic troops refluxed less than 5% of a day, but most symptomatic airmen refluxed for longer periods. Separately, this test became a useful yardstick in the investigation of chest pain [44].

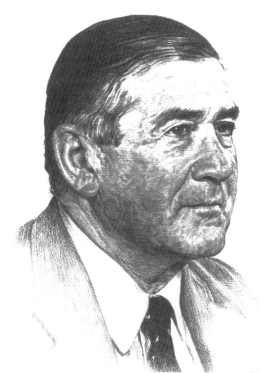

Figure 7. Ronald H.R. Belsey (contemporary).
Reproduced from the editor's private collection.

Lucius D. Hill III employed a reversed partial fundoplication [45]; his gastropexy was constructed by anchoring the plication to the median arcuate ligament in front of the aorta.

Belsey's 'Mark IV' partial fundoplication [43]

Ronald Belsey (Figure 7) devised a transthoracic approach which was a partial fundoplication [42] in the vertical plane, unlike Nissen's horizontal plication. Belsey found his fourth version was reproducible and easily taught to trainees [46].

Other diverse anti-reflux procedures

Angelchik prosthesis [47]

Jean Pierre Angelchik once assisted a urological colleague who was operating on a patient with urinary incontinence. The procedure required a silicone gel-filled U-shaped prosthesis to be slung around the bladder neck. Angelchik regarded gastro-oesophageal reflux as an example of gastric incontinence, so he designed a similar prosthesis to surround the cardia. The procedure was easily performed either by open or laparoscopic means. Angelchik's prosthesis encircled the cardia before being tied. It worked well in some, though by no means in all patients. Firm fibrosis around the collar, and migration to above and below the diaphragm reduced its popularity. According to Durrans and colleagues [48], an unacceptable 17.1% of prostheses had to be removed within 15 months. More serious complications since has caused the operation to be abandoned.

Diversion of gastric and duodenal juices from the stomach

Oesophagitis and oesophageal ulcers have been known to be related to digestive juices since the time of Quincke [49] in 1879. The acid-peptic element of reflux material has been known since Winkelstein [50] in 1935. Studies on pH have shown acid reflux coinciding with oesophageal pain or heartburn described by Tuttle and Grossman [51] in 1958.

Bile and pancreatic juices were evaluated in animal and patient studies. Royston and colleagues [52] applied the principle of diversion of duodenal contents away from the oesophagus in patients. They employed the Roux-en-Y gastrojejunostomy and added a vagotomy to protect the jejunum from stomal ulceration (Figure 8). Washer and colleagues [53] showed in 53 severe reflux-strictured patients relief for many could be obtained, with no mortality, by Roux-en-Y duodenal diversion. They, therefore, demonstrated that before the advent of firm fibrosis, reflux oesophagitis could be reversed by depleting duodenal juice from the gastric chyme.

Though successful, diversion procedures and vagotomy are rarely used today because a small number of patients became severely affected by a gastric 'dumping' syndrome, a rare complication notoriously hard to treat. Should the vagotomy be incomplete, stomal ulceration and its complications would follow [54].

Early laparoscopic operations

As in other surgical procedures, the principles in laparoscopic surgery are the same as used in open surgery. Failure to adhere to these principles has courted disaster.

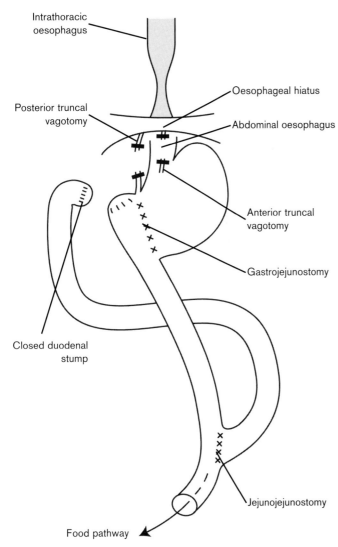

Figure 8. Duodenal juice diversion by Roux-en-Y.

In 1991, Dallemagne and associates [55] in Belgium and Geagea [56] in Canada, published their early findings using a minimal invasive approach to anti-reflux surgery.

Initial conversion rates were high: 25% in Belgium, and 10% in Canada, respectively. Today, conversion rates are below 5%. Both groups agreed that the cardia must be brought below the hiatus. The Belgians usually divided the short gastric vessels, but the Canadians usually did not. Just as in cholecystectomy, minimal invasive surgery was less painful and had a shorter hospital stay. The author of Chapter 7, Bernard Launois, informed the authors of this chapter of a rare death after one laparoscopic

repair. However, he also said 10% of the total pharmaceutical budget of Australia is spent on reflux medication. Laparoscopic anti-reflux surgery compared with long-term medical treatment has resulted in surgery being offered across the globe.

Oesophageal strictures

Reflux strictures were a huge problem before modern anti-ulcer drugs became available. Strictured gullets were historically treated in the same way as malignant strictures. They could be treated by the following:

◆ dilatation with or without anti-reflux surgery;
◆ gastric tubes;
◆ whole stomach replacements;
◆ jejunal interposition;
◆ free vascularised jejunal grafts;
◆ colon replacements;
◆ vagotomy, antrectomy and Roux-en-Y diversion.

Dilatations with or without anti-reflux surgery

Retrograde dilatation
Before quality instruments with good suction and light, oesophageal dilatation was first paradoxically safer by digital or instrumental means below the diaphragm via a gastrostomy. According to Holmes [57], in 1883 von Bergmann first published a retrograde dilatation of an oesophageal stricture. The following year he reported the work of Professor Loreta from Bologna University, who had dilated both oesophageal and pyloric strictures by this route. In 1890, Robert Abbe [58] from New York gained access by a gastrostomy from below and a cervical oesophagostomy from above, to establish safe and repeatable dilatations. Dilatation began with gum elastic bougies; recurrent strictures were split by a 'see-saw' action using the string between the cervical and gastric stomata. In 1894, von Hacker [14] employed a system of graded steel balls attached to fine strings retrieved from a gastrostomy to enable retrograde dilatation. He strongly warned about the ease of instrumental perforation immediately proximal to the stricture.

Prograde dilatation

Dilators evolved according to available endoscopes, the advent of anaesthesia or sedation, and facilities of X-Ray screening for difficult cases. These are (some are illustrated in Figure 9):

- Negus and Jackson rigid dilators;
- Moloney mercury-filled flexible tubes;
- the Eder-Puestow system, incorporating guidewires and threaded olives [59];
- Celestin graded plastic dilators mounted on guidewires;
- more modern balloon-mounted dilators which reduced the need for radiological screening.

by his American colleagues initially, until Jiannu [61] and others around 1912 to 1914, succeeded. Gavriliu [62] in 1975, added several hundred cases from Romania.

Gastric tubes, lesser curvature

Gastric tubes could also be fashioned from the lesser curvature to make a 'neo-oeosphagus'. Collis created a tube or 'neo-oesophagus' out of the lesser curvature known as the Collis gastroplasty (Figure 10) [63]. It relieved dysphagia but was ineffective against reflux.

Others realised Collis' gastroplasty was worth pursuing provided reflux was controlled. The Collis-Nissen operation emerged although neither Collis nor

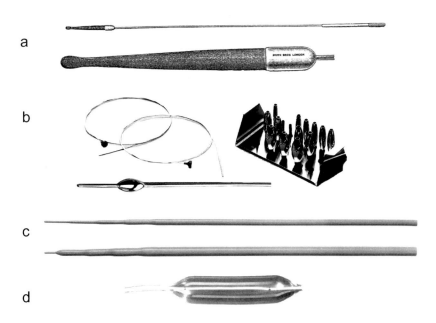

Figure 9. Some of the dilators in historical practice. a) Classical gum-elastic dilator devised by Chevalier Jackson (Down Bros London). *Reproduced with permission from B. Braun Medical Ltd.* **b) Eder-Puestow system using staff, guidewire and graded olives.** *Reproduced with permission from Olympus-KeyMed Ltd.* **c) Graduated Celestin dilators.** *Reproduced with permission from LR Celestin FRCS.* **d) Typical endoscopically inserted balloon dilator.** *Reproduced with permission from Olympus-KeyMed Ltd. (Judy Moss. Medical Photography Dept, Musgrove Park Hospital).*

Gastric tubes, greater curvature

Beck and Carrel [60] in 1905 described how a greater curvature tube could be used to replace the thoracic oesophagus from animal studies, but Beck was ignored

Nissen ever actually performed this operation! Henderson [64] in 1977, and Orringer [65] in 1978 proved it not only relieved dysphagia but also reduced reflux (Figure 11).

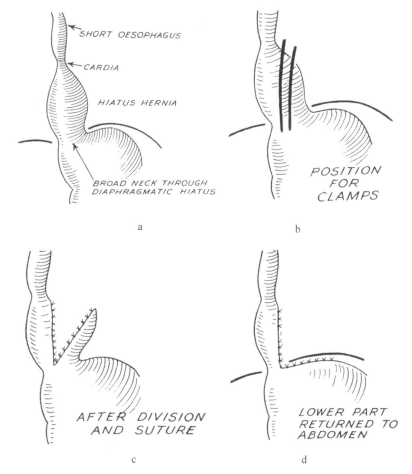

Figure 10. Original Collis gastroplasty. *Reproduced with permission from the BMJ Publishing Group. Collis JL. Gastroplasty. Thorax 1961; 16: 197-9.*

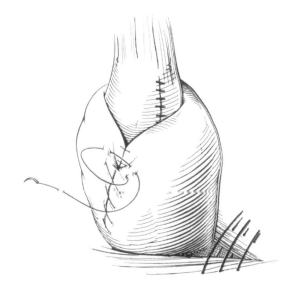

Figure 11. Collis-Nissen gastroplasty by Mark Orringer MD. *Reproduced with permission from Elsevier Science. Surgery of the Oesophagus. Jamieson GG, Ed. Churchill Livingstone, 1988: 332.*

The stages of the operation are summarised as follows:

- dilatation of the stricture;
- left thoracotomy with wide clearance around the cardia, preserving the vagus nerves and spleen;
- stapling of the 'neo-oesophagus' beside a large indwelling tube;
- fundoplication around the 'neo-oesophagus' to prevent reflux.

Orringer added a drainage procedure if either vagal nerve were cut or stretched, or if dense adhesions from previous surgery were present. This operation for a shortened oesophagus is still popular amongst thoracic surgeons today.

Whole stomach replacement

Kirschner [66] was the first to demonstrate that a mobilised stomach could reach the neck and beyond, provided it was nourished by the right gastric vessels. Figure 12 also shows his drainage of the redundant oesophagus to a jejunal loop below the stricture.

Jejunum

César Roux [67] from Lausanne, (Figure 13) achieved a huge step forward in 1907, when he resected a lye stricture of a young child mobilising a pedicled segment of jejunum from the stomach seen in Figure 14. The girl was fed by gastrostomy until the jejunal conduit was connected four years later.

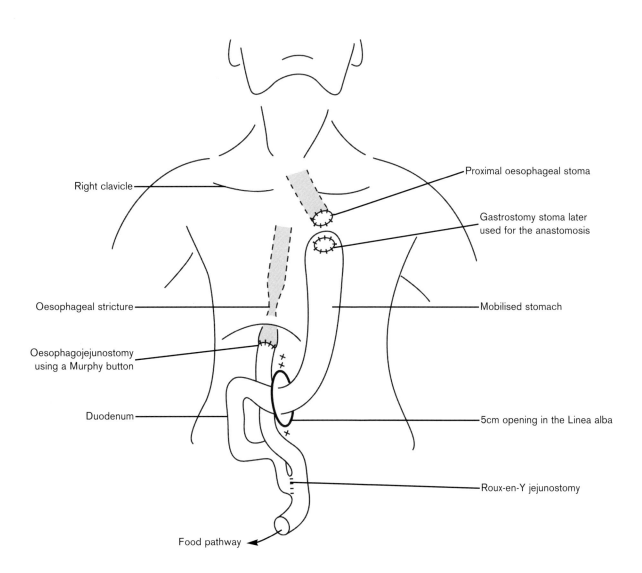

Figure 12. Kirschner's oesophageal replacement using whole stomach.

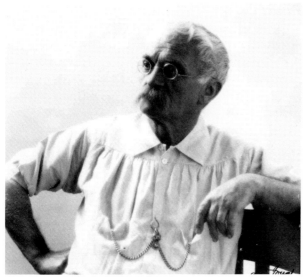

Figure 13. César Roux of Lausanne (1857-1934).
Reproduced with permission from the Institut d'Histoire de la Médecine et de la Santé, Lausanne, Switzerland.

Colon replacement

In 1911, Kelling [68] was on one occasion trying to perform a jejunal conduit to bypass a mid-oesophageal cancer, but found the mesentery too short to reach the cervical oesophagus. He was forced to insert a segment of transverse colon within a subcutaneous tunnel over the sternum. Though this was viable and the principle was established, the patient died from an unrelated cause before swallowing could be restored. Vulliet [69] succeeded in replacing a benign stricture with a length of colon. He used temporary vascular clamps on the vessels before resection and Roith [70] employed the right colon to bypass a stricture 13 years later. Subsequently, Belsey [71] and others used the left colon for benign stricture on a regular basis.

Achalasia of the cardia

(Greek 'chalasis' = relaxation, therefore 'achalasis' = failure to relax.)

The treatment of this disease was controversial in the early days, because the cause was not understood until the middle of the 20th century.

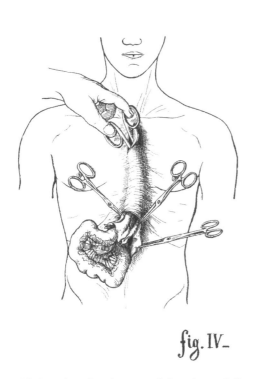

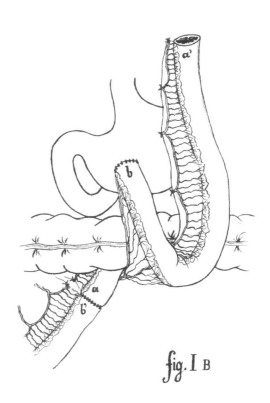

Figure 14. Roux's subcutaneous jejunal conduit. *Reproduced with permission from the Institut d'Histoire de la Médecine et de la Santé, Lausanne, Switzerland.*

Yet over 300 years ago, Thomas Willis, a founding member of the future Royal Society of London, believed the dysphagia was due to absent or poor relaxation of the muscles around the gastro-oesophageal junction. Kittle [72] quotes Willis' description in 1679 very graphically: "The patient otherwise healthful enough, …. was wont, very often, to cast up whatsoever he had eaten …. He would eat until the Oesophagus was filled up to the throat, …. nothing sliding down to the Ventricle (stomach), he cast up raw or crude whatsoever he had taken in …. I prepared an instrument for him like a rod of a whale bone with a little round button of sponge fixed to the top of it." He then started a series of dilatations with this probang for the patient whenever the dysphagia returned. Neither the clinical description, nor the treatment could have been bettered. The patient was able to swallow over the following 15 years thanks to Willis' expert repeated dilatations. According to Meade [10] Willis implied the correct explanation when he wrote that: "….. the mouth of the stomach always being closed, either by tumour or palsie, and nothing could be admitted into the Ventricle (stomach) unless it was violently opened."

Historical treatments

As dilatations were not universally successful, other methods of relieving the dysphagia had to be tried. 'Spasm' was believed the cause for a long time, but it was von Mikulicz [73] who perpetuated the misnomer of 'cardiospasm'. The explanation was not realised until 1888 when an American, Max Einhorn [74], and the German, Meltzer [75], independently suggested that 'spasm' of the cardia was not correct. According to Hertz [76] in 1915, Perry from the US and Sir Arthur Hurst from the UK coined the term 'achalasia' (failure of relaxation). Treatments included:

◆ forceful retrograde dilatation (Mikulicz-Schloffer) [77];
◆ oesophagostomy (Zaaijer) [78];
◆ oesophagogastrostomy (Heyrovsky) [79];
◆ cardioplasty (Wendel) [80];
◆ myotomy at the junction (Heller) [81].

Gottstein [82], in 1904, suggested a procedure resembling Ramstedt's procedure, but it was Ernst Heller [81] (Figure 15) in 1913, that actually put it into

practice. Heller planned to do a cardioplasty such as that devised by Heyrovsky, but at operation he found the mega-oesophagus grossly thickened and difficult. He described the oesophagus as big as "a chimney of a kerosene lamp!" He performed an anterior extramucosal myotomy parallel to the long axis of 8cm in length, which he covered with a strip of netting to prevent leakage from such a long myotomy, and did a similar myotomy posteriorly.

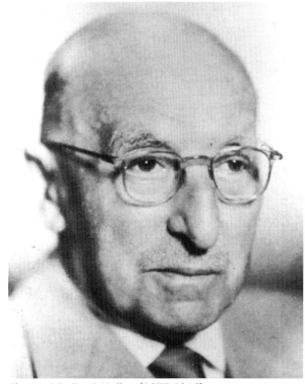

Figure 15. Ernst Heller (1877-1964). *Reproduced from the editor's private collection.*

The patient suffered from a postoperative pneumonia, from which he recovered, but was eating solid food on the eighth day. Steichen and associates [83] reported that the same patient was eating well eight years later!

The complications of cardioplasty and oesophagogastrostomy were elegantly described by Barrett and Franklin [84] in 1949. Relief of severe dysphagia would be dramatic for three to six months and then a new dysphagia, often accompanied by anaemia caused by bleeding followed because of severe reflux oeosphagitis. Conversion to myotomy rescued many of these patients.

Cardiomyotomy caught on quickly. Berg in America in 1918, followed by Rowlands in the UK in 1920 achieved success without the punishing postoperative reflux that followed the cardioplasties, and the subsequent results across the world were well recorded by Ellis and associates [85].

Many have found a single anterior seromyotomy performed laparoscopically has been satisfactory following Pinotti's [86] publication.

Oesophageal cancer

Cancer of the cervical oesophagus

First attempts at resection were made on the cervical oesophagus, because of its relative accessibility. In 1877, Czerny [87] (Figure 16) under Billroth did the first resection in a patient. At that time there was no attempt at restoring continuity, so the patient was left with a proximal cervical stoma and a distal thoracic oesophageal opening for feeding purposes. He reported: "In a case of annular carcinoma of the esophagus which caused a stricture that would not admit an esophageal sound ..... I resected a 6cm piece of the entire wall of the esophagus, and sutured the lower end into the neck." The patient died three months later from local recurrent disease occluding the lower stoma.

Billroth [88] himself resected a larger cervical oesophageal cancer including the larynx and thyroid two years later. The patient died six weeks later from mediastinitis from perforation during dilatation for feeding tube insertion. According to Mikulicz [89], by 1885 Billroth had completed nine cervical resections with five deaths; the four survivors lived between three and 12 months. Mikulicz [90] successfully excised a cervical oesophageal tumour and restored continuity with a skin tube. His patient survived for 11 months, quite remarkable for those days.

Wilfred Trotter [91] from London must have been congratulated for dogged perseverance in 1925, when he resected a cervical carcinoma. Below is the order of events:

- preliminary gastrostomy and dental clearance;
- skin flap based from the right side of the neck,

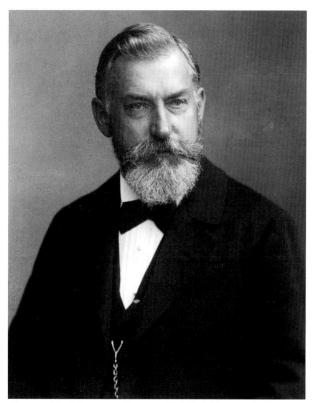

Figure 16. Vincenz Czerny (1842-1916). *Reproduced with permission from the Wellcome Library, London.*

placed behind the mobilised oesophageal tumour and sutured to the left neck;
- oesophageal tumour resected and the ends left open, similar to Czerny;
- continuity with the skin flap delayed by the need for node dissection on the left, dilatation of the lower stoma, then radiotherapy to local recurrences;
- finally, the skin tube was joined to each end of the oesophagus.

Death occurred ten years later from cordoma of the sacrum; the new oesophagus was perfect at autopsy

A revolutionary technique was introduced in 1959 by Seidenburg and Hurwith [25] involving micro-vascular expertise. A short segment of jejunum was taken from the abdomen and two anastomoses made between the internal jugular vein, and the superior thyroid artery with the mesenteric vessels. Following this, the pharynx above and the thoracic oesophagus below were joined after the vascular connection.

Remaining oesophagus

Von Ach [92] (1913) in Munich, Germany, performed a blunt transhiatal resection for mid-oesophageal cancer, via the neck and abdomen without restoring continuity, leaving a cervical oesophagostomy and a feeding gastrostomy. This could be described as two-thirds of a transhiatal oesophagectomy. This patient survived.

In 1913, Franz Torek made history with his transpleural resection [5].

Here were the stages in this historic operation:

- a preliminary gastrostomy was constructed for nourishment;
- the left chest opened, many pleural adhesions divided, and by pushing the aortic arch forward, he was able to divide oesophageal arterial branches and free the upper oesophagus;
- he carefully preserved as many vagus nerves as possible, because Sauerbruch had told him division of the vagal branches meant instant death!;
- the healthy oesophagus was divided well above the tumour and brought out of the neck, to be tunnelled to the left second intercostal space;
- the lower stump was invaginated into the stomach after removal of the tumour, retreating from the pleural cavity without drainage;
- the ribs were approximated with strong silk, the muscles with catgut and the skin with interrupted silk sutures;
- on the eighth postoperative day a rubber tube connected the cervical oesophagus to the gastrostomy permitting swallowing from mouth to stomach.

The tumour was a squamous carcinoma with node involvement. Surgery ended here because the patient refused any more treatment, but his rubber 'neo-oesophagus' worked perfectly well for 13 more years!

Torek never had an opportunity to repeat this operation, but must have been chagrined to listen to Garlock [93] present three identical resections later. Worthy of comment was the achievement of von Ach who changed from his transhiatal method to Torek's method (according to Meyer [94]), on one occasion resecting a tumour in one hour and 25 minutes! Despite Torek's publicity, there were few successes. Ochsner

and DeBakey [95] reported 17 survivors out of 58 published Torek resections, with a worrying mortality of 70%.

Rovsing [96] in 1926 was extremely aware of the dangers of infection, so he avoided colonic tubes [69, 70]. Having observed from contrast studies that both peristaltic and anti-peristaltic tubes of stomach [60, 66, 68] and intestine tend to became passive or inert after a month, illustrated by Torek's 'rubber oesophagus', he succeeded several times with a staged procedure with minimal contamination of the peritoneum. He started with a feeding gastrotomy, next a cervical oesophagostomy, then he inserted a long skin tube close to the stomata buried under an ante-thoracic flap, before finally joining the skin tube ends to the oesophageal and gastrostomy stomata.

Grey Turner [97] from Newcastle-upon-Tyne (UK) successfully emulated Rovsing's procedure with a mid-thoracic resection. The patient swallowed well after 206 days! By the end of his surgical career Turner had completed 25 resections. The operability rate was 44% and the mortality 40%. There were three long-term survivors.

While the rest of the surgical world was staying outside the chest, a remarkable Japanese surgeon paved the way for future advance. In 1933, Ohsawa [98] from Kyoto published a series started in 1925 using the whole stomach for replacement. He performed a transpleural resection with immediate anastomosis successfully in eight out of 19 resections. He did not require Sauerbruch's chamber, underwater seal drainage, or positive pressure endotracheal ventilation.

The year of 1938 heralded the beginning of transpleural resections of the cancer followed by immediate oesophagogastric anastomosis across the globe. Marshall [7] in Boston first, followed by Adams and Phemister [99] in Chicago successfully resected mid-thoracic cancers this way. Marshall's patient had node metastases and recovery was complicated by wound dehiscence, but the patient survived for nearly a year.

Adams and Phemister succeeded using general anaesthesia without an endotracheal tube, after opening the chest through the bed of the resected eighth rib. They crushed the left phrenic nerve believing that the diaphragm should be rested. Next the oesophagus and stomach were mobilised through

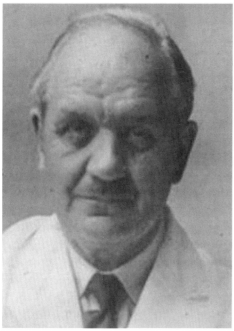

Figure 17. Ivor Lewis (1895-1982).
Courtesy of Mr. Gareth Morris-Stiff MB, BCh MD FRCS.

the enlarged hiatus and at least 10cm of oesophagus and 5cm of stomach were resected with the tumour. The gastric fundus was anchored to the posterior wall of the mediastinum before performing the anastomosis in two layers of interrupted linen. The diaphragm was closed below the anastomosis and a mushroom catheter was used as a gastrostomy feeding tube, while a De Pezzar catheter was used as an intercostal drain. The skin incision was closed with silk, and oral feeding commenced at 14 days. The first patient lived for ten years, despite coeliac node involvement.

Many contemporaries were reluctant to follow, and continued other routes for restored swallowing for some years until Ivor Lewis [1] (Figure 17) published seven operations evolving from Torek procedures to his two-incision operation in 1946:

◆ patients 1-3. These were left or right-sided Torek procedures with one 30-day death;
◆ patients 4 and 5. One-staged oesophago-gastrectomy via a left thoracotomy. One patient died on the table from a pneumothorax and pulmonary embolism;
◆ patients 6 and 7. Staged procedures using a vertical abdominal (left paramedian) incision followed by a right thoracotomy resecting the tumour and joining the oesophagus to the stomach by an oesophagogastrostomy shown in Figure 18. Both patients did well. He finished his career by doing the operation in one session afterwards. This is known today as the 'Ivor Lewis' approach and is the most used approach in the UK.

Up to 1940 the mortality after operative treatment for this disease was high and according to Ochsner and De Bakey [95], it ranged between 59-101 deaths in 191 resections. However, Sweet [100] in 1948, had a reduced mortality of 16.5% in 181 resections. After World War II was over, anaesthesia improved, antibiotics and safer blood transfusions helped to improve the outcome all over the world. Table 1 below shows the mortalities in expert hands between 1954 and 1959. Nakayama [101] showed the combination of early diagnosis, slim patients and vast skilful experience could produce an enviably low mortality.

Table 1. Mortality of oesophageal cancer [101].

Department	Year of publication	Resections	Mortality %
Garlock	1954	75	33
Sweet	1954	Middle third 120	25
		Lower third 167	12
Nakayama	1959	953	Extrathoracic 5.8
			Intrathoracic 15

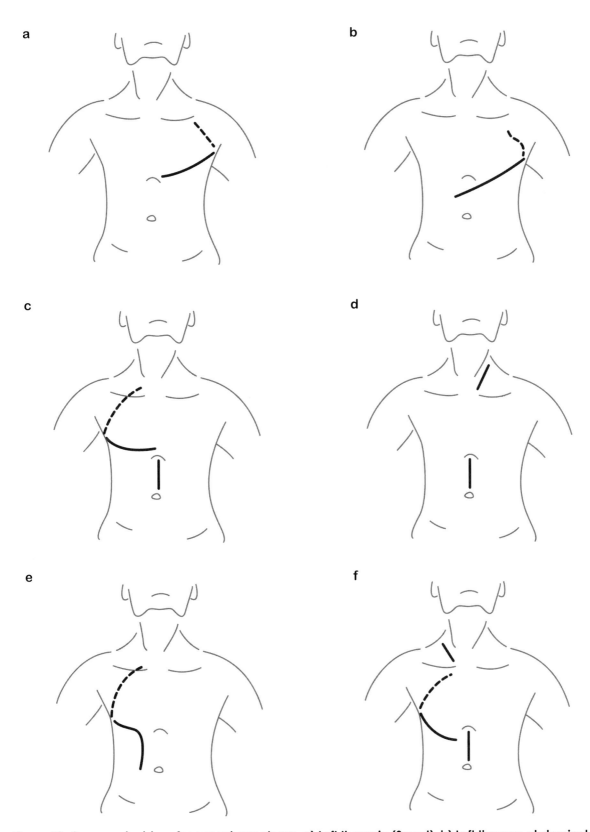

Figure 18. Common incisions for oesophagectomy. a) Left thoracic (Sweet). b) Left thoraco-abdominal (Collis-Belsey). c) Abdominal and right thoracic (Lewis). d) Transhiatal (Orringer). e) Right thoraco-abdominal (Nakayama and Wastell). f) Three stage (McKeown and Hennessey).

Churchill and Sweet [102] were usually comfortable with a left thoracotomy alone. They improved access to the stomach by opening the diaphragm, preserving the phrenic nerve. Garlock, Belsey and Collis and many others used the thoraco-abdominal route. Nakayama used a right thoraco-abdominal incision for middle third cancers and left thoraco-abdominal for lower third cancers in 1976.

McKeown [103] modified the Ivor Lewis approach, by adding a right cervical incision as a third stage. Matthews [104], in 1987, added a neck incision to the left thoraco-abdominal incision, gaining good access for the anastomosis in the neck. Most of these incisions are shown in Figure 18.

In 1988, Orringer [23] from Michigan extended von Ach's operation [92] by the same approach from the abdomen and neck, but completed the anastomosis in a similar fashion as performed by McKeown, after drawing up the stomach through the posterior mediastinum where the oesophagus used to lie. He described this as a 'transhiatal' oesophagectomy. His mortality was very low (6%) and the five-year survival rate was 22% in 130 patients. The hope for fewer respiratory complications was not realised. Wong [105] regarded it a palliative operation, and since the advent of thoracic epidural anaesthesia, the case for avoiding thoracotomy was no longer justified. Both he and Nakayama acquired huge series because of the increased prevalence of squamous cancer of the oesophagus in the Far East.

Cancer of the cardia

Arguments have taken place for years about this tumour. Is it an oesophageal tumour growing downwards, or a gastric tumour growing upwards? It is indeed an enigma, especially when it is large. According to Meyer [94], von Hacker first combined the two as a single entity, long before knowledge of the *Helicobacter* organism.

Friedrich Voelcker [106], another Billroth pupil, successfully resected a carcinoma of the cardia via an abdominal incision, after considerable downward traction on the oesophagus. The result was like an upside-down Billroth I anastomosis.

Barrett [107] coined the term 'congenital short oesophagus', because he defined the oesophagus as lined only by squamous epithelium. Cedric Bremner [108] showed in animal studies that if the lower sphincter was destroyed, the columnar epithelium extended proximally, so a 'columnar-lined oesophagus' was not congenital but an acquired condition.

In recent years there has been a realisation that the columnar-lined oeosphagus is prone to malignant change. Van der Burgh and colleagues [109] studied a group of patients who had established Barrett changes, and while they found a 30 to 40 times increased risk of cancer, they found widespread screening detected only one cancer in 180 patient years, therefore proving too costly. Because 10% of Western populations have some reflux disorder, surveillance of the minority with Barrett's oesophagus had the advantage of monitoring changes from dysplasia to cancer and a chance of cure.

Pioneers in palliation of malignant disease

Most oesophageal cancers have presented late over the centuries. Parts of the world have programmes to detect early tumours, but certainly in the Western Hemisphere, inoperable tumours all too frequently are encountered. Options for palliation have been:

- repeated dilatations;
- radiotherapy;
- laser canalisation;
- diathermy destruction;
- alcohol injections;
- chemotherapy;
- intubations.

Historically, surgical pioneers have been involved in intubation. The authors are aware of at least ten types of tubes to enable swallowing. Materials such as decalcified ivory [110], stretched de Pezzar catheters [111], silicone rubber [112] and assorted plastic tubes [113, 114] have been used.

In 1885, Charters Symonds [115] was concerned about the indignity of saliva overspill for good terminal care. He stented tumours with a boxwood funnel in

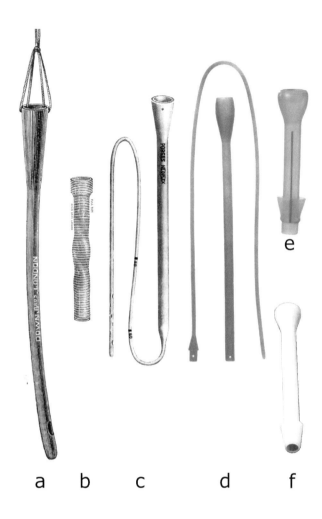

a   b   c   d   e   f

Figure 19. Assorted stents used in the palliation of oesophageal cancer. a) Symonds string suspended gum-elastic (initially boxwood) tube (Down Bros. London). b) Souttar coiled steel spiral tube inserted endoscopically (Down Bros. London). c) Mousseau-Barbin Neoplex tube placed by traction via gastrotomy (Down Bros. London). a) b) & c) *Reproduced with permission from B. Braun Medical Ltd.* d) Celestin oval polythene tube reinforced by nylon spiral placed by traction as above. e) Celestin skirted tube to deter up or down displacement inserted endoscopically. d) & e) *Reproduced with permission from L.R. Celestin FRCS.* f) Atkinson silicone rubber tube inserted endoscopically. *Reproduced with permission from Olympus-KeyMed Ltd. (Judy Moss. Medical Photography Dept, Musgrove Park Hospital).*

order to administer fluid and morphine by stomach tube. In 1927, Henry Souttar endoscopically inserted his funnelled wire tube with a spiralled stem to be gripped by the tumour when in place [116] (Figure 19). If displaced it could be cleaned, sterilised and reused!

In 1956, Roger Celestin [117] as a trainee was dissatisfied with stiff plastic tubes which often eroded through the oesophagus. After chewing and swallowing numerous breakfasts down tubes of varying diameters, he discovered an internal diameter of 11mm was the minimum diameter to permit normal food into the stomach apart from the adhesive qualities of fish. His latex-funnelled tube incorporated a stiff nylon spiral (Souttar's principle) and an added radio-opaque strip. His early tubes were inserted at operation by traction, later endoscopically by pulsion. Celestin did not advocate his tube for benign strictures, not only prey to digestive enzymes, but also prone to more reflux. Expandable stents came into use since 1993 [118]. Despite their greater cost, they were found to have a lower mortality and morbidity according to Jethwa and colleagues [119].

Conclusions

The tides have turned since the second half of the 20th century. Most foreign bodies are removed in minutes by non-surgical endoscopists, using better equipment without general anaesthesia.

Except for small uncomplicated perforations, knowledge of the options described in the chapter is still required and to be applied with urgency. The same urgency is required for damage to the oesophagus by noxious substances.

Gastro-oesophageal reflux still requires surgical attention. Some governments are aware that early effective laparoscopic surgery makes better economic sense than long-term medication. Proton pump inhibitors, safe dilatation and timely anti-reflux surgery have all reduced the number of tough reflux strictures today.

Achalasia remains uncommon, but is easily managed by balloon dilatation in the frail and laparoscopic myotomy for the robust; very few require open surgery.

Despite some surveillance programmes of columnar-lined or 'Barrett's oesophagus' patients today, most cancers are diagnosed far too late in the Western Hemisphere. It is still not understood why carcinoma of the lower third and cardia has trebled in the last 20 years. Topical ablation of the Barrett epithelium by laser is still under revue. Minimal invasive surgery of established cancer shows no advantage over open oesophagectomy so far.

There is now no room for prima donnas in oesophageal surgery; curative surgical treatment emerges from effective teamwork. This team includes radiologists, oncologists, anaesthetists, dedicated nurses, as well as the technically gifted heirs of our surgical pioneers.

Biographical footnote on Rudolf Nissen

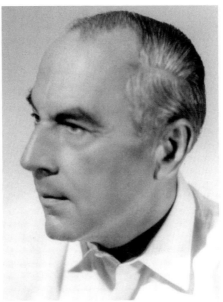

Figure 20. Rudolf Nissen (1896-1981).
Reproduced with permission from the Nissen family and Professor Liebermann-Meffert.

This remarkable man was one of three children born in Neisse, which was situated in Prussia after 1742 before becoming part of Germany. (This town is now part of Poland since the end of World War II). His father Franz was a busy surgeon, so all the children were brought up in a hectic surgical atmosphere in his father's hospital, and it was no surprise that Rudolf followed in the family tradition.

His school education was mainly in the classics in a strict Catholic school, with little exposure to modern languages. He was an artist, a peace lover and adored his native countryside.

When he left school aged 17 he joined the Army in World War I. Though attached to a casualty station he himself succumbed to several injuries, the worst being severe lung contusion. At the end of that war he entered formal medical studies in Marburg and Breslau (now Wroclaw in Poland.). After six months in internal medicine, he spent a year studying pathology under Professor Ludwig Aschoff in Freiburg.

Aged 25 he found himself at the University Hospital in Munich on the surgical staff under the newly arrived Professor Ferdinand Sauerbruch, who soon noticed the high quality of research and hard work from this young trainee. Sauerbruch took Nissen into his entourage when promoted to work in the elite Charité Hospital in Berlin. During this critical period Nissen performed several 'firsts':

- in 1930, he performed the first successful pulmonary lobectomy for tuberculosis;
- in 1931, he performed the first successful pneumonectomy for a chronic lung abscess sequel to a car accident;

◆ in 1933, he performed the first surviving total colectomy with ileorectal anastomosis for familial polyposis, without ileostomy.

With his metaphorical star in the ascendant, he was absolutely horrified by the surrounding political unrest, the economic unrest, and the anti-Semitic behaviour of the National Socialist Party under Adolf Hitler. As his mother was Jewish he resigned his post with a heavy heart partly because of the political atmosphere inside and outside the University Hospital, and partly because not even the celebrated Sauerbruch could guarantee protection. He married his wife Ruth on May 24th 1933.

Sauerbruch supported his successful application to the post of Head of Surgery in Istanbul. This is where in 1937 he made the discovery of his famous anti-reflux junction between the oeosphagus and the residual stomach resembling a Witzel gastrostomy. His five-year contract ended in 1938. He did not renew this as it was obvious that another world war was imminent. He emigrated to America in 1939, and at first his German nationality created difficulty in gaining surgical appointments.

In America he became a research fellow under Edward Churchill in the famous Massachusetts General Hospital, where he worked tirelessly on his research and his command of the English language. In 1941 he was appointed to the Jewish and Maimonides Hospitals in Brooklyn, New York, to be followed by an academic appointment in the Long Island College of Medicine. He became an American citizen. By this time his reputation had escalated and he had acquired a clientele of famous patients such as Albert Einstein.

At the end of World War II he declined several chairmanships in Germany, but because of both clinical and research possibilities, and the bonus of being able to resume speaking and writing in his native language, he accepted the Headship of the Department of Surgery in Basle, Switzerland. He did not remain in an 'Ivory Tower' in Basle, but welcomed all surgical colleagues and trainees around him to integrate postgraduate surgical education throughout the canton (province). Furthermore, he became a Swiss citizen, and settled permanently in Basle.

He abhorred unnecessary chatter in the operating theatre; he was a meticulous technician and combined this with shrewd clinical judgement. It was during the late '50s and early '60s he perfected his famous fundoplication with his bright young colleague Mario Rossetti. At first it was combined with gastropexy, but that was abandoned as unnecessary. The majority of modern anti-reflux surgical operations today, especially laparoscopic operations, are modified from the original Nissen-Rossetti fundoplication illustrated in this chapter.

He was a world surgeon not just in the political sense because of his German, Turkish, American and finally Swiss citizenships, but because of his international surgical reputation. He retired in 1967 to continue private practice for a short time, but more especially to complete the writing of the books and articles on his life's work. He was loyal to his staff at all levels and especially to the residual band of co-trainees who had also worked for Sauerbruch. He visited the latter once in 1948. He continued his love of poetry and the classics and, while physically capable, his love of skiing and hiking in his cherished Swiss mountains.

Dorothea Liebermann-Meffert MD FACS
Walford Gillison FRCS

References

1. Lewis I. The surgical treatment of carcinoma of the oesophagus, with special reference to a new operation for growths in the middle third. *Br J Surg* 1946; 34: 18-31.

2. Nuland SB. The past is prologue: surgeons then and now. *J Am Coll Surg* 1998; 186(4): 457-65.

3. Sauerbruch F. Uber die Ausschaltung der schädlichen Wirking des pneunothorax bei intrathorakalen Operationen. *Zentralb Chir* 1904; 31: 146-9.

4. Brauer L, Petersen P. Üeber eine wesentliche Vereinfachung der künstlichen Atmung nach Sauerbruch. *Z Physiol Chem* 1904; 41: 299-302.

5. Torek F. The first successful case of resection of the thoracic portion of the oesophagus for carcinoma. *Surg Gynec Obstet* 1913; 16: 614-7.

6. Rowbotham ES, Magill IW. Anaesthetics in the plastic surgery of the face and jaws. *Proc Roy Soc Med (Anes)* 1921; 14: 17-27.

7. Marshall SF. Carcinoma of the esophagus: successful resection of the lower end of esophagus with re-establishment of esophageal gastric continuity. *Surg Clin N Am* 1938; 18: 643-8.

8. Lassen HCA. A preliminary report on the 1952 epidemic of poliomyelits in Copenhagen. With special reference to the treatment of acute respiratory insufficiency. *Lancet* 1953; 1: 37-41.

9. Modlin IM. *A Brief History of Endoscopy.* Milano: Arti Grafiche Pizzi, 1999: xi.

10. Meade RH. *History of Thoracic Surgery.* Springfield, Illinois, USA: Charles C. Thomas, 1961.

11. Cheever DW. *Two cases of oesophagotomy for removal of foreign bodies.* Boston: James Campbell, 1867.

12. Enderlen E. Ein Beitragzur Chirurgie des hinteren Mediastinum. *Dtsch Z Chir* 1901; 61: 441-95.

13. Edmondson JM. History of the instruments for gastrointestinal endoscopy. *Supplement to Gastrointestinal Endoscopy* 1991; 37: 2: S27-S56.

14. Hacker von V. Erfahrung über die Enterfernung von Freundkörpen mittelst der Oesophagoskopy. (mit Demonstration der entfertern Freund Körper.) *Vehr Dtsch Ges Chir* 1898; 27: 144-8.

15. Liebermann-Meffert D, Brauer RB, Stein HJ. Boerhaave's syndrome: the man behind the syndrome. *Diseases of the Esophagus* 1997; 10: 77-85.

16. Barrett NR. Report of a case of spontaneous perforation of the esophagus successfully treated by operation. *Br J Surg* 1947; 35: 218-9.

17. Menguy R. Near-total oesophageal exclusion by cervical oesophagostomy and tube gastrostomy in the management of massive esophageal perforation: report of a case. *Ann Surg* 1971; 173: 613-6.

18. Abbott OA, Mansour KA, Logan WD Jr., *et al.* Atraumatic so-called spontaneous rupture of the esophagus. *J Thorac Cardiovasc Surg* 1970; 59: 67-83.

19. Seybold WD, Johnson MA III, Leary WV. Perforation of the esophagus. *Surg Clin N Am* 1950; 30: 1155-83.

20. Blalock J. Primary esophagectomy for instrumental perforation of the esophagus. *Am J Surg* 1957; 94: 393-7.

21. Postlethwait RW. Colonic interposition for esophageal substitution. *Surg Gynecol Obstet* 1983; 156: 377-82.

22. Constanzo J, Noirclerk M, Jouglard J, *et al.* New therapeutic approach to corrosive burns of the upper gastrointestinal tract. *Gut* 1980; 21: 370-5.

23. Orringer MB. Transhiatal esophagectomy without thoracotomy for carcinoma of the thoracic esophagus. *Ann Surg* 1984; 200: 282-90.

24. Yudin S. The surgical construction of 80 cases of artificial esophagus. *Surg Gynecol Obstet* 1944; 78: 561-85.

25. Seidenburg B, Hurwith AJ. Immediate reconstruction of the cervical oesophagus by a re-vascularised jejunal segment. *Ann Surg* 1959; 149: 162-71.

26. Tucker G. Cicatricial stenosis of the esophagus, with particular reference to treatment by continuous string, retrograde bougienage with the author's bougie. *Ann Oyto Rhinol Laryngol* 1924; 3: 255-87.

27. Kiviranta VK. Corrosion carcinoma of the esophagus: 381 cases of corrosion and nine cases of corrosion carcinoma. *Acta Otolaryngol (Stockh)* 1952; 42: 89-95.

28. Jackson C. Esophageal stenosis following caustic alkalis. Necessity for the compulsory labelling by Grocers. *JAMA* 1907; 55(22): 1857-8.

29. Paré A. *Labor improbus omnia vincit.* Translated from JP Malgaignes. Oeuvres Complètes. Paris 1840. Springfield, IL: Charles C. Thomas, 1960.

30. Bright K. Account of a remarkable misplacement of the stomach. *Guy's Hosp Rep* 1836; 1: 598-603.

31. Bowditch HI. *A treatise on diaphragmatic hernia.* Jewett Thomas and Co., 1853 (from the Library of ED Churchill MD).

32. Scudder CL. A case of non-traumatic diaphragmatic hernia operation and recovery. *Trans Am Surg Assoc* 1912; 30: 428-47.

33. Allison PR. Reflux esophagitis: sliding hernia and anatomy of repair. *Surg Gynec Obstet* 1951; 92: 419-31.

34. Nissen R. Die transpleurale resektion der kardia. *Dtsch Zeitschr Chir* 1937; 249: 311-6.

35. Mansour KA, Burton HG, Miller JI, *et al.* Complications of intrathoracic Nissen fundoplication. *Ann Thorac Surg* 1981; 32: 173-8.

36. Polk HC Jnr, Zeppa R. Fundoplication for complicated hiatal hernia. *Ann Thorac Surg* 1969; 7: 202-10.

37. Donahue PE, Bombeck CT. The modified Nissen fundoplication: reflux prevention without gas-bloat. *Chir Gastroenterol* 1977; 11: 15-22.

38. DeMeester TR, Attwood SEA. Gastroesophageal reflux disease, hiatus hernia, achalasia of the esophagus and spontaneous rupture. *Maingot's Operations.* Volume I, 9th edition. Schwartz SI, Ellis H, Eds. Norwalk, Connecticut, USA: Appleton & Lange, 1989; section v: 513-45.

39. Lind JF, Burns CM, MacDougal JT. Physiological repair hiatus hernia - manometric study. *Arch Surg* 1965; 91: 233-6.

40. Toupet A. Technique d'oesophago-gastroplastie avec phrénogastropexie applique dans la cure radicale des hernies hiatale et comme complément de l'operation d'Heller dans les cardiospasms. *Mem Acad Chir* 1963; 89: 394-409.

41. Watson A, Jenkinson LR, Ball CS, Barlow AP, Norris TL. A more physiological alternative to total fundoplication for the surgical correction of resistant gastro-oesophageal reflux. *Br J Surg* 1991; 78: 1088-94.

42. Spencer J. Use of prolonged pH recording in gastro-oesophageal reflux. *Br J Surg* 1968; 55: 864-8.

43. Baue AE, Belsey RH. The treatment of sliding hiatus hernia and reflux esophagitis by the Mark IV technique. *Surgery* 1967; 62: 396-404.

44. DeMeester DR, Johnson LF. The evaluation of objective measurements of gastroesophageal reflux and their contribution to patient management. *Ann Surg* 1976; 56: 39-53.

45. Kramer SJM, Aye RW, Hill LD. The Hill Repair: A Definitive Anti-reflux Procedure. In: *Surgery of the Esophagus, Stomach and Small Intestine,* 5th edition. Wastell C, Nyhus LM, Donahue PE, Eds. Boston: Littlle, Brown and Company, 1995; chapter 17: 215-8.

46. Belsey RHR. Personal communication.

47. Angelchik JP, Cohen R. A new surgical procedure for the treatment for gastro-esophageal reflux and hiatal hernia. *Surg Gynec Obstet* 1979; 148: 246-8.

48. Durrans D, Armstrong CP, Taylor TV. The Angelchik anti-reflux prosthesis - some reservations. *Br J Surg* 1985; 72: 525-7.

49. Quincke H. Ulcus oesophagei ex digestione. *Dtsch Arch Klin Med* 1879; 24: 72-80.

50. Winkelstein A. Peptic oesophagus: a new clinical entity. *JAMA* 1935; 104: 906-9.

51. Tuttle SG, Grossman MI. Detection of gastro-esophageal reflux by simultaneous measurement of intraluminal pressure and pH. *Am J Physiol* 1958; 33: 225-7.

52. Royston CMS, Dowling BL, Spencer J. Antrectomy with Roux-en-Y anastomosis in the treatment of peptic oeosphagitis with stricture. *Br J Surg* 1975; 62: 605-7.

53. Washer GF, Gear MWL, Dowling BL, Gillison EW, Royston CMS, Spencer J. Randomised prospective trial of Roux-en-Y duodenal diversion versus fundoplication for severe reflux oesophagitis. *Br J Surg* 1984; 71: 181-4.

54. Herrington JL, Sawyers JL. Rebound acid secretion after duodenal diversion. In: *Surgery of the Esophagus, Stomach, and Small Intestine,* 5th edition. Wastell C, Nyhus LM, Donahue PE, Eds. Boston: Littlle, Brown and Company, 1995; chapter 43: 542-4.

55. Dallemagne B, Weerts JM, Jahaes C, Markiewicz S, Lombard R. Laparoscopic Nissen fundoplication: preliminary report. *Surg Laparosc Endosc* 1991; 1: 138-43.

56. Geagea T. Laparoscopic Nissen fundoplication: preliminary report of ten cases. *Surg Endosc* 1991; 5: 170-3.

57. Holmes T. On operative dilatation of the orifices of the stomach. *Br Med J* 1885; February 21: 372-3.

58. Abbe R. Relief of oesophageal stricture by a string saw. *Ann Surg* 1893; 17: 489-90.

59. Yamamoto H, Hughes RW Jr, Schroeder KW, Viggiano TR, DiMagno EP. Treatment of benign esophageal stricture by Eder-Puestow or balloon dilators: a comparison between randomized and prospective nonrandomized trials. *Mayo Clin Proc* 1992; 67: (3) 228-36.

60. Beck C, Carrel A. Demonstrations of specimens illustrating a method of formation of a pre-thoracic esophagus. *Ill Med J* 1905; 7: 461.

61. Jiannu A. Gastrostomie und Öesophagoplastik. *Dtsch Z Chir* 1912; 118: 383-90.

62. Gavriliu D. Aspects of esophageal surgery. *Curr Prob Surg* 1975; 12 (10): 1-64.

63. Collis JL. Gastroplasty. *Thorax* 1961; 16: 197-99.

64. Henderson RD. Reflux control following gastroplasty. *Ann Thorac Surg* 1977; 24: 206-12.

65. Orringer MB. Combined Collis gastroplasty-Nissen fundoplication operation for reflux oesophagitis. *Surgical Rounds* 1978; 1: 10-9.

66. Kirschner M. Ein neues Verfahren der Oesophagoplastik. 44th congress of the German Surgical Society, April 9th, 1920: 606-63.

67. Roux C. L'Oesophago-jéjuno-gastrotomie, nouvelle opération pour rétrécissement infranchissable de l'oesophage. *Semaine Méd (Paris)* 1907; 27: 37-40.

68. Kelling G. Oesophagoplastik mit Hilfe des Quercolon. *Zentralbl Chir* 1911; 38: 1209-12.

69. Vulliet TH. De l'oesophagoplastie et de ses diverse modifications. *Sem Med* 1911; 31: 529-30.

70. Roith O. Die einzeitige antethorakale Oesophagaplastik aus dem Dickdarm. *Zentralbl Chir* 1923-1924; 183: 419-23.

71. Belsey RHR. Reconstruction of the oesophagus with the left colon. *J Thorasc Cardiovasc Surg* 1965; 49: 33-55.

72. Kittle CK. The History of Esophageal Surgery. In: *Surgery of the Esophagus, Stomach, and Small Intestine,* 5th edition. Wastell C, Nyhus LM, Donahue PE, Eds. Boston: Littlle, Brown and Company, 1995; 35.

73. Mikulicz von JV. Small contributions to surgery of the alimentary tract. (1) Cardiospasm and its treatment. (2) Peptic ulcer of the jejunum. (3) Operative treatment of severe forms of invagination of the intestine. (4) Operations on malignant growths of the large intestine. *Boston Med Surg J* 1903; 148: 608-11.

74. Einhorn M. A case of dysphagia with dilatation of the oesophagus. *Med Rec* 1888; 34: 751-3.

75. Meltzer SG. Ein Fall von Dysphagie nebst Bemerkungen. *Berl Klin Wochenschr* 1888; 25: 140-2.

76. Hertz AF. Achalasia of the Cardia. *Q J Med* 1915; 8: 300-8.

77. Mikulicz von JV. Zur Parthologie und Therapie des Cardiospasmus. *Dtsch Med Wochenschr* 1904; 30: 17 and 50.

78. Zaaijer JH. An address on the surgery of the oesophagus and lungs. *Lancet* 1929; 1: 909-14.

79. Heyrovsky H. Casuistik und Therapie der idiopatiscen Dilatation der Speisröbre. Oesophafgofastroanastomose. *Arch Klin Chir* 1913; 100: 703-5.

80. Wendel W. Zur Chirurgie des Oesophagus. *Archiv Klin Chir* 1910; 93: 311.

81. Heller E. Extra-mukose Cardiaplastik beim chronischen Cardiospasmus mit Dilatation des Oesophagus. *Mitt Grenzeb Med Chir* 1914; 27: 141-9.

82. Gottstein G. Die operative Behandlung des Cardiospasmus. *Zentralbl Chir* 1904; 31: 1362-4.

83. Steichen FM, Heller E, Ravitch MM. Achalasia of the esophagus. *Surgery* 1960; 47: 846-76.

84. Barrett NR, Franklin RH. Concerning the unfavourable late results of certain operations performed in the treatment of Cardiospasm. *Br J Surg* 1949; 37: 194-202.

85. Ellis FH, Kiser JC, *et al.* Esophagomyotomy for esophageal achalasia: experimental, clinical, and manometric aspects. *Ann Surg* 1967; 166: 640-56.
86. Pinotti HW. First development of cardiomyotomy by video-laparoscopy: a new perspective in the achalasia treatment. *ISDE News* 1991; 10: 8.
87. Czerny V. Neue Operation. *Zentralbl Chir* 1877; 4: 433-4.
88. Billroth T. Total Extirpation des Ganzenoesophagus vom Pharynx bis Sternum; ein total Extirpation de Ganzenlarynx mit des GanzenSchildrusse. *Vehr Deutch Ges Chir* 1879; 8: 7-9.
89. Mikulicz-Radecki J von. Über eine eigenartige symmetrische Erkrankung der Thränen - und Mundspeicheldrüsen, in Beiträge zur Chirurgie. *Festschr fur T Billroth.* Stuttgart, 1892: 610-30.
90. Mikulicz-Radecki J von. Ein Fall von Resection des carcinomatösen Oesophagus mit plastischem Ersatz des excidirten Stückes. *Prag Med Wochenschr* 1886; 11: 93-4.
91. Trotter W. (Reported by Pilcher R.) Carcinoma of the cervical oesophagus. *Lancet* 1937; 1: 73-6.
92. Ach V. Beitrage zur Oesophaguschirurgie. *Munch Med Wochenschr* 1913; 60: 1115-17.
93. Garlock JH. The surgical treatment of the thoracic esophagus. *Surg Gynec Obstet* 1938; 66: 534-8.
94. Meyer W. Resection of cardia for carcinoma. *Ann Surg* 1915; 62: 693-709.
95. Ochsner A, De Bakey M. Surgical aspects of carcinoma of the esophagus. *J Thorac Surg* 1941; 10: 401-55.
96. Rovsing T. The technique of my method of ante-thoracic oesophagoplasty. *Surg Gynecol Obstet* 1926; 43: 781-4.
97. Turner GG. Excision of the thoracic oesophagus for carcinoma with construction of an extra-thoracic gullet. *Lancet* 1933; 2: 1315-16.
98. Ohsawa T. The surgery of the oesophagus. *Jpn Chir* 1933; 10: 682-91.
99. Adams WE, Phemister DB. Carcinoma of the lower thoracic esophagus. *J Thorac Surg* 1938; 7: 621-32.
100. Sweet RH. Late results of surgical treatment of carcinoma of the esophagus. *JAMA* 1954; 155: 422-5.
101. Nakayama, K. Erfahrungen bei etwas 3000 Fallen von Esophagus and Kardiacarcinoma. *Langenbeck Arch Klin Chir* 1960; 295: 81-90.
102. Churchill ED, Sweet RH. Transthoracic resection of tumours of the stomach and esophagus. *Ann Surg* 1942; June: 897-917.
103. McKeown KC. The surgical treatment of carcinoma of the oesophagus. *Proc Roy Soc Med* 1974; 67: 5389-95.
104. Matthews HR, Steel A. Left-sided subtotal oesophagectomy for carcinoma. *Br J Surg* 1987; 87: 1115-17.
105. Wong J. Transhiatal oesophagectomy for carcinoma of the thoracic oesophagus. *Br J Surg* 1986; 73: 89-90.
106. Voelcker F. Ueber extirpation der Cardia vegen Carcinoms. *Verh Dtsch Ges Chir* 1908; 37: 126.
107. Barrett NR. Chronic peptic ulcer of the oesophagus and esophagitis. *Br J Surg* 1950; 38: 175-82.
108. Bremner CG, Lynch VP, Ellis FH. Barrett's esophagus: congenital or acquired? An experimental study of esophageal mucosal regeneration in the dog. *Surgery* 1970; 68(1): 209-16.
109. Van der Burgh A, Dees J, Hop WCJ, van Blankenstein M. Oesophageal cancer is an uncommon cause of death in patients with Barrett's oesophagus. *Gut* 1996; 39: 5-8.
110. Leroy, d'Etoilles De. *Lavacherie de L'Oesphagotomie.* Bibliothèque Nationale de Bruxelles, Bruxelles, 1845.
111. Guisez J. L'Intubation caoutchouée oesophagienne. *Presse Méd* 1914; 22: 85-8.
112. Atkinson M, Ferguson R. Fibreoptic endoscopic palliative intubation of inoperable oesophagogastric neoplasms. *Br Med J* 1977; 1: 266-7
113. Mackler SA, Mayer RM. Palliation of esophageal obstruction due to carcinoma with a permanent intra-luminal tube. *J Thorac Cardiovasc Surg* 1954; 28: 431.
114. Mousseau MM, Le Forrestier J, Barbin J, Hardy M. Place de intubation a demeure dans letraitement palliatif du cancer de l'oesophage. Society National Francais de Gastro-Enterology, Séance du 11 Mars 1956. *Arch Mal Appardia* 1956; 45: 208-14.
115. Stebbing GF. Sir Charters Symonds, KBE, MS, FRCS. *Guys Hospital Report* 1933; 83: 259-64.
116. Souttar HS. A method of intubating the oesophagus for malignant stricture. *Br Med J* 1924; 1: 782-3.
117. Celestin LR. Permanent intubation in inoperable cancer of the oesophagus and cardia. A new tube. *Ann Roy Coll Surg* 1959; 25: 165-70.
118. Knyrim K, Wagner HJ, Bethge N, Keymling M, Vakil NA. Controlled trial of an expansile metal stent for palliation of esophageal obstruction due to inoperable cancer. *New Engl J Med* 1993; 329: 1302-7.
119. Jethwa P, Lala A, Powell J, *et al.* A regional audit of iatrogenic perforation of tumours of the oesophagus and cardia. *Aliment Pharmacol Ther* 2005; 21: 479-84.

Chapter 5

The arrival of bariatric surgery

Henry Buchwald MD PhD FACS

Professor of Surgery and Biomedical Engineering

Owen H. and Sarah Davidson Wangensteen Chair in Experimental Surgery Emeritus

University of Minnesota, Minnesota, USA

Introduction

The history of obesity is ancient. The history of successful therapy for this disease by bariatric surgery is recent; indeed, barely more than 50 years and what a turbulent and imaginative half century of progress. It started from innovative and empiric beginnings to a specialty that in the early 21st century encompasses a major share of general surgery procedures, as well as expansion and maturation of laparoscopic techniques.

Obesity and morbid obesity

Historical perspectives

Obesity is often considered a 'modern' phenomenon - an affliction of abundance. Certainly, epidemic obesity in Western society is a current manifestation, representing one of the major health problems of the US and other nations. Yet, evidence of obesity can be found in earliest written history and even in prehistoric times.

The Venus of Willendorf (Figure 1), an 11-cm-high limestone statuette, dated to 24,000 to 22,000 BC, has become almost a talisman for students of obesity.

The particular limestone used to carve this statuette is not found in Willendorf, Austria. Therefore, either the limestone was transported to Willendorf and carved there with Stone Age flint tools, which most scholars consider unlikely, or this portable carving was transported to Willendorf by Paleolithic wanderers who considered it important enough to carry on their travels. Similar female figures, with individual characteristics, of the Paleolithic period have been found from France to Turkey, and to the steppes of Russia [1].

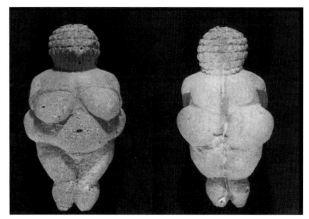

Figure 1. Venus of Willendorf, 24,000 to 22,000 BC.

From this time of migratory hunters and gatherers, we have male figures in sculpture or in engraved images, all of which are lean. Yet, the Venus figures are all corpulent. It has been conjectured that these Venuses were fertility symbols; they are obese however, but not pregnant. Another interpretation is that these Venuses were symbols of ideal femininity or of female beauty, with the lack of a face suggesting universality. Conjecture, again, would assign to these figures the role of a goddess of plenty.

Careful inspection of the Venus of Willendorf shows typical characteristics of progressive obesity: the thighs that meet, the iliac crest fat roll, the huge buttocks and the dimples at the armpits. The overall figure is pear-shaped and originally was designated 'la Poire'. These physical characteristics are all graphic depictions of obesity we are familiar with. It is plausible that the artists who made the Venuses did them from life or memory, and had actually seen nude obese women. In which case we could reasonably assume that obesity existed at least as long as 26,000 years ago.

Obese figurines are found throughout Europe from the Neolithic period (8,000 BC to 5,500 BC) [2]. Egyptian stone reliefs and mummies (3,000 BC to 1,500 BC) give evidence of obesity. Etruscan sarcophagi (400 BC to 300 BC) depict markedly obese men [3]. Pre-Colombian figures from the New World show knowledge of obesity. The Romans wrote about Dionysius, Tyrant of Heracleia (4th century BC), and Magas, King of Cyrene (3rd century BC), who were monstrously obese. In the Book of Judges of the Old Testament, Eglon, the evil king of Moab, was slain by Ehud: "Eglon was a very fat man", so that after the knife thrust by Ehud, "the fat closed upon the blade, so that he could not draw the dagger out of his belly" [4]. In more recent history, numerous leaders have been described as possessing Falstaffian proportions: William the Conqueror; Charles le Gross; Louis le Gross; Humbert II, Count of Maurienne; Henry I, King of Navarre; Henry III, Count of Champagne; Conan III, Duke of Brittany; Sancho I, King of Leon; Alphonse II, King of Portugal; and Louis XVII [2].

Obesity was recognised in Greco-Roman times as more than an ideal or an aberration, but as a state detrimental to health and longevity. Hippocrates (?460 BC to 355 BC) stated that "sudden death is more common in those who are naturally fat than in the lean" [2]. Greco-Roman traditions also hold that obesity was a cause of infertility in women and of dysmenorrhoea. Galen (130-200) defined two types of obesity: moderate or natural and immoderate or morbid. The previously cited Dionysius suffered from Pickwickian syndrome (a Dickensian reference derived from the 'fat boy' who constantly fell asleep in *The Pickwick Papers*); so that Dionysius' servants probed him with long needles to keep him awake.

In about 400 and for the next century, Arabic medicine came to the forefront. Ibn Sina, westernised to Avicenna (980-1037) (Figure 8, Chapter 15), published more than 100 books. In his *Canon of Medicine*, he devotes an entire chapter to obesity, which he regarded as a health hazard. Citing the disadvantages of obesity, Avicenna writes: "Severe obesity restricts the movements and manoeuvres of the body. It compresses blood vessels causing their narrowness. Breathing passages are obstructed and the flow of air is hindered leading to nasty temperament. The very obese are at risk of fatal rupture of a blood vessel as blood flows through. Such a situation is preceded by shortness of breath and palpitation... On the whole these people are at risk of sudden death, ... They are vulnerable to stroke, hemiplegia, palpitation, diarrhoea, fainting, ... Any physical effort they make will weaken them..." [5]

In the 17th century, Sangye Gyamtso, the Regent of Tibet, composed *The Blue Beryl*, a commentary on an ancient Chinese text, in which he noted that overeating causes illness and shortens lifespan [6]. In 1829, Wadd published his *Comments on Corpulency, Lineaments of Leanness*, in which he describes a series of clinical cases of severe obesity and notes that sudden death is not uncommon in the corpulent: "A sudden palpitation excited in the heart of a fat man has often proven as fatal as a bullet through the thorax." [7]

Quetelet, a Belgian, in 1835 quantified weight as a function of height and established the Quetelet Index (QI), better known today as the body mass index (BMI): weight in kilograms divided by height in metres squared [8]. As early as 1901, the life insurance industry equated obesity, and the central distribution of weight, with ill health and decreased longevity. This recognition, driven by economic pressures, preceded widespread attention to obesity and serious efforts at obesity management by 20th-century practitioners of medicine.

Where do surgeons enter into the history of obesity and obesity therapy? Hua Toh, a 3rd-century Chinese surgeon, described acupuncture in the pinna of the ear to reduce appetite and treat obesity. In the Talmud, it is told that Rabbi Eleazar underwent an operation: he was given a soporific potion and was brought to a marble house, his abdomen was opened, and a number of baskets of fat were removed [9]. The Roman historian, Pliny, mentions that a similar operation was performed on the obese son of the consul, Lucius Apronius. Anecdotally, Dr. John H. Kellogg (1852-1943), who with his brother William were pioneers of boxed grain cereals, was rumoured to have removed a small section of a patient's intestine when certain disease processes were not cured by a vegetarian diet. Weight loss by panniculectomy was used by 20th-century surgeons well before the introduction of gastrointestinal surgery for obesity in 1953.

Incidence and demography

Obesity history affords perspective on the past and what in that past heralded the present; current obesity incidence and demography defines what has come about in our time and what may come to pass in the future. Today, in many parts of the world, obesity is a fast-spreading epidemic. The most recent incidence and demographic statistics, though startling, may well underestimate the actual problem and its expanding threat to global health.

In the US, the National Center for Health Statistics has been the primary source of obesity prevalence data. According to a summary provided by Flegel *et al*, of the National Health Examination Survey of 1960 to 1962 (NHES I) and the National Health and Nutrition Examination Surveys of 1971 to 1974 (NHANES I), 1976 to 1980 (NHANES II), and 1988 to 1994 (NHANES III), the prevalence of obesity (body mass index [BMI] $\geq30kg/m^2$) has increased geometrically - from 12.8% in 1962 to 22.5% in

1994 - in the 20- to 74-year-old age-adjusted population [10]. In a more recent (2002) NHANES IV report, this number increased to 27% [11]. This staggering statistic translates to the fact that approximately one of every four individuals 20 to 74 years old is obese. Further, in the last 20 years, the number of obese individuals in the US has nearly doubled. Combining these calculations with an analysis by Monteforte and Torkelson [12] and with the 2000 United States Census [13], about 50 million of US adults are obese (BMI $\geq30kg/m^2$). Of these, over 15 million have a BMI $\geq35kg/m^2$ and over six million a BMI $\geq40 kg/m^2$.

These data apply to adults in the US. In children and adolescents, overweight (BMI $\geq25kg/m^2$) and obesity are defined by a sex- and age-specific BMI at or above the 95th percentile on growth charts prepared by the Centers for Disease Control and Prevention. The NHANES trends over the past three decades (1960s to 1990s) show that the percentage of overweight or obesity (BMI $\geq$95th percentile) in children (6 to 11 years old), increased from 4% in 1965 to 13% in 1999; in adolescents (12 to 19 years old), from 5% in 1970 to 14% in 1999. These increases were similar among girls and boys. Other analyses would place the number of overweight children and adolescents at 25% [14]. Unfortunately, overweight children are highly likely to grow into overweight adults [15].

According to the Worldwatch Institute, the number of overweight people is approximately equal to the number of underweight people - 1.1 billion each [16]. Of all of the world's nations, the percentage of overweight is highest in the US at over 60% [17]. However, overweight people are in excess of 50% in Russia, the UK, and Germany; 20% in Colombia, Brazil, Italy, Austria, and Switzerland; and even 10% in China. Europeans often wish to believe that overweight and obesity are products of the American way of life. This conjecture may be true, but, if so, this way of life has undergone globalisation and has firmly taken root in most countries of Western Europe, with overweight incidence rates of 10% to 25%. In Australia, 41% of adult men and 23% of adult women are overweight. In the Federated States of Micronesia, 80% of women age 40 to 49 years old are overweight and over 50% are obese. Up to 70%

of women and 65% of men on the island of Nauru in Micronesia are overweight [18].

Obesity - the disease

Overweight may not be healthy; obesity is definitely detrimental to good health; and morbid obesity (BMI ≥40kg/m^2 or BMI ≥35kg/m^2 in the presence of obesity comorbidities) is a disease [19, 20]. Certainly, there are multifactorial origins for morbid obesity, but once the BMI values defining this entity are reached, physicians must recognise that we are dealing with a disease: a life-shortening, incapacitating, malignant disease [21-24]. Yet, for society, and even for the medical community, acceptance of morbid obesity as the progenitor of certain comorbid diseases may be easier to accept than to define morbid obesity *per se* as a disease. Coronary heart disease and peripheral arterial occlusive disease were recognised clinical disease entities for decades before their causative mechanism - atherosclerosis - was regarded as a disease. Nevertheless, atherosclerosis is itself a disease of multifactorial origins that can be identified and independently treated. The same is true for obesity; in particular, morbid obesity.

Comorbidities of morbid obesity affect essentially every organ system: cardiovascular (hypertension, atherosclerotic heart and peripheral vascular disease with myocardial infarction and cerebral vascular accidents, peripheral venous insufficiency); respiratory (asthma, obstructive sleep apnoea, obesity-hypoventilation syndrome); metabolic (type 2 diabetes, impaired glucose tolerance, dyslipidaemia); musculoskeletal (back strain, disc disease, weight-bearing osteoarthritis of the hips, knees, ankles, and feet); gastrointestinal (cholelithiasis, gastro-oesophageal reflux disease, fatty metamorphosis of the liver [steatohepatitis], cirrhosis of the liver, hepatic carcinoma, colorectal carcinoma); urinary (stress incontinence); endocrine and reproductive (polycystic ovary syndrome, increased risk of pregnancy and foetal abnormalities, male hypogonadism, cancer of the endometrium, breast, ovary, prostate, and pancreas); dermatologic (intertriginous dermatitis); neurological (pseudo-tumour cerebri, carpal tunnel syndrome); and psychological (depression) [25, 26].

As well as being a medical problem in most of Western society, morbid obesity is also a social and economic problem [27-29]. Derision of the obese is one of the last publicly condoned, legally permitted prejudices. Disdain for the obese starts in the earliest social contacts of preschool children and continues through childhood and adolescence into adulthood [30-32]. This negative attitude is exhibited by people at all levels of education and income, possibly even more so in the higher socioeconomic strata of society. Indeed, many healthcare providers share this attitude [33, 34]. Studies have shown that institutions of higher learning are biased against the obese [35]. Corporate advancement to executive leadership positions is denied to them [36]. Even in buying a house or renting an apartment, obesity is a liability [37].

A direct consequence of social bias is economic disadvantage, well documented by Narbro in Sweden [38], Hughes and McGuire in the UK [39], by Lévy *et al* in France [40], by Segal *et al* in Australia [41], by Swinburn *et al* in New Zealand [42], and by Colditz in the US [43].

Pioneers of bariatric surgery

Genealogy

Bariatric surgery can be classified into four categories: malabsorptive procedures, malabsorptive / restrictive procedures, restrictive procedures, and others. The evolution of bariatric procedures and the emergence of new techniques is a function of the cost/benefit ratios for the various operative interventions. Factors to be considered in this ratio are the efficacy of weight loss (usually, stated as percent excess weight loss), lasting weight loss obtained, operative mortality and peri-operative morbidity, long-term morbidity, quality-of-life achieved, and financial burden of the procedure, as well as reversibility to provide a safe retreat from a potential iatrogenic catastrophe.

Malabsorptive procedures

By the early 1950s, years of clinical observation had taught physicians that the shortened gut led to massive weight loss. Though he never published on his procedure, Victor Henrikson of Gothenberg, Sweden, has often been credited for performing an intestinal resection, specifically for the management of obesity, in the early 1950s [44]. In 1953, Dr. Richard L. Varco, of the Department of Surgery at the University of Minnesota, performed the first jejuno-ileal bypass (Figure 2) [45]. This operation consisted of an end-to-end jejuno-ileostomy with a separate ileocaecostomy for drainage of the bypassed segment (Figure 3).

Varco did not publish this innovation. In 1954, Kremen, Linner and Nelson published a research article on nutritional aspects of the small intestine in dogs [46]. In the discussion section, they described a patient upon whom they had performed an end-to-end jejuno-ileal bypass for reduction of body weight. These authors, also from the University of Minnesota, can be credited with the first case report publication in bariatric surgery.

After a hiatus of some years, in 1963, Payne, DeWind, and Commons published the results of the first clinical program of massive intestinal bypass for the management of morbidly obese patients [47]. In a series that they had initiated in 1956, they described bypassing nearly the entire small intestine, the right colon, and half of the transverse colon in ten morbidly obese female patients. Intestinal continuity was restored by a T-shaped end-to-side anastomosis of the proximal 37.5cm of jejunum to the mid-transverse colon. Although weight loss was dramatic, electrolyte imbalance, uncontrolled diarrhoea, and liver failure proved prohibitive and required eventual reversal of the bypass [48]. To be accurate, this procedure was originally designed by Payne and associates to lead to unlimited weight loss requiring a second operation to restore additional intestinal length and weight equilibrium when ideal body weight was obtained; however, all patients in their series, following their second operation, regained their previously lost weight [49].

There were several other noteworthy steps in the development of the jejuno-ileal bypass. In the mid-1960s, Sherman et al [50], along with Payne and DeWind [49], proposed abandonment of anastomosis to the colon and, instead, restoration of intestinal

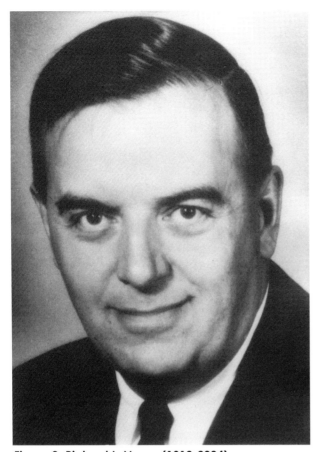
Figure 2. Richard L. Varco (1912-2004).

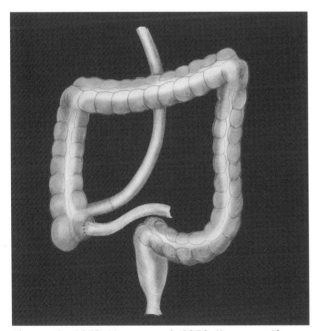
Figure 3. 1953 Varco and 1954 Kremen, Linner, Nelson: jejuno-ileal bypass with end-to-end jejuno-ileostomy with ileocaecostomy. *Reproduced with permission from Obesity Surgery. Buchwald H, Buchwald JN. Evolution of operative procedures for the management of morbid obesity 1950-2000. Obes Surg 2002; 12: 705-17.*

continuity proximal to the ileo-caecal valve by end-to-side jejuno-ileostomy. The aim of this less radical bypass was to achieve an eventual balance between caloric intake and body caloric needs, eliminating the necessity for a second operation and minimising postoperative side effects. Along this path, in 1962, Lewis, Turnbull, and Page [51], reported an end-to-side jejunotransverse colostomy (similar to that of Payne and DeWind), in which the proximal 75cm of jejunum was anastomosed to the transverse colon. As in Payne's series, significant complications eventually required reversal of these bypasses [48]. In 1966, Lewis, Turnbull, and Page described 11 patients in whom they performed an end-to-side jejuno-caecostomy, a procedure that foreshadowed implementation of a less radical approach [52]. Completing this evolution, Payne and DeWind entirely abandoned bypass to the colon in 1969 [49]. In a series of 80 morbidly obese patients, Payne and DeWind established what was to become a standard for the end-to-side jejuno-ileostomy procedure: anastomosis of the proximal 35cm (14in) of jejunum to the terminal ileum, 10cm (4in) from the ileocaecal valve. This operation became the most commonly used bariatric procedure in the US (Figure 4).

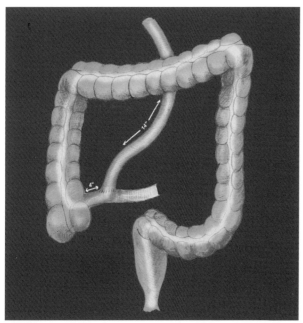

Figure 4. 1969 Payne and DeWind: jejuno-ileal bypass with 35 to 10cm (14 to 4") end-to-side jejuno-ileostomy. *Reproduced with permission from Obesity Surgery. Buchwald H, Buchwald JN. Evolution of operative procedures for the management of morbid obesity 1950-2000. Obes Surg 2002; 12: 705-17.*

This product of operative evolution allowed for significant weight loss with moderate long-term side effects and complications, and did not require a second restorative operation. It was given the colloquial designation of the '14 to 4"' operation.

Although Payne and DeWind's classic jejuno-ileal bypass was widely adopted, nearly 10% of patients did not achieve significant weight loss, possibly due to reflux of nutrients into the bypassed ileum [48]. Thus, Scott et al [53], Salmon [54] and Buchwald and Varco [55] independently returned to the original Varco and Kremen procedure of an end-to-end anastomosis to prevent reflux into the terminal ileum. In all of these end-to-end operations, the ileocaecal valve was preserved in order to decrease postoperative diarrhoea and electrolyte loss, the appendix was removed, and the jejunal stump was attached to the transverse mesocolon or the caecum to avoid intussusception [48]. Scott drained his bypassed segment into the transverse or sigmoid colon [53], Salmon into the mid-transverse colon [54], and Buchwald and Varco into the caecum near the ileocaecal valve [55]. In addition to producing significant weight loss, the Buchwald and Varco procedure, in which 40cm of jejunum was anastomosed to 4cm of ileum, proved valuable in the management of obese hyperlipidaemic patients. Three months postoperatively, patients showed an average decrease in cholesterol of 90% and a reduction in average triglycerides of 96% [55].

Next followed a series of modifications, rarely performed by others than the primary authors. Forestieri et al [56], Starkloff et al [57], and Palmer and Marliss [58] created various modifications at the jejuno-ileal anastomosis to prevent reflux into the bypassed segment without the necessity of dividing and separately draining it. Cleator and Gourlay [59] described an ileogastrostomy for drainage of the bypassed small intestine, and Kral [60] shortened the proximal intestinal segment back to the ligament of Treitz in a duodeno-ileal bypass modification.

Unfortunately, the jejuno-ileal bypass was associated with many complications: diarrhoea, electrolyte imbalance, gas-bloat syndrome, oxalate kidney stones, arthralgias, pustular eruptions, and mental disturbances. Many of these problems were attributed to the long segment of bypassed small intestine. Though isoperistaltic, it was stagnant, allowing for overgrowth of anaerobic bacteria and elaboration of bacterial toxins. Thus, the jejuno-ileal bypass was phased out with the emergence of malabsorptive/restrictive surgery or the gastric bypass procedure. Curiously, even today in Russia, the original jejuno-ileal bypass is still being performed by some surgical practitioners.

Malabsorptive surgery was not dead, however, but reappeared in a modified form in the late 1970s. The modern malabsorptive procedures share a key trait: no limb of the small intestine is left without intraluminal flow. The enteric limb has the flow of food, and the biliary or biliopancreatic limb contains the flow of either bile or bile and pancreatic juice. In 1978, Lavorato *et al* performed a standard end-to-side jejuno-ileal bypass; however, they anastomosed the proximal end of the bypassed segment of the

small intestine into the gallbladder, thereby, diverting bile into the bypassed limb [61]. In 1981, a similar operation was published by Eriksson [62]. These bilio-intestinal bypasses have not been widely performed, and the modern malabsorptive operative era began with the Scopinaro (Figure 5) biliopancreatic diversion.

At present, thousands of biliopancreatic diversions have been performed, particularly in Italy, mainly by Dr. Scopinaro, beginning with his initial series of 18 patients, reported in 1979 [63]. His current biliopancreatic diversion (Figure 6) consists of a horizontal partial gastrectomy (leaving 200-500ml of proximal stomach), closure of the duodenal stump, gastrojejunostomy with a 250cm Roux limb, and anastomosis of the long biliopancreatic limb to the Roux limb 50cm proximal to the ileocaecal valve, creating an extremely short common channel [64].

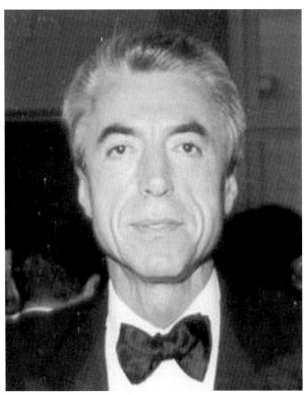

Figure 5. Nicola Scopinaro.

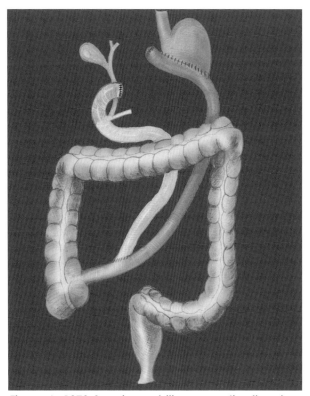

Figure 6. 1979 Scopinaro: biliopancreatic diversion. *Reproduced with permission from Obesity Surgery. Buchwald H, Buchwald JN. Evolution of operative procedures for the management of morbid obesity 1950-2000. Obes Surg 2002; 12: 705-17.*

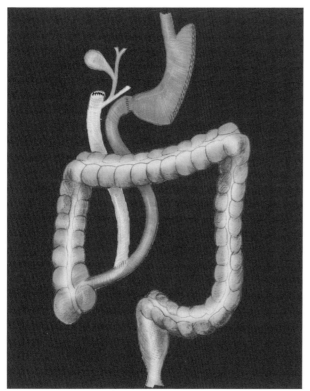

Figure 7. 1998 Hess and Hess: biliopancreatic diversion with duodenal switch with division of the duodenum. *Reproduced with permission from the American College of Surgeons. Buchwald H. Overview of bariatric surgery. J Am Coll Surg 2002; 194: 367-75.*

More than a decade later, the biliopancreatic diversion was modified into the duodenal switch in the US and in Canada. Hess and Hess, a father and son team in Ohio in the US, deviated from the Scopinaro procedure by:

- making a lesser curvature gastric tube (approximately 100ml in volume) with a greater curvature gastric resection, rather than performing a horizontal gastrectomy;
- preserving the pylorus;
- dividing the duodenum, with closure of the distal duodenal stump; and
- anastomosing the enteric limb to the post-pyloric duodenum (Figure 7) [65].

Marceau *et al*, in Canada performed a similar operation but cross-stapled the duodenum distal to the duodeno-ileostomy without dividing it [66]. The duodenum, however, unlike the stomach, does not

tolerate cross-stapling, and these patients displayed disruption of the staple line with regaining of their weight. There have been several modifications of the Hess and Hess procedure as the operation has gained world prominence, and it is being performed by both open and laparoscopic surgical techniques.

Malabsorptive/restrictive procedures

Gastric/restrictive procedures were introduced by the man often designated the 'father of bariatric surgery' - Edward Mason, who had completed his training at the University of Minnesota and performed his seminal work at the University of Iowa (Figure 8). In the original Mason and Ito gastric bypass, the stomach was divided horizontally and a loop (not a Roux) gastrojejunostomy was created between the proximal gastric pouch and the proximal jejunum (Figure 9) [67].

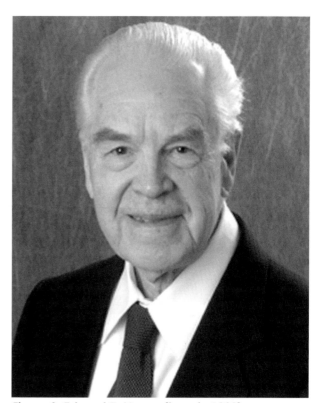

Figure 8. Edward E. Mason (born in 1920).

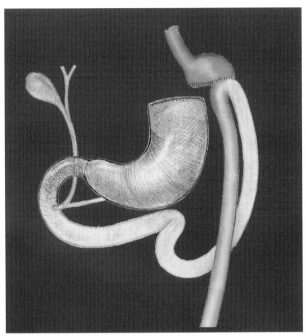

Figure 9. 1967 Mason and Ito: gastric bypass with gastric transection with loop gastrojejunostomy. *Reproduced with permission from Obesity Surgery. Buchwald H, Buchwald JN. Evolution of operative procedures for the management of morbid obesity 1950-2000. Obes Surg 2002; 12: 705-17.*

The size of the upper pouch and the size of the outlet stoma dictate the restrictive aspect of the gastric bypass. Distention of this upper pouch by food causes the sensation of satiety by mechanisms as yet undetermined. The original upper gastric pouch of Mason's was 100ml to 150ml with a stoma 12mm in diameter. Later, Mason and Printen reduced the pouch size to ≤50ml to increase weight loss, and, by including the acid-secreting mucosa in the distal stomach, to reduce ulcer formation [68].

The bariatric surgery tradition not only started in Minnesota but continued with other Minnesota surgeons. Alden, in 1977, modified the Mason divided stomach hand-sewn gastric bypass by the introduction of a horizontal staple line without gastric division and a loop gastrojejunostomy [69]. This simple gastric bypass modification changed bariatric surgery and established the gastric bypass as the dominant operation in this field. That same year, the evolution to the modern gastric bypass, was introduced by Griffen *et al* by their introduction of the Roux-en-Y gastrojejunostomy in place of the loop gastrojejunostomy (Figure 10) [70].

The Roux gastric bypass had the advantages of avoiding tension on the gastrojejunostomy and of preventing bile reflux into the upper gastric pouch [71]. Incidentally, Griffen was also a product of the University of Minnesota.

Over the next several years, variations of the Roux gastric bypass were introduced. Torres, Oca, and Garrison stapled the stomach vertically rather than horizontally, a modification that in many hands has become the standard method for preparing the upper gastric pouch [72]. Linner and Drew reinforced the gastrojejunal outlet with a fascial band [73]. Torres and Oca again achieved a first with their modification of their vertical Roux non-divided gastric bypass and the creation of a long Roux limb for individuals who had failed their original procedure [74]. The long-limb Roux gastric bypass was later popularised as a primary operation for the super-obese by Brolin *et al* [75]. Salmon combined two procedures: a vertical banded gastroplasty and a distal Roux gastric bypass [76], and, in 1989, Fobi introduced his Silastic ring vertical gastric bypass [77]. This first innovation by Fobi created a small vertical pouch drained by a gastrojejunostomy and having a restrictive Silastic ring proximal to the

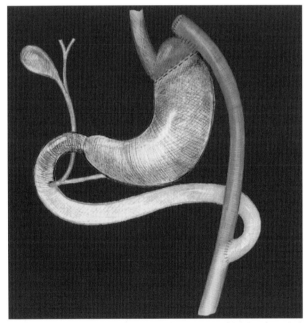

Figure 10. Griffen: gastric bypass with horizontal gastric stapling with Roux-en-Y gastrojejunostomy. *Reproduced with permission from Obesity Surgery. Buchwald H, Buchwald JN. Evolution of operative procedures for the management of morbid obesity 1950-2000. Obes Surg 2002; 12: 705-17.*

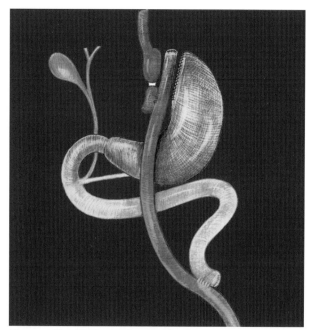

Figure 11. 1991 Fobi: gastric bypass with vertical gastric division and interposed Roux gastrojejunostomy and proximal Silastic ring. *Reproduced with permission from Obesity Surgery. Buchwald H, Buchwald JN. Evolution of operative procedures for the management of morbid obesity 1950-2000. Obes Surg 2002; 12: 705-17.*

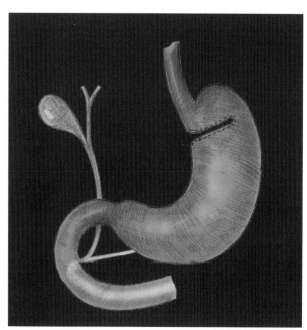

Figure 12. 1971 Mason and Printen: gastroplasty with partial gastric transection and greater curvature conduit. *Reproduced with permission from Obesity Surgery. Buchwald H, Buchwald JN. Evolution of operative procedures for the management of morbid obesity 1950-2000. Obes Surg 2002; 12: 705-17.*

gastrojejunostomy outlet. Fobi later modified this procedure by dividing the stomach and interposing the jejunal Roux limb between the gastric pouch and the bypassed stomach to ensure maintenance of the gastric division (Figure 11) [78].

In a further variation, Vassallo *et al* performed a distal biliopancreatic diversion with no gastric resection and a transient vertical banded gastroplasty constructed with a polydioxanone band that was absorbed within six months [79].

In 1994, Wittgrove, Clark and Tremblay reported their results with laparoscopic Roux gastric bypass, introducing the anvil of their end-to-end stapler endoscopically [80]. This procedure was modified by de la Torre and Scott by their introduction of the anvil of the stapler intra-abdominally to allow greater precision in anvil placement and to avoid oesophageal complications [81]. Schauer, among others, further modified and simplified the laparoscopic procedure by using the side-to-side gastrointestinal stapler to form the gastrojejunostomy [82]. Finally, Higa *et al*, in 1999, to avoid the relatively high incidence of gastrointestinal anastomotic leaks in laparoscopic procedures, described a technique for hand-sewing the gastrojejunostomy laparoscopically [83].

Restrictive procedures

In the 1970s and 1980s, bariatric surgery was simplified by the introduction of purely restrictive gastric operations: gastroplasties, gastric partitioning, banded or ringed vertical gastroplasties, and gastric banding. The restrictive operations can be performed more rapidly than a gastric bypass and are more physiological, since no part of the gastrointestinal tract is bypassed or re-routed.

The primary name in gastric restrictive surgery is, once again Edward Mason, who, in association with Printen, performed the first restrictive procedure in 1971. They divided the stomach horizontally from lesser curvature to greater curvature, leaving a gastric conduit at the greater curvature - all performed without the benefit of stapling (Figure 12).

This procedure was unsuccessful in maintaining weight loss [84]. In 1979, Gomez introduced the horizontal gastric stapling modification of the divided gastroplasty and, in addition, reinforced the greater curvature outlet with a running suture [85]. Although Gomez did many of these procedures, they, too, did not result in lasting success. Similarly, the gastric partitioning operation of Pace *et al* (1979) was unsuccessful, since the partitioning created by the removal of several staples from the middle of the stapling instrument was followed by widening of the gastrogastrostomy outlet [86]. To overcome this problem, in 1979, LaFave and Alden performed a total gastric cross-stapling and a sewed anterior gastrogastrostomy; this operation also had poor weight loss in the long term [87].

In 1981, Fabito was the first to perform a vertical gastroplasty by employing a modified TA-90 stapler and reinforcing the outlet with seromuscular sutures [88]. That same year, Laws was probably the first to use a Silastic ring as a permanent, non-expandable support for the vertical gastroplasty outlet (Figure 13) [89].

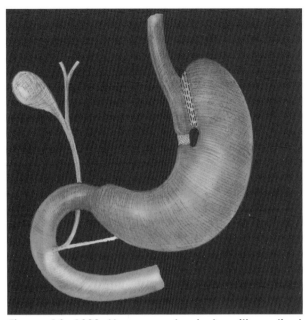

Figure 14. 1982 Mason: gastroplasty with vertical banded gastroplasty. *Reproduced with permission from Obesity Surgery. Buchwald H, Buchwald JN. Evolution of operative procedures for the management of morbid obesity 1950-2000. Obes Surg 2002; 12: 705-17.*

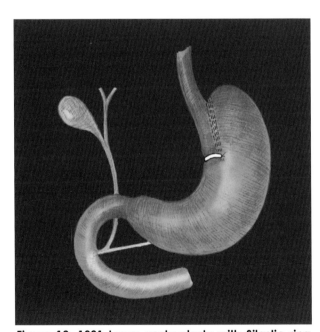

Figure 13. 1981 Laws: gastroplasty with Silastic ring vertical gastroplasty. *Reproduced with permission from Obesity Surgery. Buchwald H, Buchwald JN. Evolution of operative procedures for the management of morbid obesity 1950-2000. Obes Surg 2002; 12: 705-17.*

In 1980, Mason performed his last gastroplasty variation - the vertical banded gastroplasty [90]. This procedure involved a novel concept: namely, making a window, a through-and-through perforation in both walls of the stomach, with the end-to-end stapling instrument just above the crow's foot on the lesser curvature. This window was used for the insertion of a standard TA-90 stapler to the angle of Hiss to create a small stapled vertical pouch. The lesser curvature outlet was banded with a 1.5cm wide polypropylene mesh collar through the gastric window and around the lesser curvature conduit (Figure 14). Subsequently, in 1986, Eckhout, Willbanks, and Moore employed the Law's Silastic ring vertical gastroplasty together with a specially constructed notched stapler to avoid the window of the Mason vertical banded gastroplasty [91]. The non-reactive, narrow Silastic ring also prevented the formation of granulation tissue, which was fairly routinely induced by the polypropylene mesh of the Mason gastroplasty. Finally, in 1994, Hess and Hess [92], and in 1995, Chua and Mendiola [93], performed the vertical banded gastroplasty laparoscopically.

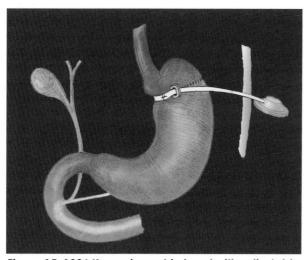

Figure 15. 1986 Kuzmak: gastric band with adjustable Silastic band. *Reproduced with permission from the American College of Surgeons. Buchwald H. Overview of bariatric surgery. J Am Coll Surg 2002; 194: 367-75.*

Gastric banding is the least invasive of the gastric restrictive procedures; a small pouch and a small stoma are created by a band around the upper stomach. The stomach is not cut or crushed by staples and no anastomoses are made. The precursors of gastric banding are found in the fundoplication procedure of Tretbar *et al* (1976) [94] and the mesh wrapping of the entire stomach by Wilkinson (1980) [95]. Wilkinson *et al* (1978) [96], Kolle (1982) [97] and Molina and Oria (1983) [98] initiated actual gastric banding. Their bands were placed during open surgery and were not adjustable, similar to the 'gastro-clip' of Bashour and Hill (1985) [99]. In 1986, Kuzmak introduced the inflatable Silastic band connected to a subcutaneous port, which is used for the percutaneous introduction or removal of fluid to adjust the calibre of the gastric band (Figure 15) [100].

In 1992-1993, Broadbent *et al* [101] and Catona *et al* [102] were probably the first to perform gastric banding laparoscopically, and in 1993, Belachew *et al* [103] and Forsell *et al* [104] were the first to perform adjustable gastric banding laparoscopically. Niville *et al* reported placing the posterior aspect of the band at the distal oesophagus and, thereby, constructing an extremely small (virtual) anterior gastric pouch [105]. Cadiere *et al* (1999) reported the world's first laparoscopic gastric banding executed robotically [106].

Other procedures

Non-malabsorptive and non-restrictive approaches to the management of morbid obesity have been, and are being, attempted. In 1974, Quaade *et al* described stereotaxic stimulation and electrocoagulation of sites in the lateral hypothalamus. In three of five patients receiving unilateral electrocoagulation lesions, there was a statistically significant but transient reduction in caloric intake and a short-term reduction in body weight [107].

In the late 1990s, electrical stimulation of the stomach was introduced into the armamentarium of bariatric procedures. The first innovator of this approach was Cigaina, who in an animal model was able to create gastric paresis and weight loss by antral electrical stimulation (Figure 16) [108]. Several gastric stimulation approaches are currently being tested in clinical trials. These systems consist of an electrode or electrodes placed into the wall of the stomach, connected to a pacer, usually in a subcutaneous pocket, programmed to deliver bipolar pulsations to the stomach.

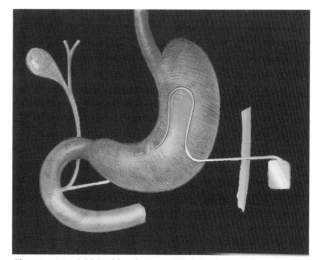

Figure 16. 1999 Cigaina: gastric electrode bipolar pulsation. *Reproduced with permission from Obesity Surgery. Buchwald H, Buchwald JN. Evolution of operative procedures for the management of morbid obesity 1950-2000. Obes Surg 2002; 12: 705-17.*

Other pioneers and pioneer societies

There are many pioneers who have contributed to the rich specialty of bariatric surgery; for the most part, they have been associated with the two major societies in this field: the American Society for Bariatric Surgery (ASBS) and the International Federation for the Surgery of Obesity (IFSO).

On April 28th-29th, 1977, the first Gastric Bypass Workshop was organised by Dr. Mason and sponsored by the University of Iowa's College of Medicine and the Department of Surgery at the Memorial Union in Iowa City [109]. Total attendance amounted to 66 people, the meeting lost money, but enthusiasm was strong for an annual meeting of bariatric surgeons. On May 24th-25th, 1978 a second Iowa meeting was held and an annual tradition was started. By 1983, this fledgling society was known as the Bariatric Surgery Colloquium and on June 3rd, 1983, by unanimous acclaim of the membership, a new national society was formed under the name of the American Society for Bariatric Surgery (ASBS). In 1987, for the first time, this meeting of bariatric surgeons was held in a city other than Iowa City, namely, in St. Louis. Since then, the ASBS has had its annual meeting in June in major US city locations. At its 2005 meeting in Orlando, Florida, registrants numbered 2,098, the meeting certainly was a financial success, and the Society had been accorded a major role in American surgery.

The list of Presidents of ASBS can be found in Table 1. Many have been mentioned as pioneers in the evolution of bariatric procedures. All have contributed dominantly to the field. Possibly four deserve additional notice (Figure 17). George S.M. Cowan, Jr., has been a continuous motivator in ASBS and a founder of IFSO; he gave rise to an organised series of lecture courses for beginning and advanced bariatric surgery at both of these societies. Mervyn Deitel, together with Cowan, started the first journal exclusively dedicated to bariatric surgery in 1991. The journal was named *Obesity Surgery* and under the continuing editorship of Deitel has achieved an extremely high impact rating among all surgical journals. Walter J. Pories gave voice to the fact that bariatric surgery, in particular gastric bypass, cures

Table 1. ASBS Presidents.	
Edward E. Mason, MD, PhD	1983-1985
John D. Halverson, MD	1985-1987
J Patrick O'Leary, MD	1987-1989
Cornelius Doherty, MD	1989-1990
George S.M. Cowan, Jr., MD	1990-1991
John H. Linner, MD	1991-1992
Boyd E. Terry, MD	1992-1993
Otto L. Willbanks, MD	1993-1994
Mervyn Deitel, MD	1994-1995
Alex M.C. Macgregor, MD	1995-1996
Kenneth G. MacDonald, MD	1996-1997
S Ross Fox, MD	1997-1998
Henry Buchwald, MD, PhD	1998-1999
Latham Flanagan, Jr., MD	1999-2000
Robert E. Brolin, MD	2000-2001
Kenneth B. Jones, Jr., MD	2001-2002
Walter J. Pories, MD	2002-2003
Alan C. Wittgrove, MD	2003-2004
Harvey J. Sugerman, MD	2004-2005
Neil E. Hutcher, MD	2005-2006

type 2 diabetes mellitus [110]. And, Harvey J. Sugerman, in addition to many scientific contributions, notably the effects of compartmental compression syndrome [111], was elected as the Editor-in-Chief of the ASBS official journal, incorporated in 2004, under the name of *Surgery for Obesity and Related Diseases* (SOARD).

A unique feature of ASBS is its Allied Health Section consisting of nurses, dieticians, social workers, psychologists, and other interested parties involved in the multidisciplinary team caring for the bariatric surgery patient. A prime mover in this area has been Georgeann Mallory, who in 1966 undertook the position of Executive Director of ASBS.

National societies in bariatric surgery soon sprang up all over the world based on the US model. In 1995,

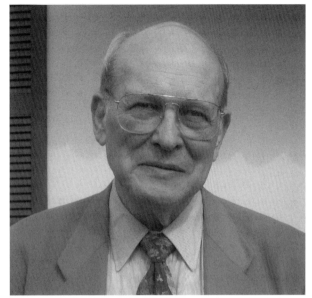

George Cowan.

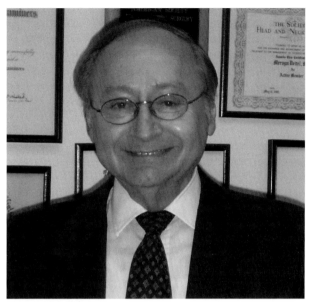

Mervyn Deitel.

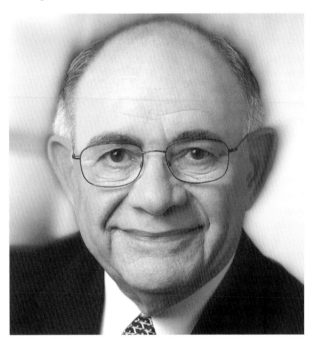

Walter Pories.

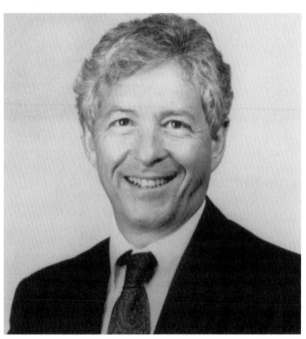

Harvey Sugerman.

Figure 17. Some of the key pioneers in the evolution of bariatric surgery.

on the initiation of Cowan, Deitel, and Scopinaro, five bariatric societies from the US, Italy, Australia/New Zealand, the Czech Republic, and Mexico formed a world body to encourage communication and education in bariatric surgery and to hold an annual congress. This group was given the name of the International Federation for the Surgery of Obesity (IFSO). At present, IFSO is composed of 32 associations, including 36 countries: Argentina, Australia/New Zealand, Austria, Belgium/ Netherlands/Luxembourg, Brazil, Chile, Czech Republic, Egypt, France, Germany, Greece, Hungary,

India, Israel, Italy, Japan, Kuwait, Mexico, Panama, Paraguay, Peru, Poland, Portugal, Romania, Russia, Spain, Switzerland, Turkey, Ukraine, United Kingdom, United States/Canada, and Yugoslavia. In addition to several countries in Europe, annual meetings of IFSO have now been held in, or scheduled for, Brazil, Japan, Australia, and Argentina. Through 1995-2006, there have been nine Presidents of IFSO (Table 2) (Figure 18).

Conclusions

Bariatric surgery is not surgery for the over indulgent or the wealthy. At the time of writing this chapter, it is the treatment of choice for the morbidly obese, the single therapy that not only causes marked weight reduction but resolves or markedly improves about 80% of the serious comorbidities of this disease [112]. Further, it has been clearly demonstrated

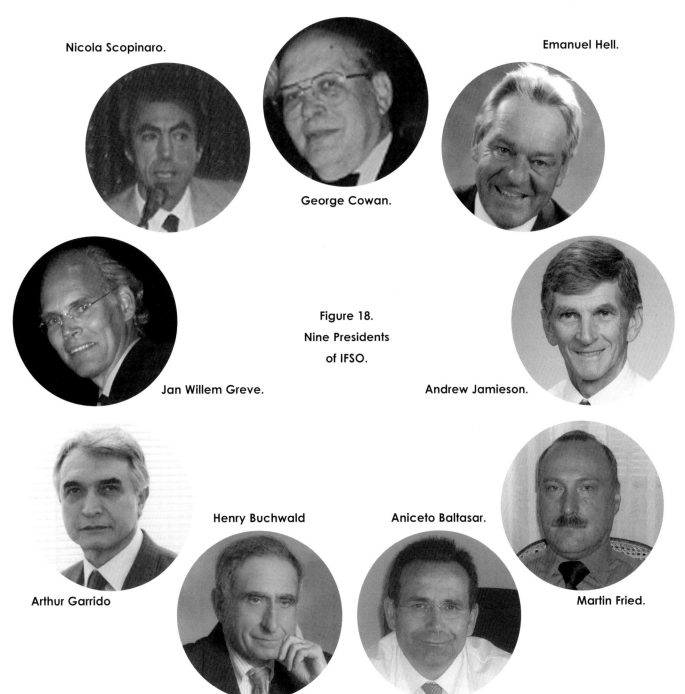

Nicola Scopinaro.

George Cowan.

Emanuel Hell.

Figure 18. Nine Presidents of IFSO.

Jan Willem Greve.

Andrew Jamieson.

Arthur Garrido

Henry Buchwald

Aniceto Baltasar.

Martin Fried.

Table 2. IFSO Presidents.		
Nicola Scopinaro, MD	Italy	1995-1997
George S.M. Cowan, Jr. MD	USA	1997-1999
Emanuel Hell, MD	Austria	1999-2000
Andrew C. Jamieson, MD	Australia	2000-2001
Martin Fried, MD	Czech Republic	2001-2002
Aniceto Baltasar, MD	Spain	2002-2003
Henry Buchwald, MD, PhD	USA	2003-2004
Arthur B. Garrido, Jr., MD	Brazil	2004-2005
Jan Willem M. Greve, MD	Netherlands	2005-2006

that bariatric surgery increases life expectancy [113]. Finally, it is cost-effective; in less than five years the medical costs of the morbidly obese not undergoing bariatric surgery exceeds that of comparable bariatric surgery patients [114].

In the first decade of the 21st century, bariatric surgery is in its prime. While it may continue to expand with new procedures, new applications in the management of disease (e.g. type 2 diabetes mellitus, gastro-oesophageal reflux disease), and into an epoch of hybrid therapy with drugs in the management of obesity, it may also be at its zenith, only to decline to become a historical footnote. Evolution of a field or discipline is inevitable (e.g. surgical therapy of Crohn's disease). Rise and decline of an exciting era is common (e.g. surgical therapy of peptic ulcer disease). What will happen to bariatric surgery?

Most of the pioneers of bariatric surgery are alive. Only posterity, and possibly shifts in perspective, will determine who in bariatric surgery will have the stature of Billroth, Kocher, Halsted, and Wangensteen. History in bariatrics is being written.

Biographical footnote on Nicola Scopinaro

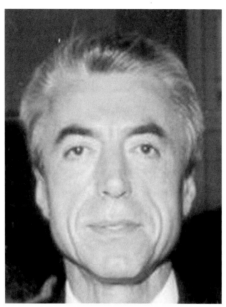

Figure 19. Nicola Scopinaro.

Nicola Scopinaro is an Italian Renaissance man of the 20th-21st centuries. He was born in Castagneto Carducci, Italy, on March 6th 1945, in the aftermath of World War II. His father was Professor of Medicine at the University of Genoa (a post he attained at the exceptional age of 36). When Nicola was 13 to 14 years old, he took pleasure in debating with his father, taking first one side of an argument and then the other. His mother prepared her second son, Nicola, for school at a very tender age, so that by the age of five he was able to read and write, had memorised about 500 verses, knew some of the history of England, and spoke a bit of Latin. He soon learned thousands of verses and undertook a life of work, study, and exploration to live up to his reputation of being a prodigy.

Scopinaro's academic career has been centered at the University of Genoa Medical School, from which he graduated in 1969, and where he rose through the ranks to become Professor of Surgery in 1992. At Genoa, he specialised in angiology in 1971, in vascular surgery in 1973, and in general surgery in 1978. For most of his professional life, his career has been centered on the surgical therapy of morbid obesity.

After a brief and very disappointing experience with the jejuno-ileal bypass, Scopinaro conceived the biliopancreatic diversion (BPD) procedure in 1973, and after two years of experimental physiological studies in dogs on the various anatomic and functional aspects of the gastrointestinal tract, he performed the first BPD in humans on May 12, 1976 (see earlier in the Chapter). In April of 2000, he performed the first laparoscopic BPD. He has also performed and studied the Roux-en-Y gastric bypass procedure as a possible alternative, in certain situations, to the BPD.

Throughout this time period, Scopinaro continued in his physiological studies of the gastrointestinal tract and has published extensively his theories on the relative metabolism of lean body mass, fat and viscera, and their individual influence on caloric consumption, weight loss, and weight stabilisation. His clinical and investigative publications number more than 400. He is an ambassador for the BPD, and he is a frequently invited international speaker. He has maintained the largest series of BPD cases (nearly 3,000), and has published the longest-term results for this procedure.

Scopinaro has been well recognised for his work in bariatric surgery. He was Chairman of the First International Symposium on Obesity Surgery, held in Genoa in 1980, and of the nine subsequent annual meetings of this symposium. When the International Federation for the Surgery of Obesity was created in Stockholm in 1995, Scopinaro, a founding member, was elected its first President. After two years, Scopinaro left this office and was elected Honorary President of the Federation. He is also President of the European Chapter of IFSO, constituted in 2005.

In his private life, Scopinaro is a daredevil and risk taker with the same dedication to achievement he has brought to his professional life. He skis for speed, he frequently crashes his sports cars, his scuba diving is hazardous, he pilots planes and occasionally crashes them, and he has driven long distance endurance treks across the African desert. As a skydiver, he has won five consecutive Italian championships, and in 1976 gave Italy the only medal it has ever achieved in a World Championship. In 1977, both of his canopies failed to open and he hit the ground at 100km/h. With 13 fractures and internal bleeding, he stayed in hospital for six months but before he could properly walk, he went skydiving again at the very site of his injury. The next year, he won one more Italian Sky Diving Championship. It is not surprising he has undergone over 20 orthopaedic operations in his life.

Scopinaro has had two short-lived marriages; he has one daughter, and two grandchildren. He currently enjoys a long-lasting relationship with a highly independent professional woman.

Biographical footnote on Edward Mason

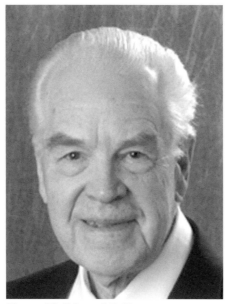

Figure 20. Edward E. Mason.

Edward E. Mason, Ed to his friends and associates, was born in the backseat of a taxi on October 10th 1920, in Boise, Idaho, an under-populated western state of the US of highly conservative convictions. At age one, his family moved to Moscow, Idaho, where his father taught journalism and his mother taught him, and his class mates, how to read. When he was nine, the family moved to Iowa, which was to remain his home, except for his eight years of surgical training at the University of Minnesota under Owen H. Wangensteen. He married Dordana Fairman of Kansas City in 1949, and the Masons with their three boys and one girl, their grandchildren, and great-grandchildren, frequently return to the Minnesota north woods and Canadian boundary waters for summer canoe trips.

During World War II, Mason completed his schooling as a Naval Officer and worked in a tuberculosis sanatorium during his last year of medical school. After internship, he was assigned to the Veteran's Administration Hospital in Wadworth, Kansas, where he did his first published research on streptomycin therapy for tuberculosis.

The years between 1945 and 1953 at the University of Minnesota were critical to Mason's intellectual development. The training program at Minnesota, responsible for the education and orientation of many of the leading American surgeons of the second half of the 20th century, was unique and world renowned for educating an academic surgeon not only in the principles of surgical diseases and in technical skills but in the performance of basic and clinical research. A Wangensteen graduate was, by definition, an investigator, and one of the most versatile of Wangensteen's pupils was Ed Mason.

On joining the Faculty of the Department of Surgery of the University of Iowa in 1953, Mason called in all of the patients diagnosed with an inoperable, giant, ventral hernia, and he prepared them for surgery by therapeutic pneumoperitoneum over six weeks before repair. Subsequently, two of his operated patients gained weight and disrupted his repairs. Influenced by Dr. Arnold Kremen, who with Linner and Nelson published the first paper on jejuno-ileal bypass surgery, Mason performed two intestinal bypass procedures for the management of morbid obesity. He was disappointed with the results and turned his attention to other fields including renal dialysis, thyroid and parathyroid surgery, splenorenal shunting for bleeding oesophageal varices, as well as basic laboratory work on serum and urinary enzymes as indices of muscle or renal cell damage.

With the help of Chikashi Ito, who came to work with Mason from Sopporo, Japan, Mason started a three-year study in the animal laboratory of gastric bypass for the management of morbid obesity in 1965. They demonstrated that if sufficient acid-secreting stomach as well as the antrum were bypassed, gastrin secretion was sufficiently inhibited so that ulcers did not occur in the gastrojejunostomy stoma or the duodenum. In 1966, based upon what Mason had learned from Wangensteen about weight loss after short-loop, retrocolic, gastrojejunostomy for treating peptic ulcer disease, he started clinical gastric bypass. These pioneer efforts, subsequently modified by others, have resulted in hundreds of thousands of gastric bypass procedures throughout the world and, in particular, in the US.

In 1971, Mason essentially abandoned the gastric bypass procedure, in spite of its success, and set off in a new direction with the use of horizontal gastroplasty for morbid obesity. This eventually led to the vertical banded gastroplasty, using a measured pouch of less than 20ml, and controlling the outlet at a calculated 11 to 12mm diameter by a 1.5cm-wide strip of Marlex mesh. Thus, another major surgical innovation for the treatment of patients with morbid obesity was introduced into the management armamentarium. For a period of time, vertical banded gastroplasty surpassed the gastric bypass in numbers, but has, in recent years, lost its appeal for many surgeons and has given way to the laparoscopic adjustable gastric band.

Earlier in the chapter the origins of the American Society for Bariatric Surgery are summarised, which was incorporated in Iowa in 1983, and had its origins in the bariatric surgery conferences initiated in Iowa City by Mason in 1976. In 1986, Mason began a computerised National Bariatric Surgery Registry, which later had a name change from National to International or the IBSR, which continues under his direction. In his latter years, Mason has returned to the laboratory from where his clinical innovations originated. He is studying the roles of various gut hormones, e.g. GLP-1, gastrin, and obestatin, on obesity mechanisms and, most interestingly, on type 2 diabetes mellitus.

Mason in his 80s remained extremely active, swimming and walking daily, as well as intimately involved in his specialty of bariatric surgery, where his many contributions have earned him the accolade of 'the father of bariatric surgery'. Mason will remain an inspiration to the many surgeons who have followed in his footsteps.

References

1. Whitcombe CLCE. Women in prehistory. The Venus of Willendorf. 2000. Available from: URL: http://witcombe.sbc.edu/willendorf/willendorfdiscovery.html. Accessed September 2, 2002.

2. Bray GA. Historical framework for the development of ideas about obesity. In: *Handbook of Obesity.* Bray GA, Bouchard C, James WPT, Eds. New York, NY: Marcel Dekker, Inc.; 1997: 1-30.

3. Giugliano D. Endocrinology and art: the obese Etruscan. *J Endocrinol Invest* 2001; 24: 206.

4. The Bible. King James version. Grand Rapids (MI): Zondervan Publishing House, 1995; Judges 3: 17-22.

5. Avicenna. *Canon of Medicine.* 400.

6. Nathan B. Vignettes from history. A medieval medical view on obesity. *Obes Surg* 1992; 2: 217-8.

7. Wadd W. *Comments on corpulency, lineaments of leanness. Memoirs on Diet and Dietetics.* London: John Ebers, 1829.

8. Quetelet A. *Sur l'homme et le development de ses facultes, ou essai de physique sociale.* Paris: Bachelier, 1835.

9. Kottek SS. On health and obesity in Talmudic and Midrashic lore. *Israel J Med Sci* 1996; 32: 509-10.

10. Flegel KM, Carroll MD, Kuczmarski RJ, Johnson CL. Overweight and obesity in the United States: prevalence and trends, 1960-1994. *Int J Obes* 1998; 22: 39-47.

11. The National Center for Health Statistics NHANES IV Report - available at www.cdc.gov/nchs/product/pubs/pubd/hestats /obes/obese99.htm2002. Accessed September 9, 2004.

12. Monteforte MJ, Torkelson CM. Bariatric surgery for morbid obesity. *Obes Surg* 2000; 10: 391-401.

13. Population Estimates Program, Population Division, US Census Bureau. Resident Population Estimates of the United States by Age and Sex: April 1, 1990 to July 1, 1999, With Short-Term Projection to June 1, 2000. Washington, DC: US Census Bureau, http://www.census.gov July 6, 2000.

14. Mun EC, Blackburn GL, Mathews JB. Current status of medical and surgical therapy for obesity. *Gastroenterol* 2001; 120: 669-81.

15. Breaux CW. Obesity surgery in children. *Obes Surg* 1995; 5: 279-84.

16. Worldwatch Institute. [online] available at: http://www.worldwatch.org. Accessed September 9, 2002.

17. Mokdad AH, Serdula MK, Dietz WH, Bowman BA, Marks JS, Coplan JP. The spread of the obesity epidemic in the United States, 1991-1998. *JAMA* 1999; 282: 1519-22.

18. World Health Organization Reports. [online] 2002. Available at: http://www.who.ch//. Accessed September 9, 2002.

19. Jung RT. Obesity as a disease. *Br Med Bull* 1997; 53: 307-21.

20. Bray GA. Obesity, a time bomb to be defused. *Lancet* 1998; 352: 160-1.

21. North American Association for the Study of Obesity (NAASO) and the National Heart, Lung, and Blood Institute (NHLBI). Clinical Guidelines on the Identification, Evaluation, and Treatment of Overweight and Obesity in Adults. The Evidence Report. NIH Publication #98-4083, Sept 1998.

22. North American Association for the Study of Obesity (NAASO) and the National Heart, Lung, and Blood Institute (NHLBI). The Practical Guide: Identification, Evaluation, and Treatment of Overweight and Obesity in Adults. NIH Publication #00-4084, Oct 2000.

23. O'Brien PE, Dixon JB. The extent of the problem of obesity. *Am J Surg* 2002; 184: 4S-8S.

24. Sugerman H. Pathophysiology of severe obesity. *Problems in General Surgery* 2000; 17: 7-12.

25. Herrara MF, Lozano-Salazar RR, Gonzalez-Barranco J, Rull JA. Diseases and problems secondary to massive obesity. *Eur J Gastroenterol Hepatol* 1999; 11: 63-7.

26. Pi-Sunyer FX. Medical hazards of obesity. *Ann Intern Med* 1993; 199: 655-60.

27. Allon N. The stigma of obesity in everyday life. In: *Psychological Aspects of Obesity: A Handbook.* Wolman BJ, Ed. New York: Van Nostrand Reinhold, 1981: 130-74.

28. Wadden TA, Stunkard JJ. Social and psychological consequences of obesity. *Ann Intern Med* 1985; 103: 1062-7.

29. Wolf AM, Colditz GA. Social and economic effects of body weight in the United States. *Am J Clin Nutr* 1996; 63(Suppl): 466S-9S.

30. French SA, Story M, Perry CL. Self-esteem and obesity in children and adolescents: a literature review. *Obes Res* 1995; 3: 479-90.

31. Stunkard AJ. T*he Pain of Obesity.* Palo Alto, CA: Bull Publishing Co., 1976.

32. Gortmaker SL, Must A, Perrin JM, Sobol AM, Dietz WH. Social and economic consequences of overweight in adolescence and young adulthood. *N Engl J Med* 1993; 329: 1008-12.

33. Blumberg P, Mellis PP. Medical students' attributes toward the obese and the morbidly obese. *Int J Eating Disord* 1985; 4: 169-75.

34. Oberrieder H, Walker R, Monroe D, Adeyanju M. Attitude of dietetics students and registered dietitians toward obesity. *J Am Diet Assoc* 1995; 95: 914-6.

35. Canning H, Mayer J. Obesity - its possible effect on college acceptance. *N Engl J Med* 1066; 275: 1172-4.

36. Klesges RC, Klem ML, Hanson CL, et al. The effects of applicant's health status and qualifications on simulated hiring decisions. *Int J Obes* 1990; 14: 527-35.

37. Karris L. Prejudice against obese renters. *J Soc Psych* 1977; 101: 159-60.

38. Narbro K, Jonsson E, Larsson B, et al. Economic consequences of sick-leave and early retirement in obese Swedish women. *Intl J Obes Relat Metab Disord* 1999; 20: 895-903.

39. Hughes D, McGuire A. A review of the economic analysis of obesity. *Br Med Bull* 1997; 53: 253-63.

40. Lévy E, Lévy P, Le Pen C, et al. The economic costs of obesity: the French situation. *Int J Obes* 1995; 19: 788-92.

41. Segal L, Carter R, Zimmet P. The costs of obesity: the Australian perspective. *Pharmacoeconomics* 1994; 5: 42-52.

42. Swinburn B, Ashton T, Gillespie J, et al. Health care costs of obesity in New Zealand. *Int J Obes* 1997; 21: 891-6.

43. Colditz GA. Economic costs of obesity. *Am J Clin Nutr* 1992; 55: 403S-7S.

44. Henrikson V. Kan tunnfarmsresektion forsvaras som terapi mot fettsot? *Nordisk Medicin* 1952; 47: 744. Translation: Can small bowel resection be defended as therapy for obesity? *Obes Surg* 1994; 4: 54.

45. Buchwald H, Rucker RD. The rise and fall of jejunoileal bypass. In: *Surgery of the Small Intestine*. Nelson RL, Nyhus LM, Eds. Norwalk, CT: Appleton Century Crofts, 1987: 529-41.

46. Kremen AJ, Linner LH, Nelson CH. An experimental evaluation of the nutritional importance of proximal and distal small intestine. *Ann Surg* 1954; 140: 439-44.

47. Payne JH, DeWind LT, Commons RR. Metabolic observations in patients with jejunocolic shunts. *Am J Surg* 1963; 106: 272-89.

48. Deitel M. Jejunocolic and jejunoileal bypass: an historical perspective. In: *Surgery for the Morbidly Obese Patient*. Deitel M, Ed. Philadelphia: Lea & Febiger; 1998: 81-9.

49. Payne JH, DeWind LT. Surgical treatment of obesity. *Am J Surg* 1969; 118: 141-7.

50. Sherman CD, May AG, Nye W. Clinical and metabolic studies following bowel bypassing for obesity. *Ann NY Acad Sci* 1965; 131: 614-22.

51. Lewis LA, Turnbull RB, Page LH. 'Short-circuiting' of the small intestine. *JAMA* 1962; 182: 77-9.

52. Lewis LA, Turnbull RB, Page LH. Effects of jejunocolic shunt on obesity, serum lipoproteins, lipids, and electrolytes. *Arch Intern Med* 1966; 117: 4-16.

53. Scott HW, Sandstead HH, Brill AB. Experience with a new technic of intestinal bypass in the treatment of morbid obesity. *Ann Surg* 1971; 174: 560-72.

54. Salmon PA. The results of small intestine bypass operations for the treatment of obesity. *Surg Gynecol Obstet* 1971; 132: 965-79.

55. Buchwald H, Varco RL. A bypass operation for obese hyperlipidemic patients. *Surgery* 1971; 70: 62-70.

56. Forestieri P, DeLuca L, Bucci L. Surgical treatment of high degree obesity. Our own criteria to choose the appropriate type of jejuno-ileal bypass: a modified Payne technique. *Chir Gastroenterol* 1977; 11: 401-8.

57. Starkloff GB, Stothert JC, Sundaram M. Intestinal bypass: a modification. *Ann Surg* 1978; 188: 697-700.

58. Palmer JA, Marliss EB. The present status of surgical procedures for obesity. In: *Nutrition in Clinical Surgery*. Deitel M, Ed. Baltimore: Williams & Wilkins, 1980: 281-92.

59. Cleator IGM, Gourlay RH. Ileogastrostomy for morbid obesity. *Can J Surg* 1988; 31(2): 114-6.

60. Kral JG. Duodenoileal bypass. In: *Surgery for the Morbidly Obese Patient*. Deitel M, Ed. Philadelphia, PA: Lea & Febiger; 1998: 99-103.

61. Lavorato F, Doldi SB, Scaramella R. Evoluzione storica della terapia chirurgica della grande obesita. *Minerva Med* 1978; 69: 3847-57.

62. Eriksson F. Biliointestinal bypass. *Int J Obes* 1981; 5: 437-47.

63. Scopinaro N, Gianetta E, Civalleri D. Biliopancreatic bypass for obesity: II. Initial experiences in man. *Br J Surg* 1979; 66: 618-20.

64. Scopinaro N, Adami GF, Marinari GM, *et al*. Biliopancreatic diversion: two decades of experience. In: *Update: Surgery for the Morbidly Obese Patient*. Deitel M, Cowan SM Jr, Eds. Toronto, Canada: FD-Communications Inc; 2000: 227-58.

65. Hess DW, Hess DS. Biliopancreatic diversion with a duodenal switch. *Obes Surg* 1998; 8: 267-82.

66. Marceau P, Biron S, Bourque R-A, *et al*. Biliopancreatic diversion with a new type of gastrectomy. *Obes Surg* 1993; 3: 29-35.

67. Mason EE, Ito C. Gastric bypass in obesity. *Surg Clin N Am* 1967; 47: 1345-52.

68. Mason EE, Printen KJ. Optimizing results of gastric bypass. *Ann Surg* 1975; 182: 405-13.

69. Alden JF. Gastric and jejuno-ileal bypass: a comparison in the treatment of morbid obesity. *Arch Surg* 1977; 112: 799-806.

70. Griffen WO, Young VL. Stevenson. CC. A prospective comparison of gastric and jejunoileal bypass procedures for morbid obesity. *Ann Surg* 1977; 186: 500-7.

71. McCarthy HB, Rucker RD, Chan EK, *et al*. Gastritis after gastric bypass surgery. *Surgery* 1985; 98: 68-71.

72. Torres JC, Oca CF, Garrison RN. Gastric bypass: Roux-en-Y gastrojejunostomy from the lesser curvature. *South Med J* 1983; 76: 1217- 21.

73. Linner JR, Drew RL. New modification of Roux-en-Y gastric bypass procedure. *Clin Nutr* 1986; 5: 33-4.

74. Torres J, Oca C. Gastric bypass lesser curvature with distal Roux-en-Y. *Bariatric Surg* 1987; 5: 10-5.

75. Brolin RE, Kenler HA, Gorman JH, *et al*. Long-limb gastric bypass in the superobese. A prospective randomized study. *Ann Surg* 1992; 21: 387-95.

76. Salmon PA. Gastroplasty with distal gastric bypass: a new and more successful weight loss operation for the morbidly obese. *Can J Surg* 1988; 31: 111-3.

77. Fobi MA. The surgical technique of the banded Roux-en-Y gastric bypass. *J Obes Weight Reg* 1989; 8: 99-102.

78. Fobi MA. Why the operation I prefer is Silastic ring vertical banded gastric bypass. *Obes Surg* 1991; 1: 423-6.

79. Vassallo C, Negri L, Della Valle A, *et al*. Biliopancreatic diversion with transitory gastroplasty preserving duodenal bulb: 3 years experience. *Obes Surg* 1997; 7: 30-3.

80. Wittgrove AC, Clark GW, Tremblay, LJ. Laparoscopic gastric bypass, Roux-en-Y: preliminary report of five cases. *Obes Surg* 1994; 4: 353-7.

81. de la Torre RA, Scott JS. Laparoscopic Roux-en-Y gastric bypass: a totally intra-abdominal approach - technique and preliminary report. *Obes Surg* 1999; 9: 492-7.

82. Schauer PR, Ikramuddin S, Gourash W, Ramanathan R, Luketich JD. Outcomes of laparoscopic Roux-en-Y gastric bypass for morbid obesity. *Ann Surg* 2000; 232: 515-29.

83. Higa KD, Boone KB, Ho T. Laparoscopic Roux-en-Y gastric bypass for morbid obesity in 850 patients: technique and follow-up. *Obes Surg* 2000; 10: 146 (abstr P34).

84. Printen KJ, Mason EE. Gastric surgery for relief of morbid obesity. *Arch Surg* 1973; 106: 428-31.

85. Gomez CA. Gastroplasty in morbid obesity. *Surg Clin North Amer* 1979; 59: 1113-20.

86. Pace WG, Martin EW, Tetirick CE, Fabri PJ, Carey LC. Gastric partitioning for morbid obesity. *Ann Surg* 1979; 190: 392-400.

87. LaFave JW, Alden JF. Gastric bypass in the operative revision of the failed jejuno-ileal bypass. *Arch Surg* 1979; 114: 438-44.

88. Fabito DC. Gastric vertical stapling. Read before the Bariatric Surgery Colloquium, Iowa City, Iowa, June 1, 1981.

89. Laws HL, Piatadosi S. Superior gastric reduction procedure for morbid obesity. A prospective, randomized trial. *Am J Surg* 1981; 193: 334-6.

90. Mason EE. Vertical banded gastroplasty. *Arch Surg* 1982; 117: 701-6.

91. Eckhout GV, Willbanks OL, Moore JT. Vertical ring gastroplasty for obesity: five year experience with 1463 patients. *Am J Surg* 1986; 152: 713-6.

92. Hess DW, Hess DS. Laparoscopic vertical banded gastroplasty with complete transection of the staple-line. *Obes Surg* 1994; 4: 44-6.

93. Chua TY, Mendiola RM. Laparoscopic vertical banded gastroplasty: the Milwaukee experience. *Obes Surg* 1995; 5: 77-80.

94. Tretbar LL, Taylor TL, Sifers EC. Weight reduction: gastric plication for morbid obesity. *J Kans Med Soc* 1976; 77: 488-90.

95. Wilkinson LH. Reduction of gastric reservoir capacity. *J Clin Nutr* 1980; 33: 515-7.

96. Wilkinson LH, Peloso OA. Gastric (reservoir) reduction for morbid obesity. *Arch Surg* 1981; 116: 602-5.

97. Kolle K. Gastric banding. OMGI 7th Congress, Stockholm, 1982: 37 (abstr 145).

98. Molina M, Oria HE. Gastric segmentation: a new, safe, effective, simple, readily revised and fully reversible surgical procedure for the correction of morbid obesity. 6th Bariatric Surgery Colloquium, Iowa City. June 3, 1983; 15 (abstr).

99. Bashour SB, Hill RW. The gastro-clip gastroplasty: an alternative surgical procedure for the treatment of morbid obesity. *Tex Med* 1985; 81: 36-8.

100. Kuzmak LI. Silicone gastric banding: a simple and effective operation for morbid obesity. *Contemp Surg* 1986; 28: 13-8.

101. Broadbent R, Tracy M, Harrington P. Laparoscopic gastric banding: a preliminary report. *Obes Surg* 1993; 3: 63-7.

102. Catona A, Gossenberg M, La Manna A, Mussini G. Laparoscopic gastric banding: preliminary series. *Obes Surg* 1993; 3: 207-9.

103. Belachew M, Legrand M, Jacquet N. Laparoscopic placement of adjustable silicone gastric banding in the treatment of morbid obesity: an animal model experimental study: a video film: a preliminary report. *Obes Surg* 1993; 3: 140 (abstr 5).

104. Forsell P, Hallberg D, Hellers G. Gastric banding for morbid obesity: initial experience with a new adjustable band. *Obes Surg* 1993; 3: 369-74.

105. Niville E, Vankeirsblick J, Dams A, Anne T. Laparoscopic adjustable esophagogastric banding: a preliminary experience. *Obes Surg* 1998; 8: 39-42.

106. Cadiere GB, Himpens J, Vertruyen M. The world's first obesity surgery performed by a surgeon at a distance. *Obes Surg* (England) 1999; 9: 206-9.

107. Quaade F, Vaernet K, Larsson S. Sterotaxic stimulation and electrocoagulation of the lateral hypothalamus in obese humans. *Acta Neurochir (Wien)* 1974; 30: 1111-7.

108. Cigaina V, Pinato G, Rigo V. Gastric peristalsis control by mono situ electrical stimulation: a preliminary study. *Obes Surg* 1996; 6:247-9.

109. Blommers TD. American Society for Bariatric Surgery: the first nine years. *Obes Surg* 1992; 2: 115-7.

110. Pories WJ, Swenson MS, MacDonald KG, *et al.* Who would have thought it? An operation proves to be the most effective therapy for adult-onset diabetes mellitus. *Ann Surg* 1995; 222: 339-52.

111. Sugerman HJ, Windsor A, Bessos M, Wolfe L. Intraabdominal pressure, sagittal abdominal diameter and obesity comorbidity. *J Intern Med* 1997; 241: 71-9.

112. Buchwald H, Avidor Y, Braunwald E, Jensen MD, Pories W, Fahrbach K, Schoelles K. Bariatric surgery: a systematic review and meta-analysis. *JAMA* 2004; 292: 1724-37.

113. Christou NV, Sampalis JS, Liberman M, Look D. Auger S, McLean AP, MacLean LD. Surgery decreases long-term mortality, morbidity, and health care use in morbidly obese patients. *Ann Surg* 2004; 240: 416-23.

114. Sampalis JS, Liberman M, Auger S, Christou NV. The impact of weight reduction surgery on health-care costs in morbidly obese patients. *Obes Surg* 2004; 14: 939-7.

Chapter 6

Gastroduodenal surgery

Dick C Busman MD PhD

Emeritus Consultant Surgeon, Leeuwarden, The Netherlands

Introduction

Whereas physicians looked after all gastric disorders before the advent of anaesthesia and asepsis, the whole picture changed after successful gastric surgery by Billroth was made public in 1881 [1]. Before this historic event, it was only when the alimentary tract became exteriorised in the form of a fistula, abscess, or open wound, that the help of a surgeon was requested.

This first successful resection of the stomach by Billroth (Figure 1) was a tremendous advance for surgical progress. For the first time surgeons were able to intrude directly into the realm of physicians to produce a potentially rapid cure that was obvious to the patient as well as the clinician. Before and since this event, the education, training and status of surgeons improved considerably, and became organised in a similar fashion to the training for physicians.

In those days, the stomach organ itself was considered crucial to every human being. Thought to be responsible for hunger, satiation after food, rejection of poisons and irritants by vomiting, it was believed to be the seat of numerous human emotions.

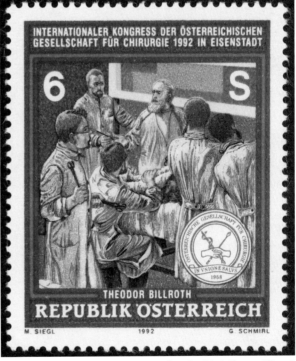

Figure 1. Operating portrait of Christian Albert Theodor Billroth (1829-1894). Detail of a painting by A. Seligmann.

Trauma

The first operations on the stomach were usually performed for direct combat injuries, stab wounds [2] and inadvertently swallowed foreign objects. Figure 2 shows the first known painting of successful operative treatment of a stab wound in 1521 on a patient named Kuntz Seytz [2, 3]. Elective operations were rare; the majority were for emergencies aptly called *operationes necessitatis*.

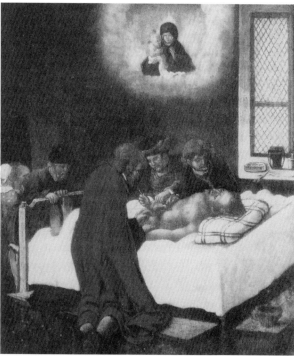

Figure 2. Operative repair of a stab wound. *Reproduced with permission from Kaden Verlag, Heidelberg. Sachs M. Geschichte der Operativen Chirurgie, Band V, 2005: 147.*

In 1602, Matthis Florian [4] successfully operated on a knife swallower. Previously this man had a trick of letting a knife disappear down his gullet, followed by a glass of beer before retrieval; however, on one occasion he failed because the knife slid into the stomach but could not be retrieved, although it could be palpated. Florian's successful operation took place seven weeks later. There were other similar stories [2, 5] where swallowed objects were removed after a sensible period of observation. This took the form of a planned operation or incision of abscesses due to inflammation of the stomach wall and abdominal wall [6].

Often, magnetic dressings were applied to bring the corresponding object nearer to the surface for excision [6].

Gastrostomies

Gastrostomies were developed to nourish people who could not swallow; for example, those with oesophageal stricture as discussed in Chapter 4, and benign and malignant diseases of the oesophagus and cardia. The medical and lay public usually appreciated that although the mortality before antiseptic surgery was high, intervention was sometimes considered the slightly better option than the usual fatal outcome of conservative measures. Such intervention was extremely distressing and painful before 1846, the time anaesthesia was introduced.

In 1849, Sedillot succeeded in creating gastrostomies in dogs, but his first patient died [7, 8]. Both the patients of Jones (1875) and Verneuil (1876) with caustic stricture survived [9, 10]. Sometimes in the first instance, a gastrorrhaphy to the abdominal wall was performed to encourage the development of adhesions. Then at the second stage, a formal gastrostomy was created [11]. This principle was similar to the technique that was advocated by Bloch for the gallbladder in 1744, described in Chapter 7, Surgery of the liver and biliary tree. The first feeding fistula was by Witzel [12] in 1891 (Figure 3).

Gastric juice

A surprising amount of physiological information was obtained from gastric juice collected from gastrostomies in animals. Réamur (1683-1757) experimented with his pet buzzard and discovered meat was not putrefied but digested by gastric juice [13]. In 1820, a chemist called William Prout demonstrated hydrochloric acid in gastric chyme [13, 14]. Soon thereafter, this was confirmed by the Germans, Tiedeman and Gmelin [13, 14].

The celebrated patient, Alexis St. Martin, an American soldier, presented with wounds both in his chest and abdomen. Miraculously, the chest wounds

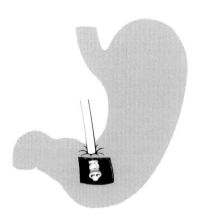 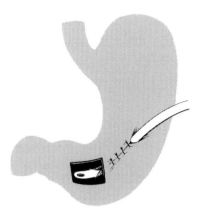 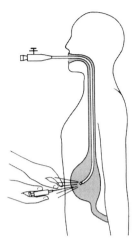

Kader fistula
Straight gastrostomy with several imbricating pursestring sutures.

Witzel fistula
Tube enters stomach after being buried in a seromuscular canal.

PEG catheter
Schematic representation of percutaneous endoscopic gastrostomy. Endoscopically, the stomach is apposed to the abdominal wall. A connection is made from here and a tube is introduced by manoeuvring from both sides. The procedure is usually performed by a physician gastroenterologist.

Figure 3. Three demonstrations of a gastric fistula: Kader, Witzel and the modern 'PEG' system. *Reproduced with permission from Georg Thieme Verlag, Stuttgart. Kremer K, Schumpelick V, Hierholzer G. Chirurgische Operationen, 1992: 229-30.*

healed, but the abdominal wound resulted in a persistent gastric fistula. His army doctor, William Beaumont, published the story in 1833, and was able to describe the response of the mucosa and its secretions to emotion, anxiety, stress and eating [15]. He even maintained the patient and his patient's family financially, in addition to his own for several years despite all parties being transferred to a position 2000 miles away [16]. He also suspected that gastric juice must have a 'chemical principle' apart from hydrochloric acid, to aid digestion. This principle, inactivated by boiling, was called 'pepsin' by Müller and Schwann in 1836 [17].

Many other studies were done in relation to the gastric juice, notably by Heidenhain and Pavlov, using denervated and innervated stomach pouches. Pavlov truly deserved the Nobel Prize in 1904 for his work on gastric physiology, including the innervation of the stomach. He was, however, not completely accurate on the destination of the branches of the anterior and posterior vagus nerves [16,18], later described correctly in detail by Latarjet [18] and illustrated in the 'selective vagotomies' section later.

Diseases of the stomach and duodenum

Baillie in 1793 [10] described the symptoms and pathology of gastric ulceration [19,20]. In 1829, Cruveilhier (Figure 4) made a clear distinction between gastric ulceration and cancer. So much so, that gastric ulceration is still eponymously called Cruveilhier's disease in France [21]. In 1830, Abercrombie was the first to describe duodenal ulceration as a distinct entity [7].

In the second half of the 19th century, both cancer of the stomach as well as gastric ulceration were often found in young women, while duodenal ulceration was relatively uncommon. Perforation of gastric ulcers was found sufficiently common in women under the age of 25, that abnormal uterine function was erroneously believed to be responsible [22]. At the turn of the 20th century, this appeared to alter. More duodenal ulcers occurred in young men in almost epidemic proportions between 1910 and 1950 [23-25]. At the same time gastric cancer began to affect more and more elderly people. The explanation for these shifts was not clear, but it

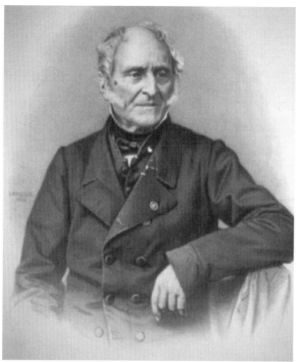

Figure 4. Jean Cruveilhier (1791-1874). *Reproduced with permission from the Musée de L'Histoire de la Médecine, Paris, France.*

was likely duodenal ulceration took place in communities of early urbanisation [23, 26].

However, since 1950, the incidence of duodenal ulceration began to decrease [27, 28], even before the arrival of the new effective ulcer-healing drugs, which are mentioned later in this chapter. Gastric cancer also began to decrease, having previously had a higher incidence. Perhaps better storage and preservation of food, especially meat products, fresh fruit and vegetables, made the difference [29, 30]. It is only in the last 20 years that the role of *Helicobacter pylori* has been highlighted as an aetiological factor in peptic ulcer disease [31, 32].

Diagnosis

In those early days, diagnoses were made on clinical grounds. Peptic ulceration or carcinoma was suspected from a history of post-prandial epigastric pain, dysphagia, vomiting, weight loss, abdominal distension, audible splashes, borborygmi, and a palpable epigastric mass such as the one that ended von Mikulicz's* life. Analysis of gastric juice was often

unspecific, and contrast studies [33] were not available until the 20th century.

Diagnostic endoscopy of the alimentary tract owed much to the pioneers who developed new ways of seeing the urinary bladder (Chapter 4, The changing tides in oesophageal surgery). Von Mikulicz [34, 35] enlisted the help of the skilled instrument maker, Leiter, to design and make the first gastroscope to enable the first views of the oesophagus and stomach mucosal linings. After von Mikulicz's departure from Vienna, Viktor von Hacker [36], another pupil from Billroth's surgical school, made further progress in this field. In 1932, Schindler [10, 37] produced a flexible gastroscope, a fine engineering feat in its day; an example of a semi-flexible instrument is shown in Figure 4, Chapter 4. Modern fiberoptic telescopes have dramatically reduced the number of contrast studies needed today and have been established as the standard diagnostic tool for gastric problems.

Resection

In 1810, Daniel Merrem, pupil of Michaelis of Marburg, successfully performed a pylorectomy or distal gastric resection in two out of three dogs [5, 10]. The application of this to patients had to wait until anaesthetic agents and antisepsis were available.

In 1874, Cavazzani [38] accidentally discovered and successfully resected a benign tumour in the abdominal wall involving the stomach without anaesthesia. Post mortem studies revealed the patient died of pulmonary tuberculosis four years later. Sadly, first attempts to perform pylorectomy in 1879 by Péan in Paris, and Rydygier from Kulm in Poland a year later, ended with fatal outcomes [5, 10]. Péan never again attempted any gastric resection [39].

The first successful distal gastrectomy took place on January 19th 1881 by Theodor Billroth [17, 39]. Billroth had the advantage of being a distinguished pathologist before embarking on his surgical career, and had access to thousands of post mortem examinations extracted from Rokitansky's material on gastric tumours and their metastases by his assistants, von Winiwarter and Gussenbauer. These assistants had previously developed gastric resection in dogs [1].

*the prefix 'von' as part of the name could be awarded in those days to people of extraordinary significance to society. It is a title that can be compared to the English 'Sir'. Five pupils of Billroth: Czerny, Eiselsberg, Hacker, Mikulicz, and Winiwarter were all granted this honorary title, but their names frequently occur without.

During the famous operation (Figures 5 and 6) on the 43-year-old Thérèse Heller, which was performed under chloroform anaesthesia, Billroth was assisted by Wölfler. The stomach had been well washed out beforehand. Careful Listerian antiseptic measures were taken excepting the carbolic spray, and all the sutures and instruments had been soaked in carbolic acid (phenol) before the operation [10]. The resection margins were close to the tumour and several lymph nodes were involved. Continuity was restored by gastro-duodenostomy, employing about 33 separate silk sutures for the anastomosis at the lesser curvature side, and 21 sutures for closing the greater curvature [40].

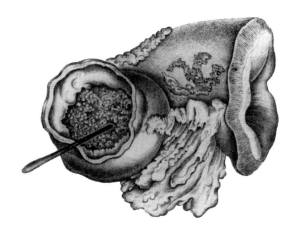

Figure 6. Resected specimen from Thérèse Heller. *Reproduced from The New Sydenham Society, London, 1891. Billroth T. Clinical Surgery. Extracts from the Reports of Surgical Practice between the Years 1860-1876.*

Medicine museum in Vienna, located in the former 'Allgemeines Krankenhaus' [1].

Billroth was aware of the importance of this operation and reported it within a week in the *Wiener Medizinische Wochenschrift*. It was described more extensively by Wölfler in 1883 together with three more cases [1]. The second and third patients did not survive because of believed duodenal kinking. Therefore, from the fourth patient onwards, Billroth decided to fashion the anastomosis to the greater curvature [41].

This kind of reconstruction, a gastroduodenostomy, developed into a standard operation. The end result was subsequently called the 'Billroth I' resection. There were many variations of which a few are shown in Figure 7.

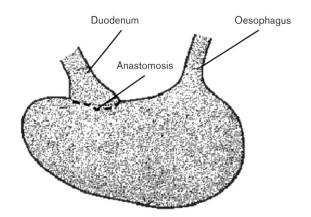

Figure 5. The first Billroth I gastrectomy.

The patient, a mother of ten children, lived for four months. A post mortem examination conducted at the patient's home by Zemann, an assistant to Heschl who was a past pupil of Rokitansky, showed diffuse metastases in the liver and omentum [17]. The specimen is still on display in the Josephinum, a small History of

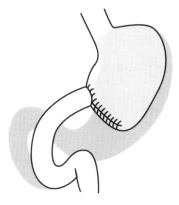

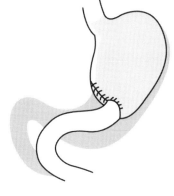

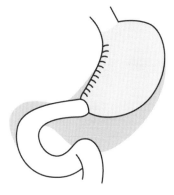

Billroth 1881, reconstruction
as in Thérèse Heller

Billroth 1881

Shoemaker 1911

Figure 7. Gastroduodenostomies (Billroth I resections). Only a few end-to-end constructions are depicted. *Modified with permission from Georg Thieme Verlag, Stuttgart. Kremer K, Lierse W, Schreiber HW. Chirurgische Operationslehre, vol 3, 1987: 146.*

In November of the same year Billroth did his famous first pylorectomy for carcinoma. Rydygier did the same operation for benign gastric ulceration with severe pyloric stenosis. He reported this to a medical journal, mentioning that this was the first operation of this kind, eliciting the editor's comment "hoffentlich auch die letzte" (let us hope also the last) [2].

Gastrojejunostomy and partial gastrectomy

Also in November of 1881, Wölfler [7, 42] performed the first gastrojejunostomy shown in Figure 8. This Figure also illustrates and enumerates several later modifications by various surgical pioneers. Von Hacker is credited with the first successful retrocolic posterior gastroenterostomy. This was for a long time the preferred procedure for ulcer disease, as well as those presenting with obstruction [7].

In January of 1885, Billroth and von Hacker [9, 43] operated upon a patient with an obstructing carcinoma of the pylorus; the patient appeared to be fragile in health, so they planned a staged operation. They started with a bypass in the form of an antecolic anterior gastroenterostomy. However, the condition of the patient on the operating table improved sufficiently for them to resect the tumour forthwith, occluding the duodenal and gastric stumps by sutures. This became

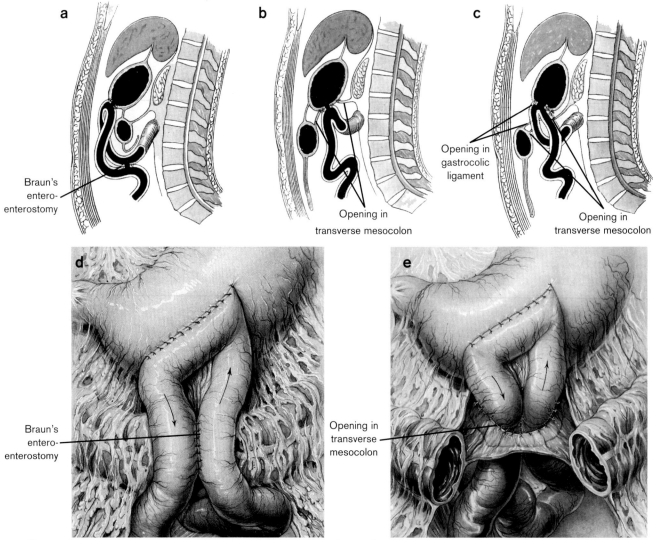

Figure 8. Gastrojejunostomy without resection of the stomach. a) & d) Antecolic anterior gastroenterostomy (Wölfler). b) Retrocolic posterior gastroenterostomy (von Hacker). c) & e) Retrocolic anterior gastroenterostomy (Billroth). *Reproduced with permission from Springer Verlag, Heidelberg. Kirschner M. Allgemeine und Spezielle Chirurgische Operationslehre, II Bauchhöhle, 1932: 120-7.*

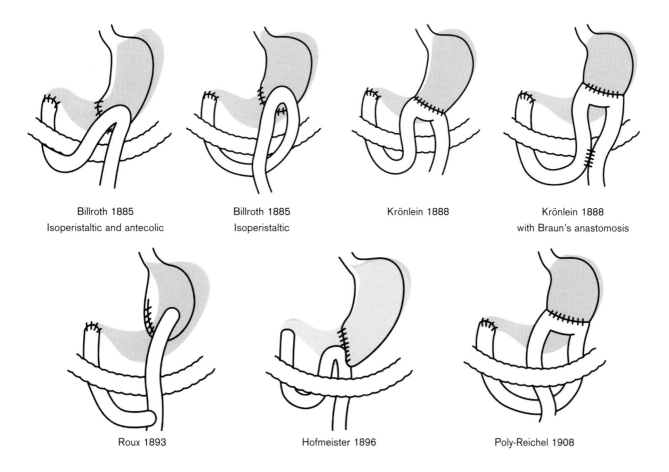

Billroth 1885
Isoperistaltic and antecolic

Billroth 1885
Isoperistaltic

Krönlein 1888

Krönlein 1888
with Braun's anastomosis

Roux 1893

Hofmeister 1896

Poly-Reichel 1908

Figure 9. Variations of partial gastrectomy and gastrojejunal anastomoses (Billroth II procedures). *Reproduced with permission from Georg Thieme Verlag, Stuttgart. Kremer K, Lierse W, Schreiber HW. Chirurgische Operationslehre, vol 3, 1987: 160.*

known as the 'Billroth II' resection [43], as reported by von Hacker [8]. Subsequently, resections were performed before making the anastomoses, as practised today.

Figure 9 shows the variations of Billroth resections. Narath [5], another pupil of Billroth, proposed calling these and other resections involving gastrojejunostomy, 'Billroth II' resections. The retrocolic Billroth II resection with anastomosis of the whole cut edge of the stomach with the jejunum was described in 1911, the 'Polya-Reichel procedure' [5, 44].

Alternatively, an anastomosis with partial connection between the stomach and jejunum was called the 'Hofmeister/Finsterer valve' [8], also shown in Figure 9, and designed in an attempt to reduce

bilious vomiting. The mortality of gastric resection in Vienna in Billroth's time was around 35-50% [10], although higher elsewhere [45], casting doubts on the feasibility of performing this operation at all. A cautious voice came from an editorial in the *British Medical Journal* in 1888: "Butlin himself was led to doubt whether resection of the pylorus was a justifiable operation.... He reported 55 patients on whom resection was performed for cancer, 41 died as a result of the operation (mortality of 70%), 13 recovered and one was untraced. Of the 10 who were followed-up, all died of recurrent cancer. None enjoyed good health at one year."

The editorial went on to say: "High risk diseases should have low risk operations. It is the brilliancy of the Vienna School of Surgery ...... that has naturally an influence on operative surgery in all countries, and has led surgeons to push surgery to its limits." Mortalities gradually decreased with increased experience, and the extent of resections increased both for carcinoma and ulceration.

Wölfler [8] performed the first Y reconstruction in 1883 in dogs and in a patient in 1893 [9], but Roux [42] from Lausanne had performed 50 cases in man by 1897; the operation became known as the 'Roux-en-Y loop'. The principle of the Roux-en-Y has since been found to be an excellent decompression manoeuvre, whether it is for a leaking duodenal stump, pancreatic duct or cyst, or a distended gallbladder (Figure 10). In addition it can be used for restoring bowel continuity after partial or total gastrectomy.

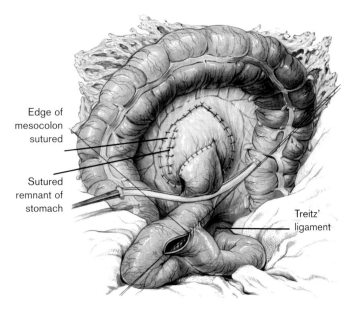

Edge of mesocolon sutured

Sutured remnant of stomach

Treitz' ligament

Figure 10. Roux-en-Y reconstruction after partial gastrectomy. (To prevent alkaline reflux the upper limb is usually much longer than depicted.) *Reproduced with permission from Springer Verlag, Heidelberg. Kirschner M. Allgemeine und Spezielle Chirurgische Operationslehre, II Bauchhöhle, 1932: 154).*

Billroth deserved credit not only for his operative achievement, but also because he founded the most famous comprehensive surgical school in his lifetime. His pupils were to become professors all over Europe and they made a tremendous impact on the development of global surgery (Figure 11) [46, 47].

Billroth will always be remembered for the honesty of his audit, and for ensuring any new procedure was thoroughly tested on animals before patients.

Billroth was Head of the Second Surgical Clinic in Vienna. The First Surgical Clinic was run by Eduard Albert, who was famous in his own right [5, 48]. Albert was a prominent teacher, traumatologist, and founder of the German Red Cross, and in addition wrote several popular textbooks on surgery. Albert was succeeded by Billroth's pupil, von Eiselsberg. Billroth himself was succeeded after his death by Gussenbauer and after him by Albert's protégé, Hochenegg. It is not surprising that the University of Vienna, staffed by so many talented pupils of both giants, as well as other illustrious men like Rokitansky, remained, together with Berlin, the most prestigious medical centre in the world until World War II.

In view of the Vienna school's modern practices of clean and near military organisation of surgical services, the German-speaking clinicians transferred surgery from operating in patients' homes to properly organised hospital surroundings [49, 50].

Ulcer complications

In 1882, von Czerny [9] excised a gastric ulcer successfully for the first time, but in 1885 he reported an operation on a patient with a perforation in 1880 who did not survive. The first survival occurred in 1892 when Heussner amazingly operated upon a patient with a gastric perforation in a patient's home, as described by Kriege [20]. In 1894, Dean [11, 20] from London, described the first successful closure of a perforated duodenal ulcer, and in 1902, Keetley [11, 20] performed the first gastrectomy for a perforated gastric ulcer.

Pyloroplasties were originally intended for pyloric stenosis. The first was described by Heinecke and von Mikulicz [9] in 1886. In 1892, Jaboulay, and later, Finney [9] in 1901, described useful pyloroplasties which took the form of gastroduodenostomies (Figure 12). Initially, both pyloroplasty and gastroduodenostomy were independent procedures for the treatment of peptic ulcer, before being used as an adjunct to vagotomy.

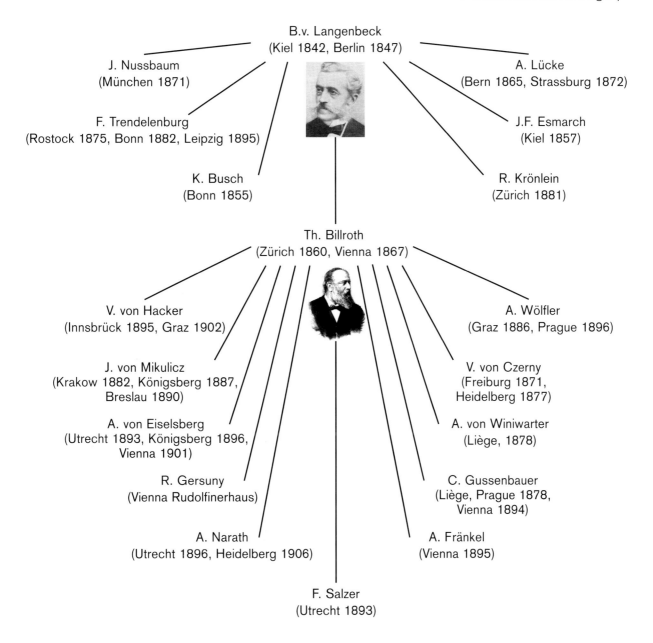

B.v. Langenbeck
(Kiel 1842, Berlin 1847)

J. Nussbaum
(München 1871)

A. Lücke
(Bern 1865, Strassburg 1872)

F. Trendelenburg
(Rostock 1875, Bonn 1882, Leipzig 1895)

J.F. Esmarch
(Kiel 1857)

K. Busch
(Bonn 1855)

R. Krönlein
(Zürich 1881)

Th. Billroth
(Zürich 1860, Vienna 1867)

V. von Hacker
(Innsbrück 1895, Graz 1902)

A. Wölfler
(Graz 1886, Prague 1896)

J. von Mikulicz
(Krakow 1882, Königsberg 1887,
Breslau 1890)

V. von Czerny
(Freiburg 1871,
Heidelberg 1877)

A. von Eiselsberg
(Utrecht 1893, Königsberg 1896,
Vienna 1901)

A. von Winiwarter
(Liège, 1878)

R. Gersuny
(Vienna Rudolfinerhaus)

C. Gussenbauer
(Liège, Prague 1878,
Vienna 1894)

A. Narath
(Utrecht 1896, Heidelberg 1906)

A. Fränkel
(Vienna 1895)

F. Salzer
(Utrecht 1893)

Figure 11. Billroth's surgical 'family tree'. Genealogy of the school of v. Langenbeck and Billroth. *Modified with permission from S. Karger AG, Basel. Gorecki P, Gorecki W. Jan Mikulicz-Radecki (1850-1905), the creator of modern European surgery. Dig Surg 2002; 19: 319. Portrait pictures: Th. Billroth, reproduced with permission from the American College of Surgeons. Schwyzer A. Theodor Billroth. Surg Gynecol Obst 1929; 48: 825; von Langenbeck, reproduced with permission from Elsevier. Absolon KB. The surgical school of Theodor Billroth. Surgery 1961; 50: 698.*

Gastrectomy and gastroenterostomy

In the US, Winslow's first pylorectomy patient died in 1884. Rodman was the first American to succeed in resection for carcinoma, and likewise, Sherick did the same in 1907 for gastric ulcer [11].

In 1897, Schlatter [51] from Switzerland performed successfully the first total gastric resection for carcinoma; it is not clear why the poor patient was detained in Schlatter's hospital ward for the remaining 14 months of his life! By 1909, Ohsawa [52] had performed 37 resections in Japan.

a

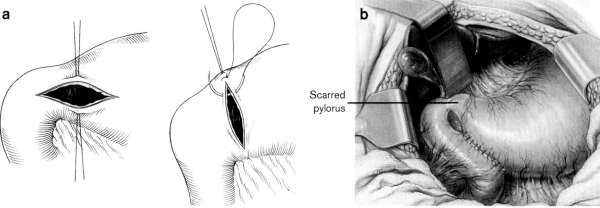

Heinecke-Mikulicz: the incision is lengthways through the pyloric muscle and is closed horizontally and vertically.

b

Scarred pylorus

Jaboulay: gastroduodenostomy avoiding the scarred area and pylorus.

c

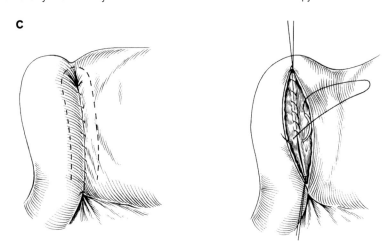

Finney: U-shaped incision through the scarred area and pylorus.

Figure 12. a) Heinecke-Mikulicz, b) Jaboulay and c) Finney pyloroplasties. *a) & c) Reproduced with permission from Georg Thieme Verlag, Stuttgart. Kremer K, Schumpelick V, Hierholzer G. Chirurgische Operationen, 1992: 235-7. b) Reproduced with permission from Springer Verlag, Heidelberg. Kirschner M. Allgemeine und Spezielle Chirurgische Operationslehre, II Bauchhöhle, 1932: 128.*

For carcinoma, gastric resection developed as the standard treatment for attempted cure, but for peptic ulceration many surgeons performed either a gastroenterostomy or pyloroplasty. These procedures appeared satisfactory at first, but gradually the reports of stomal ulceration increased, as described by Braun [7, 8] in 1899, which shifted the preference to partial gastrectomy when the mortality of resection decreased. From 1920 onwards, resection became the procedure of choice for chronic duodenal ulcer as results improved, but not everywhere at the same rate. Both Billroth gastrectomy types were used by their respective proponents, leading to heated discussions in meetings and conferences [49].

Von Haberer and Finsterer [5, 11] became pioneers for resection for ulcers with a commendable mortality below 2%. In his lifetime Finsterer had performed over 5000 gastrectomies and only 23 gastrojejunostomies. Von Haberer preferred the Billroth I resection, but others found a lower recurrence rate with their own favoured Billroth II resection. According to Nyhus [53], Harkins years later showed that at least a 75% resection of the parietal cell mass is required to prevent duodenal ulcer recurrence.

Berkeley Moynihan from the UK, and Charles Mayo [11] from Minnesota in the US, had high reputations for surgery for peptic ulcer. Moynihan's first book in 1905 on the treatment for gastric and duodenal ulceration [54] declared gastroenterostomy was "perfectly satisfactory". In support of Moynihan, Mayo said: "If anyone should consider removing half of my good stomach to cure a small ulcer in my duodenum, I would run faster than he!" [55]. Thus, gastroenterostomy remained popular in the US, though there were many champions for resection such as Crile, Lahey and others [11]. Balfour described recurrent and stomal ulceration after simple gastroenterostomy on 270 patients as early as 1926 [11].

Post-gastrectomy symptoms such as dumping and bilious vomiting were considered by some as inevitable; as a remedy some changed a Billroth II to a Billroth I reconstruction, others diverted duodenal juice using a Braun entero-enterostomy (seen in Figures 8 and 9) [9].

Complicated circumstances such as severe periduodenal inflammation or invasion of the pancreas by ulceration were overcome in various ways. Hustinx [56, 57] dissected a mucosal cylinder to ease stump closure, and von Eiselsberg [8, 9] (1895) excluded the pyloro-antral region in difficult cases, which later showed a high gastrin-mediated rebound acid production, stimulated by alkaline reflux into the excluded antrum. Finsterer [8, 9], in 1918, removed the antro-pyloric mucosa to prevent this late complication. Surgeons increasingly learned to excise a gastric ulcer to exclude cancer.

Between 1920 and 1950 in Europe including the UK, the operation of choice for peptic ulcer was between 70% and subtotal gastric resection. In the US, gastroenterostomy was practised by the majority of surgeons. However. a whole new development took place that would change gastric surgery.

Vagotomy

Although the existence and anatomy of the vagus nerves (called the pneumogastric nerves in France and Italy) was known for 2000 years, vagal function had been a mystery. Experiments on animals such as

bilateral cervical and abdominal vagotomy demonstrated the reduction of acid secretion of the stomach, according to Brodie [18] in 1814. Claude Bernard tested and proved motor action on the stomach by the vagus nerves. Pavlov added an enormous amount of knowledge on gastric secretion from his animal pouch studies. Thus, the concept of vagotomy was considered for ulcer patients, as duodenal ulceration was often, although not invariably, associated with hypersecretion.

The first attempted vagotomy in man was probably performed by Jaboulay [18, 58], but for a different indication, namely Tabes dorsalis, it was the coeliac plexus that was ablated.

Bircher [8] performed vagotomy in 20 patients for all kinds of gastric complaints. The first surgeon to subject patients with duodenal ulcer to a vagotomy was André Latarjet (Figure 13) [59, 60], from Lyon in France, in 1922. He did in fact a selective gastric vagotomy, which he called 'énervation gastrique' and in most cases added a drainage procedure to it in the form of a gastroenterostomy. However, the majority of his patients had other indications for vagotomy, which he called 'gastropathie vago-sympathique'.

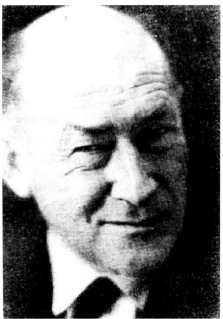

Figure 13. André Latarjet (1877-1947). *Reproduced with permission from the American College of Surgeons. Waisbren SJ, Modlin IM. The evolution of therapeutic vagotomy. Surg Gynecol Obst 1990; 170: 260.*

Latarjet's anatomical description of the vagus nerves and his operative technique were of such a high standard, that the 'principal anterior and posterior nerves' serving the antral muscle pump were named after him. All this, however, was revived only half a century later [58]. His operation did not become popular and his own publications concerning vagotomy ceased in 1923 [18].

Dragstedt

Lester Reynold Dragstedt (Figure 14) [61] at the University of Chicago was trained as a physiologist under the famous oesophageal cancer surgeon, Phemister. Phemister [61] wanted him to be a surgically trained physiologist and said: "I can make a surgeon out of a physiologist provided he can make surgeons more physiological."

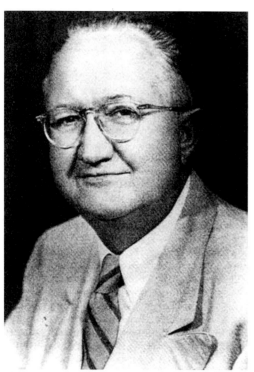

Figure 14. Lester Reynold Dragstedt (1893-1975). *Reproduced with permission from the American College of Surgeons. Waisbren SJ, Modlin IM. The evolution of therapeutic vagotomy. Surg Gynecol Obst 1990; 170: 269.*

Dragstedt conscientiously repeated many historic experiments, including Pavlov's, on the vagus nerves and stomach with a high degree of scrutiny. He was fascinated by the observation that the gastric mucosa did not digest itself, so he reinvestigated the question of the 'living principle', already addressed by John Hunter and Claude Bernard [16, 61]. He found that gastric secretion mostly accompanied food intake and that hypersecretion in the fasting state was often associated with duodenal ulceration. He postulated that duodenal ulcers should heal after bilateral vagotomy in man, but it was difficult to use animals as experimental models because they seldom developed ulcers.

By chance, a 35-year-old man was admitted to his hospital with duodenal ulceration following several severe haemorrhages. The patient refused a standard subtotal gastrectomy because his father had died from the operation, and his brother still suffered from severe sequelae after a gastrectomy. Before the patient discharged himself, Dragstedt was forced to consider vagotomy as a last resort [18, 55].

On January 18th 1943 he performed a bilateral supra-diaphragmatic vagotomy and after that, the patient was immediately relieved of pain and the bleeding ceased. True to his physiological principles, Dragstedt postoperatively instilled each day a test dose of hydrochloric acid down the oesophagus into the stomach and duodenum (a study which had been shown to trigger the ulcer pain), until it no longer produced pain. He was able, therefore, to conclude that the ulcer had healed in ten days.

He performed six vagotomies in 1943, 16 in 1944, and 60 in 1945. About one third of these patients developed some degree of gastric stasis requiring a drainage procedure [18]. As a result he changed to sub-diaphragmatic vagotomy with added gastro-enterostomy, and later a Heinecke-Mikulicz pyloroplasty (Figure 12) to his operations. Many patients had scarred or stenosed pylorus sphincters from the ulceration, so pyloroplasty was an appropriate addition to vagotomy. Later, Weinberg [62] modified this from a two-layered to a one-layered wider pyloroplasty.

The so-called Dragstedt operation proved effective, easily performed, and relatively safe. As a result, vagotomy became increasingly popular in the US over the next ten years. Not everybody was satisfied with this new operation. Disadvantages of vagotomy included more recurrences compared with gastrectomy, significant dumping (later found to be associated with the drainage procedure), diarrhoea and bile vomiting. Though these side effects were difficult to manage, they also occurred after gastrectomy.

In 1952, a study committee on ulcer treatment of the American Gastroenterological Society still recommended a gastrectomy or gastroenterostomy in preference to vagotomy [16, 61]. In the same year, however, Pollock [63], following the Leeds-York trial which incorporated 1524 patients, reported that truncal vagotomy and drainage (TV & D) had a mortality of only 1%, and a low recurrence rate of 3%. This coincided with the increased popularity of vagotomy in the UK and US.

Surgeons in mainland Europe were less convinced about the need to change to vagotomy, so partial gastrectomy remained the favoured operation. The introduction of the Dragstedt operation was more gradual; however, vagotomy was employed when recurrent ulceration occurred after gastrectomy.

The 'combined operation', truncal vagotomy and antrectomy (TV & A) was even more effective, having a lower mortality and lowest recurrence rates [64, 65]. This version of vagotomy became the most recommended operation in the US.

Selective vagotomies (Figure 15)

The unpleasant dumping and diarrhoea occurring after truncal vagotomy in an unpredictable number of patients made surgeons realise that truncal vagotomy denervated all of the fore and mid-gut supplied by the vagus. This stimulated exploring the concept of selective gastric vagotomy.

In 1948, Jackson [66] and Franksson [67] experimented with selective gastric vagotomies, but their findings did not attract much attention. A decade later, Griffith and Harkins tried an even more selective, partial gastric vagotomy on dogs, much like the later proximal gastric vagotomy, but did not publish any clinical studies [55,61]. In the early '70s the results of several randomised trials comparing truncal and selective vagotomy were disappointing. A more selective vagotomy did not reduce the side effects substantially, but produced a slightly lower recurrence rate, probably because of a more thorough dissection around the oesophagus [68]. These selective vagotomies could be compared with Latarjet's operation but still needed a drainage procedure, which caused certain side effects.

In 1963, Holle and Hart [69] from Munich devised a 'selective proximal vagotomy', restricted to the acid-secreting part of the stomach, but always added a 'form und functions gerechte' (adapted to 'form and function') pyloroplasty to it. They claimed their pyloroplasty had fewer side effects, others were not convinced.

It was not long afterwards, that Johnston in Leeds [70] in 1969, and independently, Amdrup [71] in Copenhagen, published within months of each other, a near identical selective vagotomy sparing the motor nerves of Latarjet to the antrum and pylorus, without a drainage procedure. They called this procedure 'highly selective vagotomy' (HSV), based on anatomical landmarks or 'parietal cell vagotomy' (PCV), since it attempted denervation of the parietal cell mass alone.

This latest version of vagotomy spread rapidly across the world especially in Europe. It had the appeal of being the ideal operation [68], as it was relatively safe and had few side effects. Although technically demanding, it soon became the standard operation in many hospitals. It could also be applied in case of complications. The only disadvantage demonstrated in some centres was a higher recurrence rate compared with TV & A. However, recurrence after HSV quite often seemed mild [72, 73], even before powerful anti-secretary drugs became available. Highly selective vagotomy was not accepted in some centres, either because of the lack of technical skill, or cynical disbelief, or because the hierarchy believed the teaching of resection of the stomach was paramount.

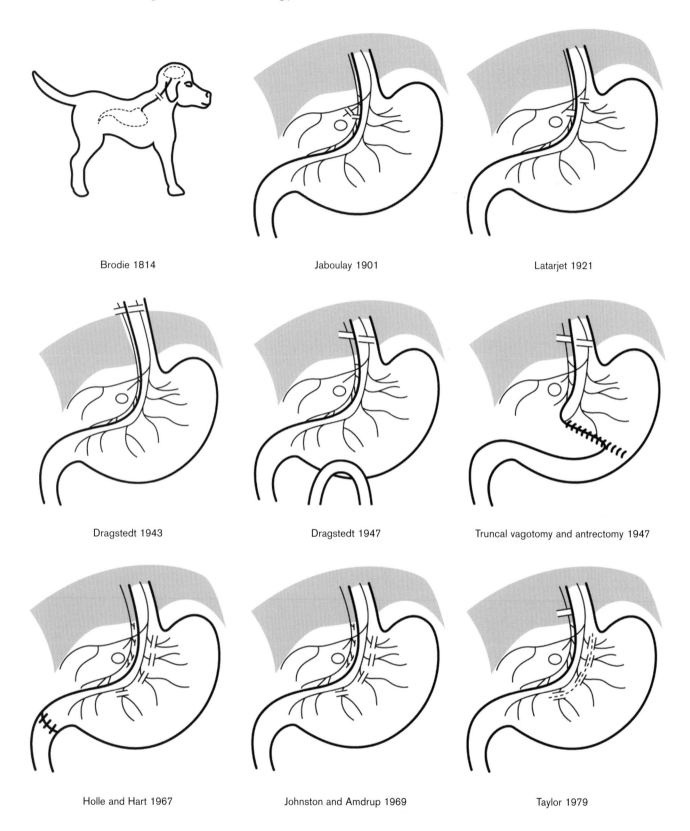

Brodie 1814   Jaboulay 1901   Latarjet 1921

Dragstedt 1943   Dragstedt 1947   Truncal vagotomy and antrectomy 1947

Holle and Hart 1967   Johnston and Amdrup 1969   Taylor 1979

Figure 15. Diagram to show the evolution of vagotomy. *Reproduced with permission from Excerpta Medica, Inc. Waisbren SJ, Modlin IM. Lester R. Dragstedt and his role in the evolution of therapeutic vagotomy in the United States. Am J Surg 1994; 167: 356.*

Methods were developed to test the completeness of the vagotomy [73] using on-table tests such as the Grassi pH measurement, the Burge motility test, or the Kusakari congo-red secretory tests. Postoperatively, the Kay histamine, the pentagastrin or the Hollander insulin tests were used.

Decline of ulcer operations

Attempts to find out which was the gold standard operation were undertaken [74, 75], but the results were inconclusive. HSV seemed to have the best reputation, but the need to operate for duodenal ulceration dramatically [26, 68] decreased for three reasons:

◆ the global incidence, especially in the Western World, of peptic ulceration, including perforation, has decreased steadily since 1960 [28]. The reason for this decline is not clear;

◆ the introduction of powerful inhibitors of gastric secretion such as the histamine-2 receptor-antagonists (H_2RA), bismuth preparations and later proton-pump inhibitors, took place in the late '70s and '80s. Relapses occurred frequently after stopping these drugs in 90% of patients within one year, so maintenance treatment was necessary for some time. Bismuth preparations were historically effective; only later was it understood, that they had antibiotic properties [76];

◆ in 1983, a renewed discovery was made by Barry Marshall (Figure 16) [76, 77], a young doctor at Warren's Institution in Australia. He investigated the previously neglected *Helicobacter pylori* organisms (HP), which had for years been seen in the gastric mucosa, but were thought to be contaminants or harmless commensal organisms. Marshall found them in about 50% of asymptomatic people and in 90-100% of patients with duodenal ulceration. These bacteria secrete urease, a phenomenon that proved helpful later, as the basis of a diagnostic test. Initially, these bacteria could not be cultured, but just by chance Marshall discovered how to grow them by extended incubation during a prolonged Easter weekend. Eradication with antibiotics now became possible, and so peptic ulceration seemed an infectious disease that could be cured without

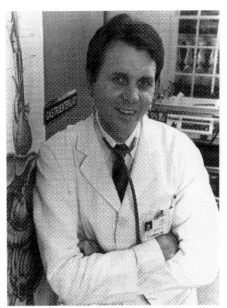

Figure 16. Barry Marshall. *Reproduced with permission from Liitle Brown & Co., London. Le Fanu J. The Rise & Fall of Modern Medicine, 1999: 235.*

the need for maintenance therapy. Operations for peptic ulceration have become a rare event today. Warren and Marshall were awarded the Nobel Prize for medicine in October 2005 for their work on *Helicobacter pylori*.

Research has shown that the prevalence of the *Helicobacter* infection in the Western World has decreased even before known effective drugs against HP became available on the market. HP has probably always been with mankind for many centuries [32], but the mechanism of ulceration is not well understood. Its presence is inversely related to gastro-oesophageal reflux disease and cardia carcinoma, which are now on the increase [31], as discussed in Chapter 4.

Early gastric cancer (EGC)

Although the German surgeon, Konjetski [46], had already described superficial early gastric cancer in 1938, since the '60s of the last century, the Japanese have defined their concept of early gastric cancer (EGC), which is cancer limited to the mucosa and submucosa [78]. The prevalence of gastric carcinoma in

Japan, and some other countries such as China, Iceland, Korea and Chile is up to ten times higher than in the Western World.

In 1962, the Japanese Society for Gastroenterology [78] developed a detailed classification system on the basis of macroscopic (obtained by fiberoscopy) and microscopic criteria for EGC [79].

An extensive endoscopic and advanced radiological screening program resulted in a yield of EGC in up to 40% of diagnosed cancers [79] in Japan. These were treated by total and sub-total gastrectomy with extensive lymph node block dissection. This policy accomplished a great improvement, often in the order of 80-95% survival after five years. The most important factor influencing survival was lymph node involvement [80].

On the basis of these far superior results compared with Western centres, trials have been conducted along Japanese lines comparing D_1 resections, which require lymph node clearance within a 5cm radius of the tumour, with D_2 resections requiring a much more extensive radical lymph node clearance [81, 82]. In randomised controlled trials in Western centres [82], so far there has been no significant increased survival for the high price of increased mortality and morbidity after the D_2 operation. It is speculated that gastric carcinoma in Europe and the US is a different cancer from the Japanese one, but no convincing scientific proof exists. The relatively low prevalence of gastric cancer in the West makes the economic case for mass screening and surveillance less tenable.

Zollinger-Ellison syndrome

This syndrome, described in 1955 by Zollinger and Ellison, as well as by others before them [10, 17], is characterised by very severe and atypical ulceration anywhere in the upper gastrointestinal tract. It is caused by abnormally large quantities of gastrin secreted by single, multiple, benign or malignant tumours, which may or may not have gastrin-secreting metastases. They are mostly localised in the area of the pancreas and duodenum. It also can be part of the Multiple Endocrine Adenopathy I syndrome [83]. Diagnosis is now made by measuring fasting serum gastrins, and sometimes including a secretin test [83] to exclude other causes of hypergastrinaemia. Treatment consists of: removal of all the solitary gastrin-secreting tumour if possible; removal of the target organ, namely the whole stomach by total gastrectomy; or by prescription of high-dose drugs like histamine-receptor antagonists or proton-pump inhibitors during the patient's lifetime. This is discussed in greater detail in Chapter 8.

Conclusions

Now well over 100 years have passed since Billroth's first gastrectomy. In many ways the pendulum has swung back in favour of physicians, admittedly mostly those who have the manual dexterity to use a gastroscope to see what only the surgeons saw. They can cauterise, cut tumour tissue with a laser, inject sclerosants for bleeding, as well as prescribe powerful drugs, and obtain a cure. Today, physicians treat and cure most patients with peptic ulceration, although an occasional patient presents as a surgical emergency due to self-neglect or complications induced by steroids, alcohol, or non-steroidal anti-inflammatory drugs.

Cancer of any portion of the stomach and cardia are still a challenge for Billroth's successors. More and more cancers are being seen earlier and even treated with the help of minimally invasive surgery. Perhaps it may take another 100 years before the gastric surgeon hangs up his scalpel forever.

Biographical footnote on Billroth

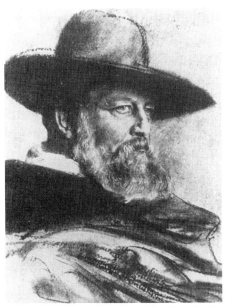

Figure 17. Billroth (1829-1894).
Reproduced with permission from Elsevier.
Rutledge RH. In commemoration of
Theodor Billroth on the 150th anniversary of
his birth. Surgery 1979; 86: 688.

Christian Albert Theodor Billroth [84] (Figures 17 and 18) was born on the 26th of April 1829 in the village of Bergen on the Baltic Sea island of Rügen, the oldest of five brothers. His father, of Swedish descent, was a pastor, who died when Theodor was only five years old. His mother, who came from Berlin, then moved to the mainland town of Greifswald, where she was supported by family and friends. Theodor was a mediocre student (in his own judgement) [85], who was inclined toward music and disliked sciences, mathematics and languages. Music was to become his great passion and source of inspiration, joy and energy, even in times of dejection. He wanted to become a musician, but his mother succeeded, with a little help from friends and family (Baum and Seifert) [85, 86], in directing him into the study of medicine. His first semester was 'lost' to music, but in 1849, he followed Wilhelm Baum, who became Professor and Chairman of the Department of Surgery in Göttingen, and he developed the self-discipline to get down to his studies. He studied in Greifswald and Göttingen and during the last year in Berlin from where he graduated in 1852. Although he became the icon of gastric resection, ironically he wrote his doctoral thesis (in Latin) [87] on the effects of vagotomy (*nervus pneumogastricus*) on the respiratory system in the pigeon in 1852 ("De natura et causa pulmonum affectionis, quae nervo utroque vago dissecto exoritur") [88].

Thereafter, he travelled (in his 'Wanderjahr') to Vienna and Paris (following courses and lectures) and started a practice in Berlin. In three months he had not treated a single patient, and was understandably worried about the future. By chance, Theodor heard from a fellow student, who was an assistant of von Langenbeck, Professor of Surgery in Berlin, about a recent vacancy for which Billroth got appointed [84].

Von Langenbeck was a great surgeon who had many famous pupils like Trendelenburg, Witzel, Kocher, Esmarch, and Bier in his tutelage (Figure 11) [46]. Billroth now applied himself diligently to anatomy, histology and pathology. He became Privatdozent (lecturer) in pathology and surgery in 1856 [87, 89]. He competed with Virchow for the Chair of Pathology in Berlin, but Virchow was elected to the post [87]. Billroth subsequently decided to become a surgeon. He worked incredibly long hours as a surgeon during the day, music in the evening and studying and writing thereafter. Evidently, he required little sleep during this period [1, 90]. He married Christel Michaelis in 1858 and as an exception was allowed by von Langenbeck to live outside the clinic [85]. In 1859, he applied for the Chair in Surgery at the University of Zürich, despite Nussbaum being the favourite; Nussbaum, however, declined the post. Von Langenbeck acquired the formal appointment for Billroth in writing on December 24th for Billroth's wife to place under their Christmas tree [87].

In Zürich he published *Beobachtungsstudien* (observational studies, 1862); *die allgemeine Pathologie und Therapie in 50 Vorlesungen* (general pathology and therapeutics in 50 lectures, 1863), which had 13 reprints and was translated into many languages, including Japanese); and *Chirurgische Klinik Zürich, 1860-67*, a unique and extensive audit of his whole surgical work, describing and commenting on his failures as well as his successes (published in 1869). In this work, Billroth stated: "... do not hesitate to admit failures, as they must show the mode and places of improvement." [47] Complete honesty in a surgical audit was as rare then as it is now!

During this period, he declined surgical chairs in Rostock and Heidelberg. In 1867, he was appointed Professor of Surgery and Head of the Second Surgical Clinic in Vienna. It was quite remarkable for a German to succeed in Austria because there was some animosity between the North Germans and Austrians at that time [91]. He called himself a "North-German herring!" [1]

In Vienna he became world famous and earned the accolade of being 'the father of gastrointestinal surgery'. He was the first to perform a laryngectomy (1873), and the first to succeed in gastric resection (1981) [85]. These and other innovations were prepared carefully in the laboratory on dogs in close co-operation with his co-workers. His Billroth I and II gastrointestinal reconstructions are among the most common terms in the surgical lexicon. He attracted and moulded many good assistants who later became famous in their own right, such as von Hacker, von Winiwarter, Gussenbauer, von Mikulicz, von Czerny, von Eiselsberg, Fränkel, and Gersuny (Figure 11). [47].

Vienna provided exactly the kind of environment in which Billroth could flourish. He could practise the violin and perform with Johannes Brahms, enjoy his musical talent with Brahms and Hanslick (a well known music critic), as well as practise the highest standards of surgery and research of his day. When he had become a surgeon he said: "Surgery is my legal spouse, but music is my mistress." [1, 67] Several famous surgeons from abroad (among them Halsted) came to visit Billroth in Vienna. During this period, he wrote the following books: *Coccobacteria Septica* and *Lehren und Lernen* (teaching and learning). In total, he wrote 153 publications during his lifetime.

In 1884, Billroth's former teacher, von Langenbeck, was to retire as Head of the famous Charité Hospital in Berlin at the age of 73. He wanted Billroth to be his successor and the Berlin Faculty was unanimous in its support, which was unusual. Billroth, however, wanted to stay in Vienna where he felt happy, socially, culturally and professionally, so he politely declined [85]. Von Langenbeck was disappointed but did not give up. In an emotional way he insisted: "Aber Sie können die kaiserliche Stadt Berlin doch nicht verweigern!" ("But you can't decline the imperial city Berlin"). Billroth answered accordingly: "Es gibt nur eine wirklich kaiserliche Stadt und das ist Wien!" ("There is only one really imperial city and that is Vienna"). Von Bergmann (father of asepsis) became the successor in Berlin.

Billroth continued to teach: not only his surgical pupils - who loved him like a father - but also medical students and nurses. To promote the latter avocation, he founded the Rudolfinerhaus in Vienna for the training of nurses.

In 1887, Billroth was afflicted with pneumonia and cardiac failure; he never recovered his former health. He delegated more of his work to his well-trained pupils. He died on the 6th of February, 1894, in his beloved holiday resort of Abbazia in Italy.

His successor was Gussenbauer, but the spiritual heritage was taken over by Anton Freiherr von Eiselsberg, who became Head of the First Clinic as Albert's successor.

Billroth achieved his final wish, to be buried in Vienna close to Beethoven and Schubert [1, 5]. Witnessing the crowds of onlookers at the funeral procession, Brahms wrote: "We do not wear such open hearts nor show such pure and warm affection as he did."

The musician and the surgeon, as well as the poet that constituted the personality of Billroth are well expressed in his own words:

"Let what you observe penetrate your inmost soul, let it so warm and replenish you that your thoughts constantly refer to it, and then you will find true pleasure and delight in your intellectual labours."

Lectures on Surgical Pathology and Therapeutics, 1863.

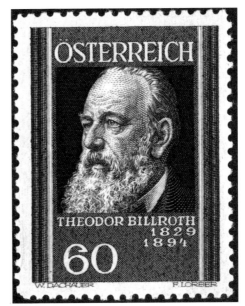

Figure 18. Theodor Billroth (1829-1894).

References

1. Rutledge RH. In commemoration of Theodor Billroth on the 150th anniversary of his birth. *Surgery* 1979; 86: 672-93.

2. Lick RF. Geschichte der Magenchirurgie. *Münch med Wschr* 1980; 122: 720-2.

3. Sachs M. *Geschichte der Operativen Chirurgie, Band V.* Heidelberg: Kaden Verlag, 2005.

4. Krafft L. Anfänge der Magenchirugie im Mittelalter, Florian Matthis - Wundarzt und Chirurg aus Brandenburg/H. *Chirurg BDC* 1992; 31: 82-4.

5. Herrington JL. Historical aspects of gastric surgery. In: *Surgery of the Stomach and Duodenum and Small Intestine.* Scott HW, Sawyers JL, Eds. Boston: Blackwell Scientific, 1991; ch 1: 1-28.

6. Miller JM. Doctor Georg Handell and the knife swallower of Halle. *Surg Gynecol Obstet* 1990; 170: 175-6.

7. Ogilvie WH. A hundred years of gastric surgery. *Ann R Coll Surg Eng* 1947; 1: 37-50.

8. Robinson JO. The history of gastric surgery. In: *The history of gastroenterology.* Chen TS, Chen PS, Eds. New York: Parthenon, 1995; ch 20: 239-46.

9. Weil PH, Buchberger R. From Billroth to PCV: a century of gastric surgery. *World J Surg* 1999; 23: 736-42.

10. Wangensteen OW, Wangensteen SD, Dennis C. The history of gastric surgery. In: *Surgery of the esophagus, stomach and small intestine*, 5th Ed. Nyhus LM, Wastell C, Donahue PE. Boston: Little Brown, 1995; ch 30: 354-85.

11. Herrington JL. Gastroduodenal ulcer. *Ann Surg* 1988; 207: 754-69.

12. Witzel O. Zur Technik der Magenfistel Anlegung. *Zbl Chir* 1891; 18: 601.

13. Wangensteen OH. The stomach since the Hunters: gastric temperature and peptic ulcer, In: *The history of gastroenterology.* Chen TS, Chen PS, Eds. New York: Parthenon, 1995, ch 11: 131-54.

14. Baron JH. The discovery of gastric acid. In: *The history of gastroenterology.* Chen TS, Chen PS, Eds. New York, Parthenon, 1995, ch 1: 3-11.

15. Wolf S. The psyche and the stomach; a historical vignette. In: *The history of gastroenterology.* Chen TS, Chen PS, Eds. New York: Parthenon, 1995, ch 2: 13-22.

16. Burden WR, O'Leary JP. The vagus nerve, gastric secretion, and their relationship to peptic ulcer disease. *Arch Surg* 1991; 126: 259-64.

17. Wangensteen OW, Wangensteen SD. Gastric surgery. In: *The rise of surgery.* Folkestone: Dawson, 1978; ch 7: 142-67.

18. Woodward ER. The history of vagotomy. *Am J Surg* 1987; 153: 9-17.

19. Herrington JL, Sawyers JL. Gastric ulcer. *Curr probl surg* 1987; 24 (12): 759-865.

20. Lau WY, Leow CK. History of perforated duodenal and gastric ulcers. *World J Surg* 1997; 21: 890-6.

21. Major R. Peptic ulcer. In: *Classic description of disease.* Springfield Ill: Thomas, 1978: 628-32.

22. Jennings D. Perforated peptic ulcer; changes in age-incidence and sex-distribution in the last 150 years. *Lancet* 1940; 255: 395-8, 444-7.

23. Susser M. Causes of peptic ulcer, a selective epidemiologic review. *J Chron Dis* 1967; 20: 435-56.

24. Grossman MI. A new look at peptic ulcer. *Ann Int Med* 1976; 84: 57-67.

25. Mendeloff AI. What has been happening to duodenal ulcer? *Gastroenterology* 1974; 67: 1020-2.

26. Thompson JC. The role of surgery in peptic ulcer. *N Engl J Med* 1982; 307: 550-1.

27. Gustavsson S, Nyrén O. Time trends in peptic ulcer surgery 1956 to 1986. A nationwide survey in Sweden. *Ann Surg* 1989; 210: 704-9.

28. Smith MP. Decline in peptic ulcer surgery. *JAMA* 1977; 237: 987-8.

29. Berkel J, Tytgat GNJ. Epidemiologie van het maagcarcinoom. *Ned Tijdschr Geneesk* 1982; 126: 1164-72.

30. Fuchs CS, Mayer RJ. Gastric carcinoma. *N Engl J Med* 1995; 333: 32-40.

31. El-Serag HB, Sonnenberg A. Opposing time trends of peptic ulcer and reflux disease. *Gut* 1998; 43: 327-33.

32. Blaser MJ. Helicobacters are indigenous to the human stomach: duodenal ulceration is due to changes in gastric microecology in the modern era. *Gut* 1998; 43: 721-7.

33. Davenport HW, Walter B. Canon's contribution to gastroenterology. In: *The history of gastroenterology.* Chen TS, Chen PS, Eds. New York: Parthenon, 1995; ch 20: 23-34.

34. Gorecki P, Gorecki G. Jan Mikulicz-Radecki (1850-1905) the creator of Modern European Surgery. *Digestive Surgery* 2002; 19: 313-20.

35. Skopec M, Zykan M. *Wiens Rolle in der Geschichte der Gastroenterologie.* Wien: Literas Universitätsverlag, 2002.

36. Stanger O. Viktor von Hacker (1852-1933) Erinnerungen an Leben und Schaffen eines bedeutenden Billroth-Schülers. *Chirurg* 2000; 71: 478-84.

37. Jones FA. Annual oration on peptic ulcer-in perspective. In: *The history of gastroenterology.* Chen TS, Chen PS, Eds. New York: Parthenon, 1995; ch 12: 155-66.

38. Cavazzani G. Extirpazione di un tumore delle pareti ventrali ed escisione di porzione delle pareti ventrali dello stomaco. *Gazzetta medica italiana, provincie Venete* 1879; 22 & 29 Marzo: 99-103, 107-13.

39. Veltheer W. History: the dawn of gastric resection. *Neth J Surg* 1981; 33: 107-14.

40. Brunschwig A, Simandi E. First successful pylorectomy for cancer; the case history. *Surg Gynecol Obstet* 1951; 92: 375-9.

41. Berns AWC. Over maagresectie. *Ned Tijdschr Geneesk* 1881; 25: 310-8.

42. Mason GR. Perspectives a century later on the 'Ansa en Y' of César Roux. *Am J Surg* 1991; 161: 262-5.

43. Meissner K. The historical review on gastric surgery by Weil and Buchberger. *World J Surg* 2000; 24: 621-2.

44. Petri G. Eugen Alexander Polya (1876-1944). *Zbl Chirurgie* 1985; 110: 46-52.

45. Butlin HT. Resection of the pylorus for cancer. *Br Med J* 1888; 1: 719.

46. Hamelmann H. The past, present and future of German Surgery. *Jpn J Surg* 1984; 14: 444-51.

47. Absolon KB. The surgical school of Theodor Billroth. *Surgery* 1961; 50: 697-715.

48. Kaiser AM. State of the art in gastrointestinal surgery 100 years ago: operations in the gastrointestinal tract in general (chapter XII) and resection of bowel carcinoma (chapter XIV). In: *Textbook of Special Surgery* (1897) by Eduard Albert (1841-1900). *World J Surg* 2002; 26: 1525-30.

49. de Moulin D. *A History of Surgery.* Dordrecht: Martinus Nijhoff, 1988.

50. Veltheer W. Heelkunde te Utrecht op het breukvlak van twee eeuwen: een onderzoek naar de lotgevallen van de universitaire kliniek in de periode van 1890 tot 1910. Thesis, Zeist, Kerckebosch, 1989

51. Sawyers JL. Gastric carcinoma. *Curr Probl Surg* 1995; 32 (2): 101-18.

52. Ohsawa T. The surgery of the oesophagus. *Jpn J Surg* 1933; 10: 593-6.

53. Nyhus LM. Personal communication to co-editor.

54. Moynihan BGA. *Duodenal Ulcer.* WB Saunders: Philadelphia, 1910.

55. Waisbren SJ, Modlin IM. The evolution of therapeutic vagotomy. *Surg Gynecol Obstet* 1990; 170: 261-72.

56. Sybrandy R. The Hustinx-closure of the duodenal stump. *Neth J Surg* 1988; 165: 40-6.

57. Kingma MJ. De primaire maagresectie bij doorgebroken maag- en duodenumzweren. Thesis, Assen, van Gorcum, 1939.

58. Skandalakis LJ, Gray SW, Skandalakis JE. The history and surgical anatomy of the vagus nerve. *Surg Gynecol Obstet* 1986; 162: 75-85.

59. Latarjet A, Wertheimer P. Quelques résultats de l'énervation gastrique. *Presse Méd* 1923; 28-Nov: 993-5.

60. Latarjet A. Résection des nerfs de l'estomach. *Bull Acad Med Paris* 1922; 87: 681-91.

61. Waisbren SJ, Modlin IM, Lester R. Dragstedt and his role in the evolution of therapeutic vagotomy in the US. *Am J Surg* 1994; 167: 344-59.

62. Weinberg JA, Stempien SJ, Movius HJ, Dagradi AE. Vagotomy and pyloroplasty in the treatment of duodenal ulcer. *Am J Surg* 1956; 92: 202-7.

63. Pollock AV. Vagotomy in the treatment of peptic ulceration. *Lancet* 1952; 2: 795.

64. Farmer DA, Smithwick RH. Hemigastrectomy combined with resection of the vagus nerve. *N Engl J Med* 1952; 247: 1017-22.

65. Edwards LW, Herrington JL. Vagotomy and gastroenterostomy - vagotomy and conservative gastrectomy. A comparative study. *Ann Surg* 1953; 137: 873.

66. Jackson RG. Anatomic study of the vagus nerves with a technique of a transabdominal selective gastric vagus resection. *Arch Surg* 1948; 57: 333-52.

67. Franksson C. Selective abdominal vagotomy. *Acta Chir Scand* 1948; 96: 409-12.

68. Donahue PE. PCV versus vagotomy/antrectomy: ulcer surgery in the modern era. *World J Surg* 2000; 24: 264-9.

69. Holle F, Hart W. Neue wege der chirurgie des gastroduodenal ulcus. *Med Klin* 1967; 62: 441-50.

70. Johnston D, Wilkinson AR. Highly selective vagotomy without a drainage procedure in the treatment of duodenal ulcer. *Br J Surg* 1970; 57: 289-96.

71. Amdrup E, Jensen HE. Selective vagotomy of the parietal cell mass preserving innervation of the undrained antrum. *Gastroenterology* 1970; 59: 522-7.

72. Johnson AG. PGV: does it have a place in the future management of peptic ulcer? *World J Surg* 2000; 24: 259-63.

73. Busman DC. Results of highly selective vagotomy. Thesis, Maastricht, Schrijen Lippertz, 1983.

74. Donahue PE, Bombeck CT, Condon RE, Nyhus LM. Proximal gastric vagotomy versus selective vagotomy with antrectomy: results of a prospective, randomised clinical trial after four to twelve years. *Surgery* 1984; 96: 585-90.

75. Hoffmann J, Jensen HE, Christiansen J, Olesen A, Loud FB, Hauch O. Prospective controlled vagotomy trial for duodenal ulcer. Results after 11-15 years. *Ann Surg* 1989; 209: 40-5.

76. Marshall BJ. *Campylobacter pyloridis* and gastritis. *J Infect Dis* 1986; 153: 650-7.

77. Le Fanu J. *The Rise & Fall of Modern Medicine*. Little Brown: London, 1999; ch 12: 177-86.

78. Sakita T, Oguro Y, Tahasu S, Fuketomi H, Miwa T, Yoshimori M. The development of endoscopic diagnosis of early carcinoma of the stomach. *Jpn J Clin Oncol* 1971; 12: 113-28.

79. Weed TE, Nuessle W, Ochsner A. Carcinoma of the stomach; why are we failing to improve survival. *Ann Surg* 1981; 193: 407-13.

80. Abe S, Yoshimura H, Nagaoka S, *et al*. Long-term results of operation for carcinoma of the stomach in T1/T2 stages: critical evaluation of the concept of early carcinoma of the stomach. *J Am Coll Surg* 1995; 181: 389-96.

81. Morris PJ, Malt RA. *Oxford Textbook of Surgery*. New York: Oxford University Press, 1994.

82. Hartgrink HH, van de Velde CJH. De behandeling van patiënten met maagcarcinoom op basis van resultaten van de Nederlandse maagkankerstudies. *Ned Tijdschr Geneesk* 2005; 149: 238-44.

83. Nyhus LM, Wastell C. *Surgery of the Stomach and Duodenum*, 4th Ed. Boston: Little Brown, 1986.

84. Roses DF. On the sesquicentennial of Theodore Billroth. *Am J Surg* 1979; 138: 704-9.

85. Schein CJ, Koch E. Autobiographic sketch of himself by T. A. Billroth. *Am J Surg* 1978; 135: 696-9.

86. Absolon KB. Theodor Billroth's formative years (1829-1894): a study in memory of the subject's 150th birthday. *Am J Surg* 1979; 137: 394-407.

87. Wolff H. Billroth in Berlin. *Zentralbl Chir* 1982; 107: 1324-6.

88. Schwyzer A. Theodor Billroth, editorial. *Surg Gynecol Obstet* 1929; 48: 823-38.

89. Schein CJ, Koch E. Mikulicz's obituary of Theodor Billroth. *Surg Gynecol Obstet* 1979; 148: 252-8.

90. Boerema I. Theodor Billroth. *Ned Tijdschr Geneesk* 1956; 100: 1313-7.

91. Rosen G. Billroth in 1870. *Surgery* 1972; 72: 337-44.

Chapter 7

Surgery of the liver and biliary tree

Bernard Launois MD FACS FRCST, (Hon) Emeritus Professor of Surgery
Department of Surgery, University of Rennes, France and University of Adelaide, Australia
Luis Ruso MD, Professor of Surgery
Department of Surgery, Hospital Maciel, University of Montevideo, Uruguay
Glyn G Jamieson MD FRCSA FRCS, Dorothy Morlock Professor of Surgery
University of Adelaide, Australia

The further you look back the easier it is to look forward!
Winston Churchill.

Surgery of the liver

Ancient history

Since the dawn of civilisation the liver has been regarded as one of the most essential organs of the human body. Medical papyri since the Egyptian physician Imhotep (ca 3000 BC) referred to diseases of the liver, including icterus, and its treatment [1, 2]. Interest by physicians further increased until the times of Hippocrates [3, 4] in the fourth and fifth centuries BC.

Hippocrates' writings bear witness to a sound knowledge of diseases of the liver. For example:

- a severe wound of the liver is deadly;
- in a bilious liver, jaundice coming on with rigor before the seventh day carries off the fever but if it occurs without fever, and not at the proper time, it is a fatal symptom;
- in cases of jaundice it is a bad symptom when the liver becomes indurated;
- when abscesses of the liver are treated by cautery or incision, if the pus which is discharged is pure and white, the patient recovers (for in this case, it is situated in the coats of the liver), but if it does not resemble oil as it flows, the patient dies;
- when the liver is filled with water and bursts into the epiploon, the belly fills with water and the patient dies.

The doctors of the Hippocratic era were indeed skilled physicians. Figure 1 shows a memorial stone, which dates from the second century BC portraying a physician palpating the liver of his patient with considerable concentration.

The legend of Prometheus depicted the importance of the liver, in a story going back into the mists of time. It prophesied not only the feasibility of liver surgery but also the concept of liver regeneration, both features confirmed many centuries later.

A beautiful painting by the Tuscan painter, Piero Cosimo, now hangs in the Strasbourg Museum. Its fine colours vividly help to illustrate the story of Prometheus and any liver surgeon will recognise the suitable position of Prometheus for a recognisable right thoraco-abdominal incision! (Figure 2).

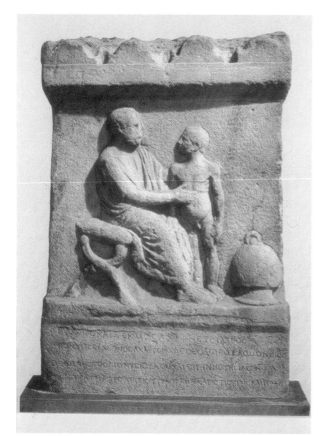

Figure 1. Stèle funéraire (memorial stone) showing clinical examination of the liver. *Reproduced with permission from the Musée de Rennes, Rennes, France.*

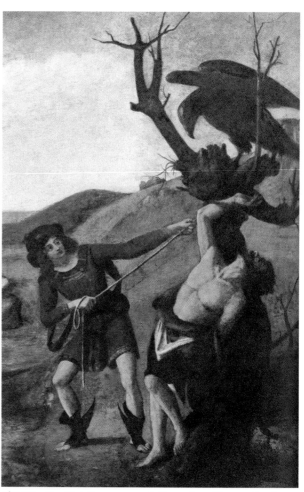

Figure 2. Strasbourg painting by Piero Cosimo. *Reproduced with permission from A. Castel, Le Grand Atelier d'Italie. Gallimard Paris, and the Art Musée, Strasbourg.*

History of liver anatomy

The history of surgery of the liver goes hand in hand with the history of liver anatomy. Four to five thousand years ago, Babylonian priests were interested in the anatomy of the liver as they used its fissures for ritual divination. Galen [5] (ca 130-200 AD) of Pergamum (Figure 1, Chapter 1) whose work was based on animal anatomy, stated the liver had several lobes. After Galen, anatomists whose science was more theoretical believed that the portal vein was an artery. Others thought that the liver was a hollow throbbing muscle and called it the 'abdominal heart'.

Vesalius [6] wrote in his historic *De Humanis Corporis Fabrica* that the lobes of the human liver

were quite unlike those of the pig or the dog. Leonardo da Vinci [7] in the 16th century made fine, although not completely accurate drawings of the liver; however, he distinctly showed the portal vein and the hepatic artery (Figure 3).

As a result of dissections on human cadavers, Ambroise Paré [8] became familiar with the concept of right and left lobes. Chapter 1 describes how many anatomists stubbornly followed Galen for centuries. Rex [9], the father of modern liver anatomy, after injection studies described not only the bile ducts, but also the network of vessels belonging to the different branches of the portal vein. However, most of his work was in animals and not in man.

Cantlie [10] in 1898 was the first to consider that the liver had a right part and a left part, divided by a plane called 'Cantlie's line', running from the fundus of the gallbladder to the terminations of the suprahepatic veins. This was confirmed by many others including Wendel [11-12] in 1921, McIndoe and Countseller [13] in 1927, Hjortsjö [14] in 1951, Elias and Patty [15], in 1952, Couinaud (Figure 4) [16] in 1954 and Tung in 1963 [17].

This anatomical knowledge was the foundation of modern liver surgery. The entire art of hepatectomy is based on a sound knowledge of the fissures: only one is visible to the naked eye. The others are hidden within the liver. Traditional anatomy commenced where the liver had been defined into two lobes by the obvious umbilical fissure.

A significant step forward was made when the vascular and biliary ducts were replaced by casts of wax, then latex and finally, synthetic resin (Figure 5).

In 1957, Couinaud [18] published a 530-page book entitled *The Liver: Anatomical and Surgical Studies.*

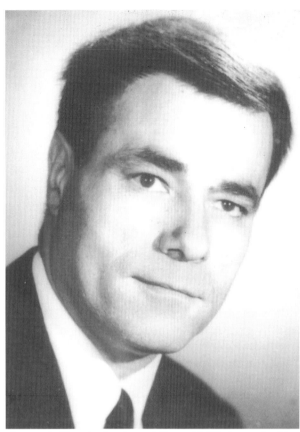

Figure 4. Claude Couinaud (born 1922). Presented by Claude Couinaud to Bernard Launois. *Reproduced from the author's private collection.*

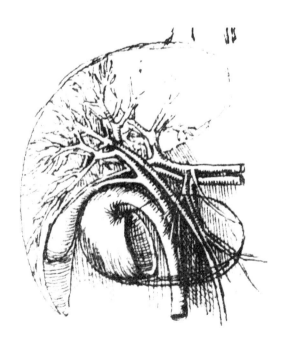

Figure 3. Anatomical drawing by Leonardo da Vinci. *Reproduced with permission from the library of Windsor Castle, by authorisation of her Majesty The Queen Elizabeth II.*

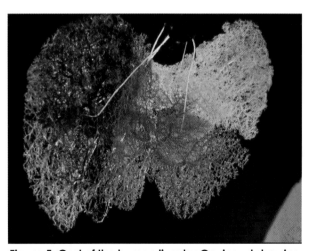

Figure 5. Cast of the human liver by Couinaud showing the ducts and vessels. The original illustration was made by Claude Couinaud and presented to the author. *Reproduced from the author's private collection.*

The book covered 140 observations made over a period of six years using similar corrosive casts. He injected a combination of acetone and polyvinyl material into the ducts and vessels from fresh cadavers. Twenty-four hours later he eroded the surrounding parenchyma with hydrochloric acid to produce the effect seen in Figure 5.

Portal segmentation through the parenchyma corresponds exactly to the branches of the portal vein. The left and right branches of the portal vein supply the right and the left 'livers', separated from each other by the main portal fissure.

The right liver is made up of two sectors, namely the right medial (anterior) sector near the main portal fissure shown in blue, and a lateral (posterior) sector shown in green, seen in Figure 5. The left liver is supplied by the left branch of the portal vein which divides into two branches at the extreme left of the hilum. A small unique branch supplies the posterior part

of the left lobe shown in yellow, while a large portal vein component (Rex's recessus), supplies the rest of the left liver shown in red, also seen in Figure 5.

The left liver is also made up of two sectors. The left medial sector is shown in red. It is comprised of two segments: the left occupies the anterior part of the left liver and the right corresponds to the quadrate lobe and is separated by the umbilical fissure. The left posterior sector lies behind the anterior left portion of the paramedial sector. Each sector is divided into two segments, except for the left posterior sector which is segment II (Figure 6).

Behind the portal vein the caudate lobe corresponds to the dorsal segment (I) or Spigelian lobe. By convention all the segments are labelled using Roman numerals, beginning at the inferior part of the liver and going around the portal vein in an anti-clockwise direction. As Ronald Malt [19] described, the segments are arranged in a spiral, like the arondissements of

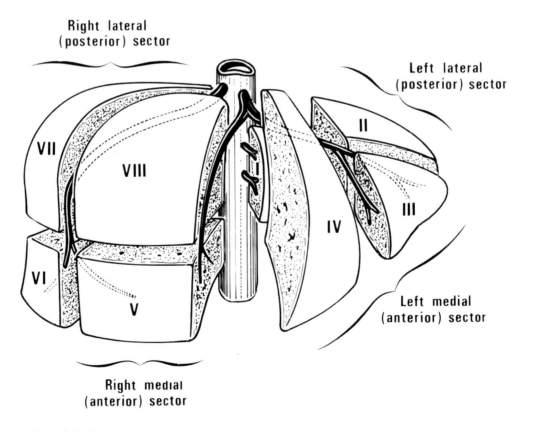

Figure 6. Surface view of the human liver showing most of the segments. *Reproduced with permission from Elsevier Scientific Inc. In: Modern Techniques of Liver Surgery. Launois B, Jamieson G. London: Churchill Livingstone, 1992.*

Paris! There are eight segments, segment VIII being the most easily seen on the superior surface (Figure 6).

Real anatomy as opposed to traditional anatomy of the liver is learnt by the surgeon in the operating theatre equipped with an ultrasound probe to recognise the portal pedicles in the liver substance and the crucial hepatic veins which essentially lie within the fissures. The right main fissure is variable in its path, as the right segments are variable in size and shape.

When the liver is removed in the mortuary, the plane of the right fissure tends to be anteroposterior. In the living patient, however, the plane of the fissure between the right medial and lateral sectors is coronal, and this means that the segments of the right medial sector tend to lie in front of the segments of the right lateral sector.

Glisson's capsule which encapsulates the liver on the outside, condenses around each derivative of the hepatic artery, duct and portal vein, known as the 'portal trinity' (Figure 7) as they enter the liver substance. Couinaud [18], aware that Valoeus described the identical fascia long before Glisson, called them 'Valoean sheaths'. There are many variations which make dissection of individual structures within the liver difficult and hazardous. He found that if the sheaths were ligated instead of the individual components, isolating a specific segment became technically simpler and safer.

Armed with this anatomical knowledge, within ten years of his anatomical findings Couinaud was able to describe several new operations for the first time. These included:

- extended left hepatectomy;
- central hepatectomy;
- right lateral sectorectomy;
- right paramedial sectorectomy and excision of segment I;
- excision of segment II;
- excision of segment III;
- excision of segment IV; and
- excision of segment VI.

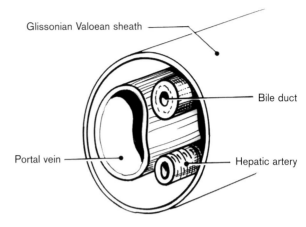

Figure 7. Couinaud's Glissonian (Valoean) sheath around a portal trinity. *Reproduced with permission from Elsevier Scientific Inc. In: Modern Techniques of Liver Surgery. Launois B, Jamieson G. London: Churchill Livingstone, 1992.*

Glisson's capsule thickens at the level of the hilum to form a plate or ceiling. This plate covering the hilum forms a demi-cylinder open toward the base. This cylinder possesses an anterior face (corresponding to the hilar plate described by Hepp and Couinaud [20]), a superior face and a posterior face. An incision is made at the junction of the hilum with the liver substance in front of the hilum, extending along to the gallbladder bed, on the right and to the umbilical fissure on the left. The incision is deepened and the liver parenchyma pushed upwards and away from the hilum, in order to expose the confluence of the hepatic structures. The hilar plate is dissected on its superior surface, with little risk of bleeding. This is the manoeuvre called 'taking down the hilar plate'. Liberation of the superior face of this demi-cylinder will mobilise together the left and right Glissonian sheaths and permit exteriorisation of the hilum, facilitating exposure of the left and the right hepatic ducts. The biliary ducts are firmly adherent to the top of the cylinder at the portal bifurcation. During secondary repairs of the biliary tree, the sclerosed hepatic pedicle can be ignored. The left bile duct lumen is opened widely with no attempt to separate it from the adherent Glissonian capsule. The anastomosis is performed to a Roux-en-Y loop of jejunum (Figure 10, Chapter 6). Credit for this major advance is owed to Jacques Hepp (Figure 18).

History of liver physiology

Like anatomy, the history of liver surgery is intimately related to knowledge of liver physiology. We know the liver is receiving 1500ml of blood per minute, 1200ml via the portal vein and 300ml through the hepatic artery.

On October 21st 1850, Claude Bernard [21-23] (Figure 8) presented to the Academy of Sciences his first communication called "The new function of sugar in the liver in man and in animals". The presence of

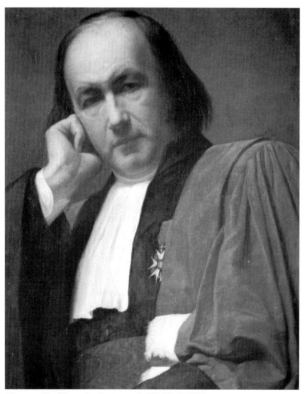

Figure 8. Claude Bernard (1813-1878). *Reproduced with permission from Musée de Claude Bernard, St. Julien-en-Beaujolais, France.*

sugar in the circulation had been known for a long time, and it was thought to have arrived there by food intake alone. In 1853, he showed on the basis of experiments on an isolated and 'washed' liver, that glucose accumulates in the liver in the form of animal starch called glycogen. He wrote: "I believe I have established the glycogenic function of the liver." [23]

We now know the liver has small reserves of sugar. After a night without food, it only contains 70-80g of glycogen. Seventy-five percent of glucose is produced by glycogenolysis and 25% by gluconeogenesis. After 18 to 24 hours of fasting, the production of glucose falls dramatically.

The role played by the liver in protein metabolism is similar; broken down protein pours in via the portal veins, mostly in the form of amino acids. These amino acids are processed to meet the needs of the liver itself, the needs of the peripheral tissues, but mostly to form muscle. Many years later it was found that changes in amino-acid metabolism brought about by porto-caval shunting were a major cause of porto-systemic encephalopathy.

The first portocaval shunt was described by Nikolai Eck [24] in a dog. He wrote: "I consider the main reason to doubt that such an operation can be carried out on human beings has been removed because it has been established that the blood of the portal vein, without any danger, could be diverted directly into the general circulation and by this means it is a perfectly safe operation." He said: "I had to postpone further experiments because I was called to join the Army!" For this work his immortality has been assured, which is interesting, as seven of the eight dogs having his fistula died and the remaining animal escaped to an unknown fate on the Russian Steppes.

In 1893, Hahn, Massen, Nenck and Pavlov [25] published an original and crucial contribution to hepatology. They created Eck fistulas in 20 dogs, and gave the animals a meat diet, which produced ataxias and convulsions quickly proceeding to death. They called the state 'meat intoxication' but now it is known as 'hepatic encephalopathy'. Autopsies showed fatty infiltration of the liver in every animal.

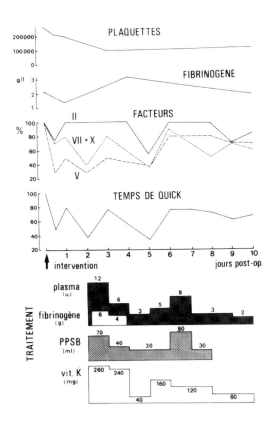

Figure 9. Biochemical chart of a patient three days after major hepatic resection. Chart of patient operated on by Bernard Launois. *Reproduced from the author's private collection.*

After major hepatic resection we have realised that albumin, both the general and specialised proteins, as well as the coagulation factors, are all affected. Figure 9 shows the state of one of the authors' patient's chemistry three days after major hepatic resection. There is a clear lowering of the levels of proteins, albumin, the coagulation factors and the 'quick time' (now known as prothrombin time). It took a full eight days for the levels to return to normal. This particular patient developed hepatic insufficiency after a right hepatectomy and removal of segment IV for carcinoma of the gallbladder.

Liver regeneration

Extensive resection of normal liver is compatible with survival and a return to full health, because of its tremendous capacity to regenerate. Recovery has been reported after 80-90% of the liver being resected. Fausto and colleagues [26] found that not only had there been a rapid increase of liver cell size (hypertrophy) but also active cell division and multiplication (hyperplasia).

Mann [27] of the Mayo clinic believed the restoration of the liver depended on the flow and quantity of portal blood flowing through the liver. The 'portal flow' orientated view held its sway until challenged by investigations originating from liver transplantation. Impressive new evidence came from research conducted between 1964 and 1972. Sceptics found no growth factor in the portal blood, but in 1973 Starzl and colleagues found that the alleged endogenous hormones from the splanchnic blood were actually insulin and glucagon [28]. Proof came from the addition of insulin to isolated liver cells taken from 17-day-old rat foetuses. This brought about cell proliferation to twice the normal rate [29].

It is clear that surgery of the liver would be impossible without a thorough knowledge of liver anatomy and basic liver physiology.

History of liver surgery including resection

Early liver surgery was limited to treatment of trauma. In 1839 Dupuytren (Figure 5, Chapter 12) wrote: "Wounds of the liver are very serious and despite most energetic treatment, the outcome is often regrettable." [30]

Liver resection

The first elective resections were attempted towards the end of the 19th century largely by the German School of Surgery. In 1888, Garré [31] reported that Bruns probably resected the first intrahepatic malignancy using cautery. The next year, Keen [32] resected a primary carcinoma in the left lobe which would now be called a left lateral segmentectomy. In his report he reviewed 76 cases from the world literature, in which 17 had resection with 13 survivors. The mortality of all the patients was 14.9%, which was very commendable for operations of that magnitude at that time.

In 1908, Hogarth Pringle [33], an Australian working in Glasgow, described a vital step in the control of bleeding in liver surgery by temporary occlusion of the portal pedicle, since known as the 'Pringle manoeuvre'.

In London, Grey Turner [34] reported two liver resections in 1923. The first was a wedge resection of a sessile adenoma of the right lobe and the second, a removal of a left lobe tumour. He employed the Pringle manoeuvre during both operations. In 1938, Ton That Tung and Meyer-May [35] successfully performed the first anatomical resection of the left lobe by first ligating the pedicle. They wrote: "We particularly stressed preliminary main ligation, rather than manual dissection of the pedicle, after opening the tissue of the liver from a Kocher clamp." In 1952, Lortat-Jacob and Robert [36] reported the first case of extended right hepatectomy, after preliminary ligation of the hilar vessels.

In the same year, Quattlebaum [37] reported three cases of major hepatic resection; the first of the three operations was an extended right hepatectomy. In his historic book *Le Foie: Études Anatomiques et Chirurgicales*, Couinaud [18] summarised all the original techniques. At that time his book seemed esoteric, but it became the basis for expanding modern liver surgery. Right hepatectomies and extended right hepatectomies became routine, but it was not until 1982 that Thomas Starzl [38] (Figure 10) published the first extended left hepatectomy since called trisegmentectomy.

Ronald Malt said: "By analogy to the lung, the two main divisions of the liver are best called the right liver and left liver. Thus, the right hepatectomy and left hepatectomy are the semantically appropriate terms for removal of those parts of the liver." [19] As any one of the anatomical segments can be removed individually, they are called 'segmentectomy'. The surgical segments of the liver are conglomerations of

anatomical segments. Thus surgical segments might preferably be called 'sectors'.

Segmentectomies

The first formal segmentectomies were done by Fredet [39], when he resected segments V and VII in 1956 (Figure 6). Champeau [40] published his mobilisation or resection of segment IV which gave surgeons good access to the upper biliary junction. After 43 years of anatomical studies, Ton That Tung [41] reported on most, if not all, of the major and minor liver resections. When three segments, for example segments IV, V and VI are removed together, it is called a trisegmentectomy. A major hepatectomy includes more than four segments.

Incisions

The first abdominal approaches usually were via a thoraco-abdominal [36] incision, but the risk of pleural effusion in cases of ascites led surgeons to prefer a solely abdominal approach. A popular incision is a bi-sub-costal (roof-top) incision [42] or even a bi-sub-costal with vertical mid-sternal ('Mercedes') incision.

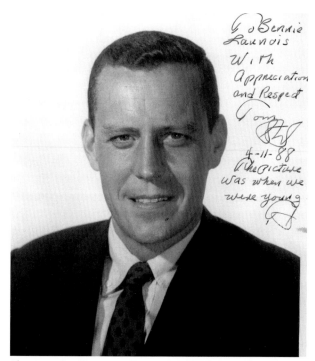

Figure 10. Thomas Starzl (contemporary). Portrait presented to Professor Bernard Launois by Dr. Starzl.
Reproduced from the author's private collection.

There were now three distinctly different approaches to the hepatic pedicles:

♦ intrafascial (extrahepatic) [36];
♦ extrafascial [18];
♦ transfissural [18] approaches including the anterior transfissural approach [18, 41-43] and the posterior or dorsal approach [44].

Methods of cutting the liver surface
Methods of cutting the liver surface are as follows:

♦ traditional blunt dissection with the handle of a scalpel or closed scissors;
♦ finger fracture dissection as described by Lin in 1958 [45, 46]. Henri Bismuth [47] employed a Kelly clamp used in gastric surgery, in combination with finger fracture resection;
♦ Foster [48] used the inner cannula of a sucker instead of finger fracture;
♦ the ultrasonic scalpel was first used by Putnam [49] following the idea of Finkelstein *et al* [50], in order to cut through the liver parenchyma.

Tumour resection

Resection of the liver was initially limited to benign tumours or solitary secondary tumours. With the help of computed tomographic (CT) scans, the indications for resection increased proportionately, to include multiple and even bilateral metastases. Liver resection and liver transplantation are the mainstay curative treatments available for hepatocellular carcinoma in normal and cirrhotic livers. The knowledge of and ability to resect individual segments, instead of removing a whole left or right liver at one time, meant repeat surgery for colonic secondaries was possible, with a better chance of cure.

Intrahepatic biliary-digestive anastomoses
These are discussed later on pages 130-131 in the section on surgery of the biliary tree.

Liver transplantation

This 'final stride' remained to be taken. Liver transplantations were at first a long catalogue of failures. Thomas Starzl [51] (Figure 10) made his first

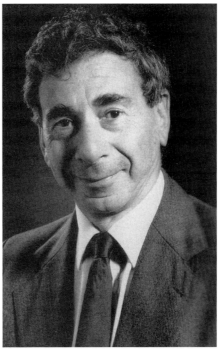

Figure 11. Sir Roy Calne (contemporary).
Reproduced with permission from the UCLA Tissue Typing Laboratory. Terasaki P. History of Transplantation: Thirty-five Recollections, 1993; 1(1).

attempts in 1963, but his early results forced surgeons back to the laboratory. Nevertheless, in the same year it was found that kidney transplantation rejection could be reversed with high doses of corticosteroids [52]. As long ago as 1899, Elie Metchnikoff published a paper entitled "Studies on the resorption of cells" in which he described the first anti- lymphocyte globulin [53]. However, the first reference to testing antisera for homograft rejection was by Woodruff [54]. The immunosuppressive effect of anti-lymphocyte serum was confirmed not only in canine renal and liver homotransplantations, but also in human renal homotransplantations [55]. Eventually in 1968, the first long-term patient liver transplant survivor of 400 days was achieved [56]. The available results of liver transplantation in the pioneer centres of Denver (Colorado) and Cambridge (UK) were poor at that time, so the main indications were for malignant tumours and tumours too large for resection. Sadly, the cancer recurrence rate was high [57], but Starzl (Figure 10) in Denver and Roy Calne (Figure 11) in Cambridge, UK, started getting significant successes in children with biliary atresia and non-malignant disease.

Post-transplant obstructive jaundice was often attributed to rejection, when in fact it was more often due to other problems, such as recurrence of viral hepatitis [57, 58], or related to the biliary anastomosis. The problem of stricturing of the biliary anastomosis used to be the Achilles' heel of liver transplantation until mastered by the early pioneers. Added to these problems, Starzl found immunosuppressive therapy involving high doses of steroids had been a frequent cause of serious or fatal opportunistic infections [57].

Storage and preservation of the liver then seemed difficult and complex until Benichou [59] showed that the techniques used in kidney transplantation could be applied to the liver for six to eight hours. At the end of the 1970s, all the disappointing results of transplantation prompted Starzl to write an article: "The Decline in Survival after Liver Transplantation". He was honest enough to admit that out of 23 consecutive patients, only six survived for more than a year [60].

Jean Borel [61] brought renewed hope when he demonstrated the immunosuppressive characteristics of a fungal metabolite - cyclosporine - in 1976. Calne used this drug in 1979 in transplant patients [62]; the early results were very disappointing because of nephrotoxicity and a high incidence of non-Hodgkin's lymphoma.

A letter hostile to transplantation was sent to all members of the Colorado Society of Nephrology, and signed by a physician from Colorado Springs in January 1980: "Because of many rumours and accusations regarding the transplant program at the University of Colorado, the senior physician asked me to write to the nephrologists in the State regarding their experience with the transplant program. He would also like to invite comments on any potentially immoral and unethical situations" [63].

This led to the Denver School of Medicine withdrawing its support for Starzl's liver transplantation programme. The Chairman of the Department of Anaesthesia, the Director of the Clinical Research Centre responsible for liver transplantation and two others were dismissed by the Dean. This signalled that the University was no longer interested in transplantation, and that cyclosporine

trials could no longer be conducted in Colorado. Starzl was forced to resign, taking effect at the end of the year. He said: "I had no place to go; I only knew where not to remain." He had previously applied to the University of California in Los Angeles, but that University had imposed so many restrictions that Starzl could not contemplate re-applying there.

In Denver, an innocent response to a journalist's question made matters worse. When someone enquired about the purported battle within the University between 'titans', Starzl asked: "Who is the other titan?" not intending to suggest he was one of them. Regrettably, exception was taken to this, so the ten beds of the historic Liver Transplantation Unit in Colorado General Hospital were converted into Administration Offices. Even the plaque commemorating the tenth anniversary of transplantation was thrown away!

Nevertheless, at the biennial meeting of the Transplantation Society in Boston on the July 4th holiday, Starzl reported how the first batch of liver recipients treated with cyclosporine, (admittedly from only one to four months) were still alive and well [64].

He was offered an appointment in Pittsburgh later that year, so Starzl drove to Pittsburgh on December 31st 1980. It happened to be the city's coldest New Year's Eve in 100 years! He was uncertain if it were a good omen or a bad one!

The four first transplant attempts in Pittsburgh died between four and 22 days, raising the possibility that the Colorado successes had been a "statistical artefact or even a fraud" [63]. One morning while driving to work, Starzl had cause to worry when he listened to a phone-in survey on a local radio station. The radio audience was being asked if the Liver Transplant Program should be closed down before any more failures occurred.

On June 30th 1981, 54 medical residents and interns unanimously signed a resolution which they brought to the Chairman of the Medical Department, declaring that liver transplantation was "an unrealistic objective and possibly an unethical pursuit" [63]. Fortunately, the next 22 liver transplants followed the happier results of the smaller Colorado series of

1980. From that moment onwards, the next 19 patients' long-term survival improved and their one-year survival rate climbed to 68% [63].

In spite of these results, the Federal bureaucrats declared this transplant programme experimental, thereby denying medical insurance for potential recipients. This provided a barrier behind which private insurance companies took refuge. The arguments by powerful institutions, such as the National Institute of Health (NIH), the Health Care Finance Administration, The Veterans Administration and Surgeon General's office followed the same pattern; if Medicare (the US Government's most powerful and pervasive healthcare provider) had decided these operations were experimental and therefore non-reimbursable, why should private companies take any other position? [63].

The solution to this financial dilemma came about when liver transplantation was submitted to a process called "Consensus Conference Review". In June 1982, a Consensus Development Conference, which was in all fairness sponsored by the National Institute of Health, the Health Care Finance Administration, the Veterans Administration, and the Surgeon General's Office, took place. After an all-night session, the 'jury' came out in favour of transplantation. Their conclusion was that liver transplantation was a service and not an experimental operation. Furthermore, the Conference submitted a list of liver diseases that were eligible for liver replacement [65].

Until 1981, transplantation of other organs, apart from kidneys, was rare. However, it soon became obvious that the numbers of liver, heart and lung transplants were going to increase. At the request of the Surgeon General of the US, a flexible protocol for multiple cadaveric organ procurement was described by the University of Pittsburgh [66]. Since then, a simplified modification has been used which entails minimal dissection of organs for transplantation, all organs being cooled *in situ* and then removed as speedily as possible by dissection in the resulting bloodless field [67].

Belzer had been interested in preservation of organs since the '60s [68]. He patiently experimented with different infusion liquids, testing the quality of preserved organs, including the pancreas. Years went by before

he and his colleagues found the final ideal perfusate for liver preservation, which they called the 'Wisconsin solution', extending viability to a whole day [69-70].

With the new development of liver transplantation, Starzl resurrected a forgotten principle which had made liver transplantation feasible in dogs as long ago as 1958. While the diseased liver was being removed and the new one implanted, it was the policy that both the vena cava returning blood to the heart from the legs, trunk, and kidneys, and the portal vein should not be clamped for longer than 30-60 minutes. Such a time limit produced a very stressful operation for the surgeon, especially in adult patients. The introduction of a veno-venous pump without the need for anticoagulants enabled surgery to be orderly, unhurried and was very much for the patient's benefit [71]. The preservation of the patient recipient vena cava, with subsequent unclamping of the recipient vena cava combined with the 'piggy back' surgical procedure, rendered the use of extracorporeal circulation unnecessary.

The shortage of donor organs for children encouraged surgeons to develop new ways to increase the pool of potentially usable organs. Henri Bismuth had the practical idea of using adult cadaveric livers, reduced in size by removing some of the parenchyma [72]. The success of this meant many more transplants were able to be carried out for children and small adults. The term 'reduced graft' for this technique was used because the liver parenchyma was reduced, yet the graft utilised all components of the hepatic pedicle, as well as the inferior vena cava. In children, this had the distinct advantage of reducing the chances of thrombosis in the small vessels.

A German group had the inspired idea of dividing the right liver from the left liver, preserving each liver with its own vessels and bile duct. It meant that a single liver from a cadaver could be divided and transplanted into two recipients (split-liver technique) [73].

The ultimate application of partial grafting was to expand the pool of donors further by the procurement of liver allografts from living donors [74, 75]. For religious reasons this was the only option in several countries. Unfortunately, in the adult, only the right liver is capable of supporting the life of one normal-sized adult [80]; the left liver being so much smaller it is suitable only for children or small adults. Furthermore, a right hepatectomy from any living donor is not without risk [76].

In 1992, a second Consensus Conference was held in Paris, where it was agreed that transplantation should be made available to all patients including those at highest risk. At the latest Consensus Conference in Lyons in January 2005, the main indications for liver transplantation are:

- post-hepatitis B cirrhosis;
- post-hepatitis C cirrhosis;
- alcoholic cirrhosis;
- hepatocellular carcinoma.

The criteria for living donor transplantation should have remained unchanged.

Surgery of the biliary tree

Ancient times

Biliary diseases have been known since ancient times. In some mummies, more than 3000 years old, found in Crete and in Egypt, gallstones had been felt through their thin abdominal walls [81]. X-rays of other mummies have confirmed identical calcified gallstones [77].

Treatment of biliary diseases had been attempted since the time of Hippocrates (c 460-377 BC) who ably described jaundice both in the presence and absence of fever [78-79]. Galen [80] (Figure 1, Chapter 1) described various humours which included the yellow bile of 'cholerics' and the black bile of the 'melancholics' and treated them symptomatically. He prescribed diets for patients suspected of gallstones, and even established that yellow bile was formed in the gallbladder [81]. According to Glenn in 1971 [81], Alexander of Tralles in the 6th century AD discovered intrahepatic gallstones in men and described ascites in patients with liver disease.

Middle ages

Arab physicians were much concerned with liver disease [82]. Rhazes or Abu Bakr Ibn Zakairay Razi

(850 and 923 AD) pointed out the importance of stones, as well as abdominal and intestinal tumours. Avicenna (Ibn Sina 980-1037) (Figure 8, Chapter 15) described the formation of biliary fistulas after drainage of abdominal abscesses. He also established that biliary fistulas were less dangerous than intestinal fistulas [83].

During the Renaissance, dissection of cadavers gradually improved knowledge of anatomy of the biliary tree, as well as the alimentary tract. Gabriel Fallopius (1523-1562), successor to Vesalius in Padua, described both urinary and gallbladder stones [82]. His contemporary, Jean Fernel [84] (1497-1558) in Paris, understood that gallstones were formed from the precipitation of bile; he recognised acholia, choluria, and the migration of gallstones through the digestive tract. In addition, he could distinguish between jaundice due to stones and to malignant disease. Shortly afterwards, Johann Schenck [82, 85] accurately described all the known clinical complications of hepatobiliary diseases. Theophile Bonet [86] in the 17th century summarised the observations on obstructive jaundice from the literature. It appeared that Fabricius (1560-1634), also known as Willem Fabry, might have extracted gallstones from an abscess in 1620. Francis Glisson [82] (1597-1677), author of *Anatomia Hepatis*, who later described the sphincter of Oddi, described a very severe attack of gallstone colic in himself "from which there is no release except by death"!

In the second half of the 17th century in Holland, Lieberger extracted a large stone from an abdominal wall abscess [87]; so also did Johannitius in 1676. Thilesius and van der Wiel described a repeated discharge of gallstones through an abdominal fistula over a period of nine years.

In 1743, Jean-Louis Petit (Figure 9, Chapter 15) [88] presented to the Académie Royale de Chirurgie in Paris, a paper with the following title: "Consideration concerning tumours produced by retained bile in the liver, sometimes mistaken for liver abscesses". It was he who introduced the term 'biliary colic', establishing the clinical treatment of it and of obstructive cholecystitis. When the gallbladder adhered firmly to the abdominal wall, he advised that it be punctured and opened in order to remove the stones. He did succeed on one occasion.

In 1761, Giovanni Morgagni (Figure 1, Chapter 15) published his famous book in which he analysed the treatment of gallstones and reported on three women with biliary fistulas, from which stones had been removed [89]. He studied the physiopathology and complications, noting a higher incidence in females. However, biliary surgery was only performed in exceptional cases such as in circumstances described by Petit and Morgagni above.

Biliary tract disease is universal. Both the meek and the famous can succumb to this affliction. Alexander the Great, Saint Ignatius of Loyola (at whose autopsy gallstones were found), Catherine of Russia and the writer, Walter Scott; all suffered attacks of acute biliary colic [90].

Unlike urological surgery, most biliary surgery had to await the advent of anaesthesia in 1846, and at least a partial degree of surgical cleanliness. The biliary tree being deeply situated in the abdomen, meant that for a long time elective surgery was regarded as 'off limits', because of the enormous risk of fatal biliary peritonitis.

Cholecystostomy

Biliary surgery started seriously on July 15th 1867, when John Bobbs of Indiana [91] (Figure 12) operated on a woman who had a large tumour, believing it to be an ovarian cyst. To his amazement, when the abdomen was opened, he found an enormous gallbladder containing stones. He opened the gallbladder, extracted the stones, and after suturing it carefully, replaced it back into the abdomen. The patient not only survived the operation but outlived her surgeon!

Theodor Kocher (Figure 14, Chapter 12) from Berne, the celebrated American gynaecologist, Marion Sims and Lawson Tait (Figure 6, Chapter 12) from Birmingham, UK, all conducted elective cholecystotomies about the same time. First, they fixed the gallbladder to the abdominal wall before extracting either pus or stones and then left it open to the exterior. They wisely went to tremendous lengths to avoid contamination of the abdominal cavity.

In Paris in 1878, Marion Sims [92] operated on a patient with longstanding jaundice and a palpable tumour in the right hypochondrium. Applying good antiseptic principles, he opened the gallbladder and extracted 60 stones. Next, he sutured the opened gallbladder to the abdominal wall as a cholecystostomy. The patient died of haemorrhage on the eighth day. This was, nevertheless, the first elective surgical procedure for obstructive jaundice. It took the wisdom of Halsted [93] (Figure 6, Chapter 10) as late as 1924 to realise the real danger of death from bleeding in jaundiced patients 11 years before the discovery of Vitamin K by Quick [94] and Dam [95] in 1935.

In the same year, Kocher [96] performed a cholecystostomy on a patient in two stages. At the first operation, he packed the wound with Lister's phenol-impregnated gauze down to the neck of the

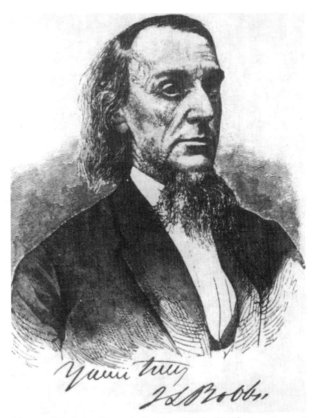

Figure 12. John Stough Bobbs (1809-1870). *Courtesy of Professor Grosfeld, Indiana University School of Medicine, Indianapolis, USA.*

mobilised gallbladder. Eight days later he emptied all the stones from the gallbladder, now surrounded by adhesions, and the patient survived.

Lawson Tait [97] (Figure 6, Chapter 12), who had already removed gallstones from a gallbladder fistula in 1869, performed his first cholecystostomy in one stage in 1879 with survival. By 1889, he had completed a total of 55 with a mortality of 5%. Understandably, he was reluctant to change to resection even though in the same year Langenbuch had performed 24 cholecystectomies.

Cholecystectomy

Experimental cholecystectomy had been successful since Zambecari [83] performed the procedure in a dog in 1680, and a medical student called Teckof [83] repeated the exercise soon after.

The story of cholecystectomy in patients occurred much later [98]. Convinced of the inadequacy of the medical treatment for biliary tract disease, Langenbuch (Figure 13) resolved to study the problem in depth and, to that purpose, rehearsed his cholecystectomy in human cadavers, as well as in dogs. On July 15th 1882, while practising Listerian principles he performed the first cholecystectomy on a man of 43 who was an alleged morphine addict because of recurrent biliary colic. According to Garrison [99], the patient smoked a cigar the next day, was up on the twelfth day and was fit to go home six weeks later. He was alleged to have been free of his addiction after the operation.

In April 1883, Langenbuch presented to the 12th German Congress of Surgery his third successful cholecystectomy [99], pointing out that the gallbladder needed to be taken out not only because it contained stones, but because he correctly believed stones would continually re-form. He published his second volume of *The surgery of the liver and gallbladder* [100] in 1897. Ironically, Langenbuch died of appendicitis shortly after giving a lecture entitled: "Treatment of Peritonitis" in 1887 [101].

Graham's [102] discovery of cholecystography in 1924 reduced the number of negative operations for suspected gallstones. The separate discoveries by Quick [94] and Dam [95] in 1935 showed that bleeding tendencies were often due to the deficiency of prothrombin in the blood caused by the lack of absorption of fat and fat-soluble vitamins in the absence of bile salts. When Vitamin K was introduced jaundice became an early indication for surgery instead of a contraindication.

Frank Glenn [103] from New York must be commended for introducing intravenous cholangiography in 1960 and percutaneous cholangiography [104] in 1962. These investigations are nowadays replaced by MRI (magnetic resonance imaging) cholangiography [105]. These valuable examinations warned surgeons of the probability of finding gallstones in the duct. A previous history of jaundice, a dilated common bile duct and a past history of pancreatitis became indications for exploring the common bile duct at operation.

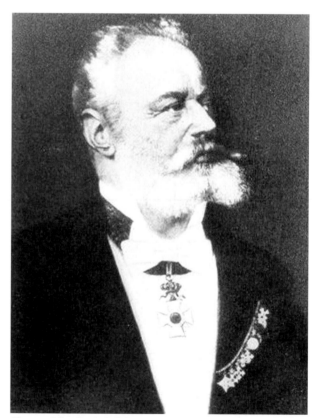

Figure 13. Carl Johann August Langenbuch (1846-1901). Presented to Bernard Launois by R. Praderi.
Reproduced from the author's private collection.

The role of intra-operative cholangiography

Operative cholangiography was introduced by Pablo Mirizzi, a surgeon from Cordoba in Argentina [106-107]. Cholangiography was soon recognised as an essential aid to hepatobiliary surgery. It was because Mirizzi was familiar with working with radiologists and cholangiography, that the technique of operative cholangiography emerged so quickly. In France, Jacques Caroli, a great hepatologist, had to lie down under the operating table in order to observe the injection of contrast media in the biliary tract [108]! Mirizzi was indeed a scholar, traveller and prolific writer. In 1981, his disciples from Cordoba celebrated the 50th anniversary of operative cholangiography which they called 'Mirrizzigraphy'. According to Praderi [83], Kerr's tube described below and operative cholangiography were the two major milestones in the history of safe and scientific biliary surgery. Ever since cholangiography began, there has been argument as to whether it should be used selectively [109] or routinely [110].

Advocates of routine operative cholangiography have traditionally recognised its value in identifying the entire intrahepatic biliary system at operation, so that unsuspected lesions are not missed. Routine cholangiography can detect unsuspected bile duct stones, as well as abnormal surgical anatomy, and thus provide early detection of bile duct injury. If the intrahepatic bile ducts are not clearly seen, either an injury to the biliary system or a tumour should be considered. Routine operative cholangiography, especially with digital fluoroscopy, has a very low false positive rate [111, 112]; likewise an extremely low false negative rate [113, 114].

The story of laparoscopic cholecystectomy

In 1983, Lukichev and colleagues [115] suggested laparoscopic cholecystectomy as surgical treatment for acute cholecystitis. However, resection of the diseased gallbladder using laparoscopic techniques was not performed until 1985 when the first laparoscopically-assisted cholecystectomy was performed by Muhe [116-117] from Boblingen in Germany, using conventional gynaecological equipment. The missing technological link that

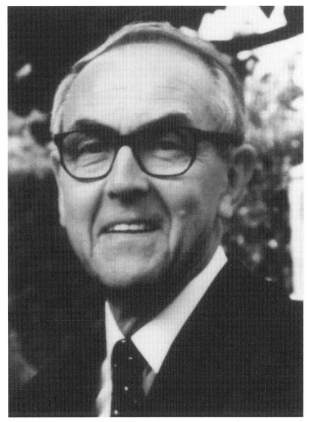

Figure 14. François Dubois (contemporary). Presented to Walford Gillison. *Reproduced from the editor's private collection.*

brought laparoscopy into mainstream general surgery was the advent in 1985 of the charged coupled device (CCD) or silicone chip solid-state image sensor and the miniature video camera.

In 1987, Philippe Mouret, a general surgeon in Lyon, performed a laparoscopy for a gynaecological problem, when he saw a gallbladder packed with stones. It was so tempting that he performed the first laparoscopic cholecystectomy under direct vision with standard surgical instruments [118].

Since 1982, François Dubois from Paris (Figure 14) was perfecting the technique of cholecystectomy through a small incision called a mini-laparotomy. He would wear a powerful light on his forehead and use especially designed self-retaining retractors [118]. However, when Dubois heard about Mouret's single success, he asked Mouret to come to Paris to demonstrate or to produce the video-recording of that operation [118]. After careful successful laparoscopic cholecystectomies improving both equipment and technique, and despite several rejections by publishing companies in 1988, he successfully published the operation over the next two years [119-120], which produced global repercussions.

By coincidence in 1989, Jacques Perissat [121] from Bordeaux showed at the World Congress of the Société Internationale de Chirurgie in Toronto, a video presentation of percutaneous lithotripsy of large gallstones immediately preceding laparoscopic cholecystectomy. Reddick and Olsen [122, 123] were the first surgeons to perform laparoscopic cholecystectomy in the US, and Alfred Cuschieri the first in the UK [124]. After some disasters by untrained surgeons in the immediate aftermath, the conversion rate to open surgery has significantly reduced, and so too the complication rate of this now routine operation.

Choledochotomy

What about stones trapped in the common bile duct? Tait crushed them with rubber-covered forceps, Kocher with his fingers, but the first successful exploration was performed by Kümmel [125] in 1884, followed by Riedel [126] in 1888, the very next year Robert Abbe [127] in New York, and Thornton [128] in London followed suit.

In 1890, Ludwig Courvoisier [129] (Figure 7, Chapter 8), the distinguished Professor of Surgery from Basel with a fine reputation in biliary surgery, published his well known monograph on the pathology and surgery of biliary ducts, based on a careful study of 187 cases of jaundice. However, the operation of the choledochotomy was not taken up universally, because of the fear of biliary peritonitis.

A cautious but safe approach was taken by Iversen [130] in 1892, who performed choledochotomy in two stages; as Kocher had done for cholecystostomy. He first packed gauze around the duct to generate adhesions, and at the second stage, he opened the common duct to remove the stones.

After graduation, Hans Kehr (Figure 15) practised surgery in a private clinic which he founded in Halberstadt, which is a small Saxon city at the foot of the Hartz Mountains. There, he managed a huge number of patients for biliary complications, with the result that he rapidly acquired an impressive reputation. By 1910, Kehr was rightly regarded as the 'father of modern biliary surgery', so he moved to Berlin where in 1913 he published his treatise of *Surgery of the Biliary Tract*, which for more than 40 years became the 'bible' for this specialty.

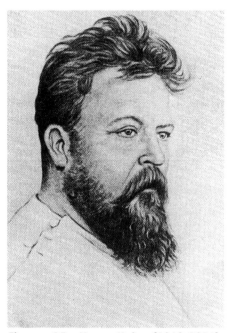

Figure 15. Hans Kehr (1862-1916). Presented to the authors by R. Praderi. *Reproduced from the author's private collection.*

Kehr is also famous for his method of resection of the gallbladder for cancer, which included partial hepatic resection [131]. He successfully resected hepatic duct tumours, aneurysms of the hepatic artery, as well as having achieved the first hepato-enteric and hepatoduodenal anastomoses, incorporating the gallbladder as a link or bridge between them.

In 1895, Kehr placed a rubber tube into the common duct via the cystic duct after completing his cholecystectomy. He gave this procedure the grand name of 'hepaticus drainage' [132-133]. According to

Gosset [134], this rapidly became popular because of its relative safety, but the credit must go to Kehr for the T-tube that was named after him, for drainage of the opened bile duct.

In 1897, instead of using the cystic duct, Quenu [135] placed a similar tube directly into the bile duct during choledochotomy. It proved that sutures in the common duct did hold, despite previous distal obstruction. All this must have been hard to determine without the assistance of cholangiography. A good drainage procedure with a rubber tube to the exterior with or without packing in those days increased postoperative safety.

Kehr and hepaticus drainage

Kehr and Quenu became adept in extracting stones through tunnels formed by drainage tubes in relatively bloodless manoeuvres. These preceded the techniques developed by Mendet [136] and Mazariello [137]. Kehr experimented with several methods of drainage in patients with biliary stones:

- the simplest one consisted of a method by which the gallbladder was not resected if the cystic duct was patent. After the stones had been extracted, the common bile duct was closed by sutures and a cholecystostomy performed to decompress the biliary tree. The common bile duct was therefore drained via the cystic duct and the gallbladder.

Other variations of hepaticus drainage included:

- the making of a lateral hole in his tube;
- the insertion of two tubes, one in the hepatic duct and the other in the common bile duct;
- additional transpapillary drainage.

Choledochotomy with closure by sutures was cautiously replaced by choledochostomy combined with tube drainage. This became very evident in two major European congresses held in 1908.

At the Second World Congress of Surgery held in Brussels, Kehr presented his historic paper on "The treatment of biliary lithiasis" [138]. At the 21st French Congress of Surgery, Délagenière and Gosset gave an up-to-date presentation of hepatic and bile duct surgery. By that stage, Kehr had operated on 280 bile ducts, William Mayo 207 [139], Mayo Robson 130 [140], Czerny 108 [83], Poppert 96 [83], Korte 74 [141] and seven French surgeons together totalled 102. Kehr had drained almost all the common bile ducts with a mortality of 4.2% [138], which was a much lower mortality than contemporary surgeons who had performed fewer drainage procedures.

As a result of these congresses, not only the majority of German surgeons, but many other eminent surgeons supported this 'safety first' policy. This group included Mayo Robson and Moynihan from the UK; Terrier, Hartmann and Pauchet from France; Halsted and the Mayo brothers from the US, amongst many others.

At one time, bile duct tubes were called Kehr tubes in mainland Europe, or Mayo-Robson tubes in the British Commonwealth. However, simple straight tubes for common bile duct drainage were difficult to keep in place, owing to the detergent properties of bile. In 1912, to prevent such slippage, Kehr designed a T-shaped tube which he called a Rummirohr drainage tube. English surgeons continued to call it a T-tube, but in South America and in France, for a long time it was still called a Kehr tube. These tubes not only protected choledochotomies, but also repairs after the increasing number of iatrogenic injuries to bile ducts.

The number of duct explorations today is very much reduced. Many more duct stones have been removed by expert endoscopists by endoscopic retrograde cholangiography (ERCP) and endoscopic sphincterotomy (ES), since the publications of Classen [142] and Kawai [143] and their respective colleagues. Petelin introduced laparoscopic choledochotomy in 1991 [144].

Biliary-digestive anastomoses

Two of Billroth's protégés performed the first cholecysto-digestive anastomosis. Alexander von Winiwarter [145], then Professor of Surgery in Liege, operated on a woman with obstructive jaundice in 1882. In order to connect the gallbladder to the intestine he performed a cholecystostomy parallel to a transverse colostomy, thinking both fistulas would inter-connect. This was not achieved because one of them closed spontaneously. The patient was operated on five more times until a successful cholecysto-jejunostomy was created 18 months later.

Before Kehr described his tube, choledochotomies often became biliary fistulas, especially in the presence of distal obstruction, either because of residual bile duct stones, or pancreatic cancer.

Biliary fistulas, when complicated by hypo-coagulation, often resulted in patients dying, just as Marion Sims' patient fared in Paris, from uncontrollable haemorrhage. Because of this risk, many decided that if a single surgical procedure was needed after the extraction of bile duct stones, it was necessary to provide a connection between the bile duct and the digestive tract.

Riedel [126] performed a cholecystectomy on a patient on July 23rd 1888, but had reason to fear the existence of stones in the common bile duct because of later jaundice. He operated again on December 8th. This time he opened the bile duct, extracted the stones and anastomosed the duct to the duodenum (choledochoduodenostomy). Tragically, the suture line leaked and the patient died of peritonitis.

Two years later in January 1890, Sprengel [146] performed a procedure recommended by Kümmel who had recently lost a patient following choledochotomy. This procedure consisted of crushing and displacing the gallstones (cholecysto-lithotripsy) through the cystic duct into and beyond the common bile duct, hoping to avoid choledochotomy. Not surprisingly, Sprengel's patient became jaundiced eight years later and required re-operation. This time, the patient had comprehensive surgery starting with a cholecystectomy, next a choledochotomy, followed by a side-to-side choledochoduodenostomy. The patient recovered and this approach became more and more popular among central European surgeons, according to Sasse [147] and Flörcken [148], who believe such patients recovered more speedily.

In 1888, a Russian surgeon, Monastyrsk [149], operated on a case of cancer of the pancreas,

performing an anastomosis of the gallbladder to the duodenum; the patient survived for two months. About the same time, Bardenheuer [150] repeated the same operation. Likewise, Terrier [151, 152] published in the following year, a case of pancreatic cancer with an enlarged gallbladder treated in this way. This significant publication preceded 'Courvoisier's rule' in the German literature (wrongly called 'Courvoisier's Law' in the English literature) [153] by one year, which is why in French medical literature it is understandably called the 'Courvoisier-Terrier rule'.

In 1887, Kappeler [154] performed a side-to-side anastomosis of the gallbladder to the jejunum, and the patient survived one year and three months. In 1888, Mayo Robson operated in the UK on a patient who had a cholecystostomy complicated by a persistent biliary fistula. He achieved a good result by converting it to a cholecystojejunostomy [140].

In 1892, Murphy had successfully performed three cholecystoduodenostomies, using his metallic button (Figure 8, Chapter 10) which facilitated the anastomosis [155]. In 1892, another of Billroth's students, Robert Gersuny performed a cholecysto-gastrostomy in a case in which the duodenum and jejunum were blocked [83]. This worked well, so that he subsequently continued to bypass the pancreas in that manner.

Transduodenal surgery

At the end of the 19th century, choledocholithotomy for stones ended with tube drainage or with a choledochoduodenostomy, depending on the preference of the surgeon. Even authors such as Langenbuch practised choledocholithotripsy, i.e. crushing stones in the gallbladder or in the bile duct, and then manoeuvring them through the papilla of Vater. Some surgeons, like Pozzi [83] and Czerny [83] had accidentally opened the duodenum and discovered they could extract impacted papillary stones through it.

In 1894, Theodore Kocher [156] wrote an article on sphincterotomy to remove supra-ampullary bile duct stones. He had performed 20 duodenotomies to retrieve stones by this route by 1899. Not only did Terrier and Kehr successfully perform duodenotomies for the same purpose, but also Charles McBurney [157] from New York (Figure 8, Chapter 12), who published a similar series in 1898.

Ampullectomies

Since the time surgeons first attempted duodenotomy, they concentrated on cancer of the ampulla of Vater, as well as removing impacted stones. Halsted [158] (Figure 6, Chapter 10) from John Hopkins, Baltimore, aware of advances in European surgery, operated on a 60-year-old woman suffering from jaundice, diarrhoea, and a bleeding disorder with an enlarged gallbladder in 1898. He resected that part of the duodenum including the tumour, re-implanted the common duct into the remaining duodenum, and simultaneously performed a cholecystostomy. Some weeks later, he removed her gallbladder and implanted the dilated cystic duct into the duodenum. The patient survived seven months before dying from widespread cancer.

In 1900, William Mayo [139] (Figure 16) operated on a 49-year-old man suffering from ampullary cancer, dividing the procedure into three stages:

- first he did a cholecystostomy to relieve the jaundice;
- at the second operation, he opened the duodenum, removed the tumour, and anastomosed the common bile duct to the duodenum before closing the duodenotomy;
- the jaundice reappeared a year and a half later, so Mayo relieved the jaundice again with another bypass in the form of a cholecysto-duodenostomy.

Ampullectomy became a swift elegant procedure which was not too difficult, although oncologically unsound. It was quickly adopted as an elective procedure at a time when biliary surgery was fraught with danger in jaundiced patients with bleeding disorders. Kausch [159] and Hartmann [160] in their publications gave an account of those ampullary tumours which had been successfully resected at the beginning of the 20th century. Others added gastroenterostomy for believed safety.

In 1908, in Uruguay, Alfredo Navarro performed an ampullectomy on a patient whose survival was confirmed by Larghero 30 years later. This particular case history was presented in Paris by Navarro's teacher, Hartmann, in 1923 [160], showing it worked occasionally.

Choledocho- and hepaticojejunostomy

At the same time that Kocher's manoeuvre, utilised for gastrectomy, was applied to biliary surgery, César Roux (Figure 13, Chapter 4), Kocher's highly valued assistant at one time, employed a jejunal loop as an adjunct to gastro-oesophageal surgery. The 'Roux' loop used in gastric surgery (Figure 10, Chapter 6) became a worldwide household name, because it allowed decompression of the biliary and pancreatic ductal systems.

The Roux-en-Y jejunostomy procedure was presented by Monprofit [161] for hepaticojejunostomies in the animal laboratory at the French Congress of Surgery in 1904. However, Dahl [162] was the first to do so in patients in 1907.

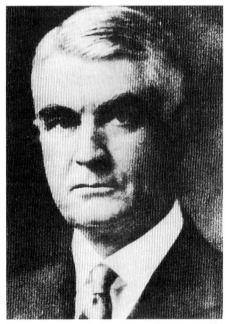

Figure 16. William Mayo (1861-1939). *Reproduced with permission from the Académie de Médecine, Paris, France.*

It was because cholangitis was often experienced after bilio-digestive anastomoses that this new measure safeguarded patients from infection caused by reflux of food. One can imagine that in those days, biliary anastomoses performed with thick Reverdin needles were far from elegant. In 1903, Maragliano [163] used Braun's jejunojejunostomy (Figure 8d, Chapter 6) below a cholecysto-jejunostomy which reduced food contamination. A single variation was created by Praderi [164] who modified previous bilio-digestive anastomoses to combine the advantages of a Roux-en-Y with the simplicity of an omega loop.

Intrahepatic biliary anastomoses

Intrahepatic biliary anastomoses were first described and attempted for irresectable cancer of the liver hilum. Kocher, in 1882, then Langenbuch and Krausch performed an external hepatostomy for seriously jaundiced patients. In 1898, Czerny [83] fixed a jejunal loop to the cut section of an external hepatostomy but his patient died. Kehr [165] successfully performed three operations of this type in 1903. He also utilised the gallbladder to relieve jaundice in one patient by performing hepatico-cholecystostomy.

Longmire [166] (Figure 17), from Stanford University, published in 1948 a technique of cholangio-jejunostomy after resection of the peripheral ends of segments II and III (Figure 6). In 1954, Dogliotti [167] described a similar procedure using the stomach (cholangiogastrostomy) instead of the Roux-en-Y jejunal loop. Couinaud and Soupault published a landmark operation: "A new procedure for an intra-hepatic biliary shunt: a left cholangiojejunostomy without sacrificing the liver" in 1957. They showed the feasibility of a bypass between the bile duct belonging to segment III to a jejunal loop accessed by the umbilical fissure [168].

When the bile confluence is obstructed by the tumour with a risk of cholangitis, septic shock and death, biliojejunal anastomoses could be attempted to relieve the obstruction [169]. Hepp (Figure 18) [170] recommended this approach if the bile duct diameters

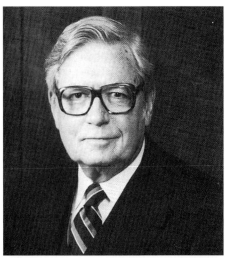

Figure 17.   W. Longmire (1913-2003). Presented to the authors by R. Praderi. *Reproduced from the author's private collection.*

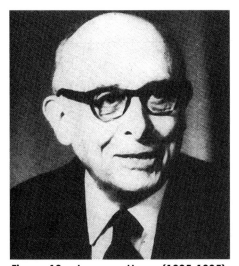

Figure 18.   Jacques Hepp (1905-1995). Presented to the authors by R. Praderi. *Reproduced from the author's private collection.*

were greater than 5mm. Nowadays, better palliation is achieved with modern internal or external stents.

Henri Bismuth and Lechaux [171] described a hepatotomy on the edge of segment V in order to find a bile duct and make a cholangio-entero-anastomosis. Prioton [172], in 1968, described splitting the main fissure to get access to the border between segments V and VIII, as the duct of segment V is usually predictable, superficial, and its volume is satisfactory. Furthermore, the authors found access to this difficult segment belonging to segment V was surprisingly easy by a posterior approach [173].

Benign biliary strictures

This subject has been of interest to surgeons, lawyers and medical defence societies ever since the Suez crisis in 1956. There was a political and military confrontation involving the new republic of Egypt, against the forces of the UK and France which precipitated the closure of the Suez Canal. Anthony Eden, the British Prime Minister of the day, had recurrent cholangitis following a cholecystectomy, complicated by stricture during the conflict; some have speculated that his illness affected his judgment. His biliary stricture was subsequently treated by further surgery by Cattell (Figure 2, Chapter 13) in the Lahey Clinic.

The first procedure used in biliary repair was the resection of postoperative strictures and an end-to-end suture proposed by Lahey and Pyrtek [174] in 1950, although it was difficult to avoid tension. The main principle was to construct an anastomosis using normal mucosa from both ends of the bile duct. Warren Cole *et al* [175] from Chicago brought up a Roux-en-Y jejunal loop to the upper end of the bile duct. They thought resection of as much sclerotic tissue is necessary, and the construction of an anastomosis should be taken well above the stricture.

In 1967, Nuboer [176] employed a mucosal graft not only to cover but also overlap a fibrotic stricture. Smith [177] in London tried to emulate this but the upper level of such a stricture was uncertain, especially as it was splinted blindly over a transhepatic tube.

In 1956, Hepp and Couinaud [87] demonstrated that Glisson's capsule is thicker at the hilum and constitutes a tough fibrous plate at the ceiling of the hilum. This plate is prolonged towards the right as the 'cystic' plate, and towards the left as the 'umbilical' plate. As mentioned in the anatomical section, the vasculobiliary pedicles are surrounded by Glisson's sheath, extending into the parenchyma. Therefore,

surgeons following Hepp and Couinaud, incised Glisson's capsule at the posterior edge of segment IV, and were able to expose the hilar plate and also the main left hepatic duct, even if previous surgery had taken place. It became possible to perform a cholangiojejunostomy (mucosa-to-mucosa), achieving a length of at least 2cm.

On the rare occasions of this approach being too difficult in a huge cholestatic liver, Champeau [40] described an extended access to the left hepatic duct via a transfissural approach either with mobilisation or resection of segment IV [186].

Cancers of the biliary tract

Gallbladder cancer, a depressing disease

Gallbladder cancer has had a sinister reputation since the first description in 1778 [178]. Blalock [179] recommended in 1924 that surgery be avoided for gallbladder cancer if the diagnosis was made before surgery. In 1954, Glenn and Hayes [180] introduced a more rational approach, which included a wedge resection of the gallbladder bed combined with regional lymphadenectomy of the whole hepato-duodenal omentum. Surgical resection for gallbladder cancer has varied from simple cholecystectomy for early limited disease, to combined cholecystectomy with resection of segments IV, V and VI if more penetrating. In more extensive disease, which may reach the hepatic confluence, resections have been successfully carried out removing the right liver and performing a hepaticojejunostomy to the left. Some have added pancreaticoduodenectomy, but the results from that have been very disappointing [181].

Bile duct cancer

Bile duct cancer has been classified into four types [182]:

- upper third cancer;
- middle third cancer;
- lower third cancer; and
- diffuse cancer.

Upper third cancers have several descriptions: for example, 'cancers of the biliary confluence', 'high bile duct cancer', 'proximal bile duct cancer', and 'hilar cholangiocarcinoma'. This type of tumour was first mentioned by Altemeier [183] but the pathology was described by Klatskin and it is often known as a Klatskin tumour [184]. The first proximal bile duct cancer resection was performed by Crayton Brown in Melbourne, Australia [185] in 1954. Tumour resection with or without hepatectomy was performed in 1979 with a resectability rate of 62% [186, 188]. In 1984, Blumgart [187] combined portal vein resection if there was venous involvement. There is a close relationship between overall resectability rates and associated liver resection rates for individual authors. Roughly, the resectability rate is often double that of the hepatectomy rate [188]. Liver transplantation has poorer results for this cancer, compared with its other indications [189].

Conclusions

After the work of Pasteur and Lister, biliary surgery developed rapidly but still remained a component of general surgery. Following the Second World War, biliary surgery progressed to being a part of surgical gastroenterology. After 1957, the landmark description of the intrahepatic anatomy of the liver by Couinaud enabled the feasibility of curative procedures, which had previously been declared impossible.

However, the performance of intrahepatic palliative bypasses (usually signalled by the onset of jaundice), first on the left liver and then on the right liver, made tremendous progress. This was further enhanced by greater knowledge of the surgical anatomy and understanding the liver parenchyma. In the 1980s, CT scanning techniques enabled the diagnosis of many liver tumours to be made, including colorectal metastases and hepatocellular carcinoma, both in the presence or absence of cirrhosis. Liver surgery had now come of age and grew rapidly. In 1985, the use of cyclosporine accelerated the progress of liver transplantation, which had previously been a dream akin to walking on the moon.

Finally, in 1989, laparoscopic cholecystectomy arrived. This has been described as key-hole surgery or minimally-invasive surgery. The learning curve from this operation unfortunately provided an increased need for repair of post-cholecystectomy biliary strictures. These strictures have now become much less frequent. Very few medical or surgical specialties have made so much progress in recent years. Hepatobiliary surgery is now a major surgical specialty with its own training programme. Hepatobiliary surgery was first an adventure but has achieved more and more so-called impossible conquests.

Biographical footnote on Jean-Louis Lortat-Jacob

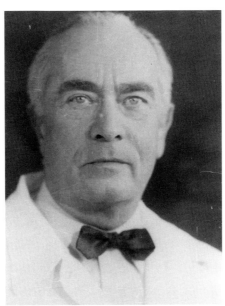

Figure 19. Jean-Louis Lortat-Jacob (1908-1992). *Reproduced from the author's private collection.*

Main institution: Hôpital Beaujon, Clichy, Paris.

His medical education was in the Faculty of Medicine in Paris; he was immediately appointed as a surgical registrar in various hospitals in Paris (1935-1940) before being appointed Chef de Clinique (Senior Registrar or Senior Resident) at the St. Louis Hospital.

At this stage in his career, Paris was occupied by German troops which meant that the advances in surgery, medicine and anaesthesia in the outside world were temporarily unavailable in France. In July 1944, he decided to resect a lower third oesophageal carcinoma by the left chest under local anaesthesia. The anastomosis was made using the famous Murphy button (see Chapter 10). A month later the patient did very well and was walking around the hospital courtyard before discharge. Precisely at this stage,

the Allied troops were fighting pitched battles with the retreating German army, and colleagues were so concerned that one said to Dr. Lortat-Jacob: "Don't let the patient be killed by a sniper!" Fortunately, the patient was not put in danger and he did survive.

Immediately after the war was over, the results of oesophagectomy were disappointing, not because of technical failure, but because of respiratory insufficiency, even with mechanical ventilation. However, postoperative survival improved as anaesthetic and postoperative care improved. As a result, Lortat-Jacob received referrals from all over France and beyond. He performed over 2000 oesophagectomies during his professional lifetime; however, not only cancer patients were referred to him, but a whole range of oesophageal disorders which included complicated and uncomplicated reflux, reflux and caustic strictures, as well as other assorted problems, such as achalasia, pharyngeal diverticulum etc. He devised his own anti-reflux operation which emphasised repair of the hiatus and increase of the acuteness of the gastro-oesophageal angle. His wife even wrote a thesis on peptic ulcer of the oesophagus.

In 1957, he described a previously unrecognised entity which he called 'endobrachyoesophage', where a significant lining of the lower oesophagus is covered by a gastric type epithelium. Exactly in the same year, Barrett published his paper on the "Lower oesophagus lined with columnar epithelium". Perhaps the simpler-to-pronounce name of 'Barrett's Oesophagus' was the reason for the eponymous name to be remembered more easily!

In 1949, he joined François de Gaudard d'Allaines' famous cardiovascular surgery team which is where Associate Professor, Charles Dubost, performed the first resection of an abdominal aortic aneurysm in the world. In 1956, he moved to Hôpital Tenon and finally to the Hôpital Beaujon in 1961 until his retirement in 1978.

Lortat-Jacob's expertise extended far beyond the oesophagus; he became a doyen of gastric cancer as well. In 1950, he described the technique of total gastrectomy which included splenectomy, resection of the tail of the pancreas and full lymph node clearance via his thoracophrenicolaparotomy approach. The mortality of total gastrectomy in his hands was no different from subtotal gastrectomy. Thus, he became an advocate of total gastrectomy 'in principle' against sub-total gastrectomy for cancer of the gastric antrum.

His repertoire also extended to the problems of portal hypertension, including portocaval, splenorenal shunts. Most significantly in 1952, he performed the first right hepatectomy extended to segment IV through a thoracophrenolaparotomy incision. He divided extrahepatically, the right hepatic duct, the right hepatic artery and right portal vein first, before dealing with the pedicles belonging to segment IV, and finally dividing the corresponding liver parenchyma.

Jean-Louis Lortat-Jacob was an elegant, precise and meticulous surgeon. He did not appear to hurry, but he was famous for employing both scissors and forceps in a 'supine' (concave sides upwards) position, which he used with great efficiency. The field of operation was invariably dry following a combination of diathermy and dividing between previously placed double ligatures. He constantly emphasised the importance of adequate exposure, and designed his own self-retaining retractors, especially for the chest. His oesophageal anastomoses were always in three layers of interrupted non-absorbable sutures.

In 1988, he celebrated his 80th birthday in the presence of Thomas Starzl who gave the first Lortat-Jacob lecture. All subsequent visiting lecturers have been very distinguished and have come from all over the world. All in all, Jean-Louis Lortat-Jacob left a huge heritage to French and world surgery lasting to the present day.

Dedication

This Chapter is dedicated to Raoul Praderi, a special friend and a great biliary surgeon who inspired us concerning the many significant events in the history of biliary surgery.

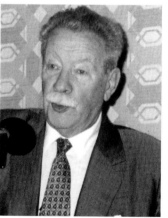

Figure 20. Raoul Praderi (born 1927). *Courtesy of Luis Ruso, MD.*

References

1. Bender GA. *Great moments in Medicine*. Detroit: Northwood Institute Press Ed, 1966: 50-5.

2. Bruns, cited by Beck C. Surgery of the liver. *JAMA* 1902; 38(17): 1063-8.

3. *Hippocratic aphorisms*. Paris: Le livre club du libraire ed, 1961.

4. Hippocrateic writings (translated by F Adams). *Great Book of the Western World*. Chicago: Encyclopaedia Britannica, 1952; Volume 10: 1-160.

5. Galen: On the natural faculties (translated by AJ Prock). *Great Book of the Western World*. Chicago: Encyclopaedia Britannica, 1952; Volume 10: 167-215.

6. Vesalius. A. *De Humanis Corporis Fabrica*. Gryphon Editions, The Classics of Surgery Library.

7. Huart P. *Leonardo da Vinci, Dessins Anatomiques (anatomie artistique, descriptive et fonctionnelles)*. Paris: Les editions Roger Dacosta, 1961: 167.

8. Paré A. *Conseiller et premier chirurgien du roi. Oevres avec les figures et les portraits tant de l'Anatomie que des instruments de chirurgie et de plusieurs monstres, le tout divisé en 26 livres. Premier livre, figure trois*. Paris: Gabriel Buon, 1575.

9. Rex H. Beiträge zur Morphologie der Säugerleber. *Morphol Jahrb* 1888; 14: 517-616.

10. Cantlie J. On a new arrangement of the right and left lobes of the liver. *J Anat Physiol* (London)(Section Proc Anat Soc Great Britain & Ireland) 1898; 32: 4-10.

11. Wendel W. Beitrage zur Chirurgie der leber. *Arch Klin Chir* 1911; 95: 887-94.

12. Wendel W. Leberlappenresection. *Arch Klin Chir* 1920; 114: 982-1000.

13. McIndoe AH, Countseller VS. A report on the bilaterality of the liver. *Arch Surg* 1927; 62: 589-611.

14. Hjortsjö CH. Topography of the intrahepatic bile duct systems. *Acta Anat* (Basel) 1951; 11: 599-615.

15. Elias H, Patty D. Gross anatomy of the blood vessels and bile ducts within the human liver. *Am J Anat* 1952; 90: 59-111.

16. Couinaud C. Bases anatomiques des hepatectomies droite et gauche réglées, techniques qui en découlent. *J Chir 5 Paris* 1954; 10: 933-66.

17. Tung TT. A new technique operating on the liver. *Lancet* 1963; 1: 192-3.

18. Couinaud C. *Le Foie: Études Anatomiques et Chirurgicales*. Paris: Masson ed, 1957.

19. Malt RA. Neoplasms of the liver. *New Engl J Med* 1985; 313: 1591-5.

20 Hepp J, Couinaud C. Abord et utilisation du canal biliaire gauche dans les réparations de la voie biliaire principale. *Presse Méd* 1956; 41: 917-8.

21. Bernard C. La Fonction glycogénique du Foie. *Comptes Rendus Hebdomadaires de l'Académie des Sciences* 1850; 31: 533-7.

22. Bernard C. Critique Expérimentale sur la glycémie. Des conditions physiologiques a remplir pour constater la présence de sucre dans le sang. *Comptes Rendus Hebdomadaires des séances de l'Académie des Sciences* (Paris) 1876; 82: 1405-10.

23. Bernard C. Sur le mécanisme de la formation du sucre dans le foie. *Comptes Rendus Hebdomadaires de l'Académie des Sciences* 1855; 61: 461-9.

24. Eck N. Kvoprosu o percvyazkie voronois veni: Predvaritelnoye soobschjenye. *Voen Med J* 1877; 130: 1-2 (translated by CC Child III). *Surg Gynecol Obstet* 1953; 96: 375-6.

25. Hahn O, Massen H, Nenck IM, Pavlov J. Die Eck's sche Fistel zwischen der unteren Hohlvene und der Pfortader und ihre Folgen fur den Organismus. *Arch Experim Path Phar* 1893; 32: 161-2.

26. Fausto N, Hadjis NS, Fong Y. Liver hyperplasia, hyperplasia, hypertrophy and atrophy and the molecular basis of liver regeneration. In: *Surgery of the liver and biliary tract*. Blumgart LH, Fong YWB, Eds. London: Saunders, 2000: 65-84.

27. Mann FC. The William Henry Welch lectures II: Restoration and pathologic reactions of the liver. *Mt Sinai J Med* 1944; 11: 65-74.

28. Starzl TE, Watanabe K, Porter KA, Putnam CW. Effects of insulin, glucagon, and insulin/glucagon infusions in liver morphology and cell division after complete porto-caval shunt in dogs. *Lancet* 1976; 1: 821-5.

29. Guillouzo A. Personnal communication.

30. Dupuytren G. *Leçons orales de Clinique Chirurgicale faites à L'Hotel-Dieu de Paris par le Baron Dupuytren*. Ballière: Paris. 1839; 6: 429.

31. Garré C. On resection of the liver. *Surg Gynecol Obstet* 1907; 5: 331-41.

32. Keen WW. Report of a case of resection of the liver for removal of a neoplasm, with a table of seventy-six cases of resection of the liver for hepatic tumours. *Ann Surg* 1899; 30: 267-83.

33. Pringle JH. Notes of the arrest of the hepatic hemorrhage due to trauma. *Ann Surg* 1908; 48: 541-9.

34. Turner GG. A case in which an adenoma weighing 2lb 3oz was successfully removed from the liver: with remarks on the subject of partial hepatectomy. *Proc R Soc Med* (part 3, Section of Surgery) 1923; 16: 43-64.

35. Meyer-May J, Ton TT. Resection anatomique du lobe gauche du foie pour cancer: Guerison opératoire et survie de 5 mois. *Mém Acad Chir* 1939; 65: 1208-16.

36. Lortat-Jacob JL, Robert HG. Hépatectomie droite réglée. *Presse Méd* 1952; 60: 549-52.

37. Quatllebaum JK. Massive resection of the liver. *Ann Surg* 1952; 137: 787-95.

38. Starzl TE, Itwatsuki S, Shaw BW, *et al*. Left hepatic trisegmentectomy. *Surg Gynecol Obstet* 1982; 155: 21-7.

39. Fredet M, Bernier E. Hépatectomie segmentaire droite réglée pour angiome caverneux du foie. *Mém Acad Chir* 1956; 62: 1060.

40. Champeau M, Pineau P. Voie d'abord élargie transhépatique du canal hépatique gauche. *Mém Acad Chir* 1964; 90: 602-13.

41. Ton TT. *Les resections majeures et mineures du foie*. Paris: Masson ed, 1979

42. Launois B, Corman J, Martineau G. Voie d'abord abdominale de la veine cave inférieure sus-hépatique *Mém Acad Chir* 1874; 100: 429-31.

43. Lai EC, Fan ST, Lo CM, Chu KM, Liu CL. Anterior approach for difficult major right hepatectomy. *World J Surg* 1996; 20: 314-7. Discussion 318.

44. Launois B, Jamieson GG. The posterior intrahepatic approach to resection of the liver. *Surg Gynecol Obstet* 1992; 174: 7-10.

45. Lin TY. Results in 107 hepatic lobectomies with a preliminary report of the use of a clamp to reduce blood loss. *Ann Surg* 1973; 177: 413-21.

46. Lin TY. A simplified technique for hepatic resection. The crush method. *Ann Surg* 1974; 180: 285-90.

47. Bismuth H. *La technique des hepatectomies*. Paris: Encycl Med Chir, 1984; *Techn Chir* 1970; 40-945: 1-16.

48. Foster J, Brennan M. Solid liver tumors. In: *Major problems in clinical surgery*. Ebert P, Ed. Philaldephia: WB Saunders, 1977: 209-34.

49. Putnam CW. Techniques of ultrasonic dissection in resection of the liver. *Surg Gynecol Obstet* 1983; 57: 474-8.

50. Finkelstein JL, Hodgson WJ, McFinney AJ, Aufses AH. Preliminary studies using ultrasonic device for endarterectomy. *Mt Sinai J Med* 1979; 46: 107-10.

51. Starzl TE, Marchioro TL, Von Kaulla N, Herman G, Britain RS, Wadell WR. Homotransplantation of the liver in humans. *Surg Gynecol Obstet* 1963; 17: 659-76.

52. Starzl TE, Marchioro TL, Waddell W. The reversal of rejection in human homografts with subsequent development of homograft tolerance. *Surg Gynecol Obstet* 1963; 117: 385-95.

53. Metchnikoff E. Etudes sur la resorption des cellules. *Annales de L'Institut Pasteur* 1899; 10: 737-89.

54. Woodruff MF, Anderson NF. Effect of lymphocyte depletion by thoracic duct fistula and administration of anti-lymphocytic serum on the survival of homografts in rats. *Nature* (London) 1963; 200: 702.

55. Starzl TE, Marchioro TL, Porter KA, Iwasaki Y, Cerilli J. Use of heterologous anti-lymphoid agents in canine renal and liver homotransplantations and in human renal homotransplantations. *Surg Gynecol Obstet* 1967; 124: 301-18.

56. Starzl TE, Groth GG, Brettschneider L, *et al.* Orthotopic homotransplantations of the human liver. *Surg Gynecol Obstet* 1968; 124: 392-415.

57. Starzl TE, Putnam CW. *Experience in hepatic transplantation*. Philadelphia: WB Saunders Company. Also in: *1969 Liver transplantation*. Philadelphia: WB Saunders Company, 1967.

58. Launois B, Corman J, Porter KA, Ryerson T, Bostroni S. Gustafsson A, Groth CG, Starzl T. Radioiodinated rose bengal kinetics in extrahepatic biliary obstruction and hepatic homograft rejection in the dog. *Surg Forum* 1972; 23: 338-9.

59. Benichou J, Halggrimson CG, Weil III R, Koep LJ, Starzl TE. Canine and human liver preservation for 6 to 18 hr by cold infusion. *Transplantation* 1977; 24: 407-11.

60. Starzl TE, Koep L, Porter K, Schroter G, Weil III R, Hartley RB, Halgrimson CG. Decline in survival after liver transplantation. *Arch Surg* 1980; 115: 815-9.

61. Borel JF, Feurer C, Gubler HU, Stachelin H. Biological effects of cyclosporin A. A new antilymphocytic agent. *Agents and Actions* 1976; 6: 468-75.

62. Calne R, Rolles K, White GJ, Thiru S, Evans DB, McMaster P, Dunn DC, Craddock GN, Henderson RG, Azzis S, Lewis P. Cyclosporin A initially as the only immunosuppressant in 34 recipients of cadaveric urgans: 32 kidneys, 2 pancreas and 2 livers. *Lancet* 1979; 2: 1033-6.

63. Starzl TE. *The puzzle people*. University of Pittsburgh Press, 1992.

64. Starzl TE, Klintmalm GBG, Porter KA, ItwatsukI S, Schroter G. Liver transplantation with use of cyclosporine A and prednisone. *New Engl J Med* 1981; 305: 266-9.

65. Schmid R. Issues in liver transplantation. *Hepatology suppl* 1984: 1-104.

66. Starzl TE, Hakala TR, Shaw BW, Hardesty RL, Rosenthal TE, Griffith BP, Iwatsuki S, Bahson HT. A flexible procedure for multiple organ procurement. *Surg Gynecol Obstet* 1984; 158: 223-30.

67. Starzl TE, Miller C, Broznick B, Makowka L. An improved technique for multiple organ harvesting. *Surg Gynecol Obstet* 1987; 165: 343-8.

68. Belzer FO, Ashby BS, Dunphy JE. 24 hour and 72 hour preservation of canine kidneys. *Lancet* 1967; 2: 536-8.

69. Jamieson V, Sundberg R, Lindell S, Laravuso R, Kalayoglu M, Southard JF, Belzer FO. Successful 24-to-50 hour preservation of the canine liver. Preliminary report. *Transplantation Proceedings* 1988; 20: 145-7.

70. Kalayayoglu M, Sollinger HW, Stratta RJ, *et al.* Extended preservation of the human liver for clinical preservation. *Lancet* 1988; I: 617-9.

71. Shaw BW Jr, Martin DJ, Marquez JM, *et al.* Venous bypass in clinical liver transplantation. *Ann Surg* 1984; 200: 524-34.

72. Bismuth B, Houssin D. Reduced-sized orthotopic liver grafting hepatic transplantation in children. *Surgery* 1984; 95: 367-70.

73. Pichmayr R, Ringe B, Gubernatis G, Hauss J, Bunzendahl H. Transplantation einer neue Spenderleber auf zwei empfengre (splitting transplantation). Eine Neue Methode in der Weiterntwicklung der Lebersegmenttransplantation. *Langenbecks Arch fur Chirurgie* 1988; 373: 127-30.

74. Raia S, Nery JR, Mies S. Liver transplantation from a live donor. *Lancet* 1989; 2: 497-511.

75. Strong RW, Lynch SV, Ong TH, Matsunami H, Koido Y, Balderspoon GA. Successful liver transplantation from a living donor to her son. *New Engl J Med* 1990; 322: 505-7.

76. Fan ST, Lo CM, Liu CL. Transplantation of the right hepatic lobe. *New Engl J Med* 2002; 347: 615-8.

77. Sheshadi W. The biliary system through the ages. *Int Surg* 1979; 64: 63-7.

78. Praderi R, Hess W. A brief history of bilio-pancreatic diseases and their treatments. In: *Textbook of biliopancreatic diseases*. Hess W, Berci G. Padova Piocin, 1997; 14(12): 2819-52.

79. Daremberg C. *Oeuvres choisies d'Hippocrate*. Paris: Labe, 1885.

80. Daremberg C. *Oeuvres anatomiques, physiologiques et médicales de Galien*. Paris: Baillière, 1954.

81. Glenn F. Biliary tract disease since antiquity. *Bull NY Acad Med* 1971; 47: 329.

82. Gohrbandt T. Anastomosen intrahepatischer gallen wedge mit dem magen und darm kanal (unter benut-zung von gumm, prothesen). *Arch Klein Chr* 1934; 179: 665.

83. Praderi R. Avicenna: one hundred years of biliary surgery. *Surg Gastroenterol* 1982; 1: 269-87.

84. Major Ralph H. *Classic Descriptions of Disease. With biographical sketches of the Authors*. Third Edition, 5th

85. Schenck J. *Observationum medicarum rararum, novarum Sumpt.* Rhodii Francoturii, 1600.

86. Bonet T. *Sepulchretum, sive anatomia practica ex cadaveribus morbo denatis.* L. Chouet Geneva, 1679.

87. Hepp J, Coinaud C. L'abord et l'utilisation du canal hapatique gauche dans les reparations de la voie biliare principale. *Presse Méd* 1956; 64: 947-8.

88. Petit JL. Remarques sur les tumeurs formées par la bile retenue dans la vésicule du fiel qu'on a souvent prises pour des abcès au foye. *Mém Acad Chir* 1743; 1: 255.

89. Morgagni GB. *De sedibus et causis morborum per anatomen, indagatis libri quinque.* Remonlimania, Venetiis, 1761.

90. Gordon-Taylor G. Gall stones and their sufferers. *Br J Surg* 1937; 25: 241.

91. Bobbs J. A case of lithotomy of the gallbladder. *Trans Med Soc Indiana* 1868; 68: 6.

92. Sims JM. Remarks on cholecystostomy in biopsy of the gallbladder. *Br Med J* 1878; 1: 811.

93. Halsted WS. *Surgical Papers.* The Johns Hopkins Press 1924; 427-62.

94. Quick AJ. The prothrombin in haemophilia and in obstructive jaundice. *J Biol Chem* 1935; 2109: 153.

95. Dam CP. The constitution of vitamin K2. *J Biol Chem* 1940; 133: 721.

96. Kocher T. Mobilsierung des duodenum und gastroduoden-ostomie. *Zentrabl Chir* 1903; 30: 33.

97. Tait L. Cholecystostomy versus cholecystectomy. *Br Med J* 1885; 1: 224.

98. Langenbuch C. Ein fall von exsterpation der gallenblase wegen chronischer cholelithiasis. *HeilungBerl Klein Wochenschr* 1882; 19: 237.

99. Garrison FH. *Introduction to the history of medicine.* 4th Ed. Philaldelphia: WB Saunders & Co, 1929: 353-4, 504-6.

100. Langenbuch C. *Chirurgie der Leber and Gallenblase.* Stuttgart: Ferdinand and Enke, 1894-1897.

101. Halpert B. Carl Langenbuch - master surgeon of the biliary system. *Arch Surg* 1932; 25: 178.

102. Graham F, et al. *Diseases of the Gallbladder and Bile Ducts.* Philadelphia: Lea and Febiger, 1928: 142-4, 399-400.

103. Glenn F, Johnson G, Pearce C. Intravenous cholangiography in biliary tract disease. *Ann Surg* 1960; 152: 91.

104. Glenn F, et al. Percutaneous transhepatic cholangiography. *Radiology* 1962; 78: 362.

105. Georgopoulos SK, Schwartz LH, Jarnagin WR, Gerdes H, Breite I, Fong Y, et al. Comparison of magnetic resonance and endoscopic cholangiopancreatography in malignant pancreatobiliary obstruction. *Arch Surg* 1999; 234: 1002-7.

106. Mirizzi PL. La colangiografia durante las operationes de las vias biliares. *Bol Soc Cir Buenos Aires* 1932; 16: 1133-5.

107. Mirizzi PL. Operative cholangiography. *Surg Gynecol Obstet* 1937; 65: 702-10.

108. Caroli J. Personal communication.

109. Huguier M, Bornet P, Charpak Y. Selective contraindications based on multivariate analysis for operative cholangiography in biliary lithiasis. *Surg Gynecol Obstet* 1991; 172(6): 470-4.

110. Hepp J, Bismuth H. Problèmes généraux de la chirurgie de la lithiase biliaire. *Enc Medico-chir* 1983; 40915: 1-16.

111. Khalili M, Philips EH, Berci G, et al. Final score of laparoscopic cholecystectomy. *Surg Endosc* 1997; 16: 1095-8.

112. Flowers JL, Zucker KA, Graham SM, et al. Laparoscopic cholangiography. *Ann Surg* 1992; 215: 209-16.

113. Stuart A, Thompson TIG, Alvord LA. Routine intraoperative laparoscopic cholangiography. *Am J Surg* 1998; 176: 632-7.

114. Kullman E, Borch K, Lindstrom E, et al. Management of of bile duct stones in the era of laparoscopic cholecystectomy: appraisal of routine operative cholangiography and endoscopic treatment. *Eur J Surg* 1996; 162: 872-80.

115. Lukichev O, Filimonov M, Zybin I. A method of laparoscopic cholecystectomy. *Kirurgia* 1983; 8: 125-7.

116. Muhe E. Personal communication to the author.

117. Underwood LA, Soper NJ. Laparoscopic cholecystectomy and choledocholithotomy. In: *Surgery of the liver and biliary tract.* Blumgart LH, Fong Y. London: WB Saunders, 2000.

118. Dubois F. Personal Communication to Editor, 2003.

119. Dubois F, Berthelot G, Levard H. Cholécystectomie par coelioscopie. *Presse Méd* 1989; 18: 180-2.

120. Dubois F. Coelioscopic cholecystectomy. *Ann Surg* 1990; 4: 5062.

121. Perissat J, Collet D, Belliard R. Gallstones: laparoscopic treatment in cholecystectomy, cholecystostomy, and lithotomy. Our own experience. *Surg Endosc* 1990; 4: 1-5.

122. Reddick E, Olsen DO, Daniel JF. Laparoscopic laser cholecystectomy. *Laser Med News Adv* 1989; 7: 38-40.

123. Reddick EJ, Olsen DO. Laparoscopic laser cholecystectomy. A comparison with minilap cholecystectomy. *Surg Endosc* 1989; 3: 31-3.

124. Cuschieri A. Laparoscopic revolution. *J Roy Coll Surg Edin* 1990; 34: 295.

125. Kümmel H. Zur chirurgie der gallenblase. *Deustch Med Wochenschr* 1890; 12: 237.

126. Riedel B. *Erfahrungen uber die gallensteinkrank beit mit une ohne ikterus.* Berlin: Hirschwold, 1892.

127. Abbe R. The surgery of gallstone obstruction. *Med Rec* 1893; 43: 548.

128. Thornton J. Removal of a calculus from the common bile duct - 2 inches long and 3½ inches in circumference - without suturing the duct. *Lancet* 1898; 2: 22.

129. Courvoisier LG. *Casnistish - Statistische beitrage zur pathologie und chirurgie der gallenwege.* Leipzig: Vogen, 1890.

130. Iversen H. In: *Gallstones, causes and treatment.* Rains AH. London: Heinemann, 1964.

131. Kehr H. *Chirurgie der gallenwege.* Stuttgart: Ferdinand Enke, 1913.

132. Kehr H. Die behandlung der kalkulosen cholangitis durch die direkte drainage der ductus hepaticus. *Munch Med Wochenschr* 1897; 44: 128.

133. Kehr H. *Bericht uber 137 gallensteinslaparotomien.* Munchen: Lehman, 1904.

134. Gosset A. Chirurgie du canal cholédoque et du canal hépatique. *Cong Fr Chir* 1908; 21: 85.

135. Quenu A, Duval P. Les angiocholites aiguës. *Congrès Soc Intern Chir* 1908; 20:(2): 453.

136. Mendet A. Technica de la extraction incruenta de los calculos en la lithiasis residual del coledoco. *Bull Soc Cir Buenos Aires* 1962; 46: 278.

137. Mazariello R. L'extraction instrumental de los calculos biliaires résiduales. *Bull Soc Arg Cir* 1966; 27: 640.

138. Kehr H. Gallensteine. *Congrès Soc Intern Chir* 1908; 20: (2), 341.

139. Mayo W. Cancer of the common bile duct. Report of a case of carcinoma of the duodenal end of the common duct with successful excision. *St Paul Med J* 1901; 3: 374.

140. Mayo-Robson A, Dobson J. *Diseases of the gall bladder and their bile ducts including gallstones.* New York: Wood, 1904.

141. Korte W. *Beitage zur chirurgie der gallenwege un der leber.* Berlin: Hirschwald, 1905.

142. Classen M, Demling L. Endoskopische Sphinkterotomie der Papilla Vater. *Dtsch Medizinische Wochenschrift* 1974; 99: 496-7.

143. Kawai K, Akssaka Y, Murakami K, Kohli Y, Nakajima M. Endoscopic sphincterotomy of the ampulla of Vater. *Gastrointestinal Endoscopy* 1974; 20: 148-51.

144. Petelin J. Laparoscopic approach to common bile duct pathology. *Surg Laparosc Endosc* 1991; 1: 33-7.

145. Winiwarter von A. Ein fall von gallenretention bedingt durch impermeabilitat des ductus choledocus anlegung einer gallen blasen darmfistel, heilung. *Prager Mediz Wochensf* 1882; 7: 201.

146. Sprengel O. Uber einen fall von extirpation der gallenblase mit anlegungeiner communication znischen ductus choledochus und duodenum. *Arch Klein Chir* 1891; 42: 550.

147. Sasse F. Ober choledochoduodenostomies. *Arch Klein Chir* 1913; 100: 969.

148. Flörcken H, Sieden E. Die nah und fernergebnissen der choledocho-duodenostomies. *Arch Klin Chir* 1923; 124: 59.

149. Monastyrsk ND. Zur frage der chirurgischen behandlung der vollstandigen undurchangikeit des ductus choledocus. *Zentrabl Chir* 1888; 15: 778.

150. Bardenheuer R. Anlegung einer gallenblasen Dumm darmfisteln. *Berlin Klein Wochenschr* 1888; 25: 877.

151. Terrier F. Remarques cliniques sur un cas d'obstruction du canal cholédoque avec dilatation de la vésicule biliaire, laparotomie. Ponction de la vésicule, cholésysto-entérostomie guérison. *Rev Chir* 1889; 9: 973.

152. Terrier F. Remarques sur deux cas, l'un de cholécysto-duodénostomie, l'autre de cholécysto-gastrotomie. *Rev Chir* 1896; 16: 169.

153. Courvoisier LG. *Casuistisch-statistische Beiträge zur Pathologie und Chirurgie der Gallenwege.* Leipzig: Verlag von FCW Vogel, 1890; XII: 376, citation 57-8.

154. Kappeler O. Die einzeithge cholecystostomie. *Korrespondiezbl Sweinzer Arste* 1889; 17: 213.

155. Murphy JB. Cholecysto-intestinal gastrointestinal, entero-intestinal anastomoses and approximation without sutures. *Med Rec* 1892; 42: 665.

156. Kocher T. Ein fall von choledoco-duodenostomia interna wegen gallen stein. *Korrespondenzbl Schweizer Arste* 1895; 1: 192.

157. McBurney C. Removal of biliary calculi from the common duct by the duodenal route. *Ann Surg* 1898; 28: 481.

158. Halsted W. Contribution to the surgery of the bile passages, especially the common bile duct. *Johns Hopkins Hosp Bull* 1900; 11: 1.

159. Kausch W. Uber gallenwege-darm, verdungen. *Arch Klin Chir* 1912; 97: 449.

160. Hartmann H. *Chirurgie des voies biliaires.* Paris: Masson, 1923.

161. Monprofit A. Du remplacement du cholédoque et de l'hépatique par une anse jéjunale. *Cong Fr Chir* 1904; 13: 380.

162. Dahl R. Eine new operation des gallennwege. *Zentrabl Chir* 1909; 36: 206.

163. Maragliano D. Cholecystenterostomies verbunden mit entero-anastomose. *Zentrabl Chir* 1903; 30: 941.

164. Praderi R, Estefan A, Gomez-Fossatti C, Mazza M. Derivations bilio-jejunale sur anses excluses. Modifications techniques du procede de Hivet-Warren. *Lyon Chir* 1973; 69: 459.

165. Kehr H. Hepato-cholangio-enterostomie. *Zentrabl Chir* 1904; 31: 185.

166. Longmire WF, Sanford MT. Intrahepatic cholangiojejunostomy with partial hepatectomy for obstuction. *Surg* 1948; 24: 264.

167. Dogliotti M. Gastrohepatoductostomies dans le traitement chirurgical des obstructions des voies voies biliaires. *Lyon Chir* 1951; 46: 353-6.

168. Soupault R, Couinaud C. Sur un procédé de derivation biliare intra-hepatique: cholangio-jejunostomie gauche sans sacrifice hepatique. (A new procedure for intra-hepatic biliary shunt: left cholangiojejunostomy without sacrificing the liver.) *Presse Méd* 1957; 65(50): 1157-9.

169. Hepp J. La place des hepatectomies dans las anastomoses biliodigestives intra-hépatiques. *Rev Int Hépat* 1960; 10: 1005-10.

170. Hepp J, Bismuth H. L'anastomose intrahépatique droite. *Ent Bichat Chirurgie* 1959; 9: 633-46.

171. Bismuth H, Lechaux JP. *Les anastomoses bilio-digestives intra-hépatiques.* Encycl Med Chir (Editions Scientifiques et Médicales). Paris: Elsevier SAS. *Techniques Chirurgicales-Appareil Digestif* 1970: 40-945: 1-16.

172. Prioton JB, Bernard JH, Serrroux B. La double cholangio-jéjunostomie périphérique. (Droite et Gauche) dans le traitement des cancers primitifs du confluent biliere supérieur. *Montpelier Chir* 1968; 14: 317-35.

173. Launois B. Transhepatic Glissonian approach to liver resection. In: *Surgery of the liver and biliary tract.* Blumgart LH, Fong Y. London: WB Saunders, 2000: 1702.

174. Lahey H, Pyrtek ILJ. Experience with operative management of 280 strictures of the bile ducts. *Surg Gynecol Obstet* 1930; 114: 25-6.

175. Cole WH, Ireneus C, Reynolds JT. Strictures of the common bile duct: studies in 122 cases. *Ann Surg* 1955; 142: 537-50.

176. Nuboer JF. Des stenoses cicatricielles des voies biliaires extra-hépatiques. *Lyon Chir* 1967; 63: 481-94.

177. Smith R. Hepaticojejunostomy with transhepatic intubation. A technique for very high strictures of the hepatic ducts. *Br J Surg* 1964; 51: 186-94.

178. Katos, Nakagawa T, Kobayashi H, Arai E, Isetani K. Formation of the common hepatic duct associated with an anomalous junction of the pancreaticobiliary ductal system and gallbladder cancer. A report of a case. *Surgery Today* 1994; 24: 534-7.

179. Blalock KA. A statistical study of 888 cases of biliary tract disease. *John Hopkins Hosp Bull* 1924; 35: 391-409.

180. Glenn F, Hayes DM. The scope of radical surgery in the treatment of malignant tumors of the extrahepatic biliary tract. *Surg Gynecol Obstet* 1954; 99: 529-41.

181. Nimura Y, Hayakaw AN, Kamiya J, Maeda S, Kondo S, Yasui A, Shionoy A. Hepatopancreatoduodenectomy for advanced carcinoma of the biliary tract. *Hepatogastroenterology* 1991; 38: 170-5.

182. Tompkins RK, Thomas D, Wile A, Longmire WP, Jr. Prognostic factors in bile duct carcinoma. *Ann Surg* 1981; 194: 487-97.

183. Altemeier WA, Gall EA, Zinninger NN, Hoxworth IP. Sclerosing carcinoma of the hepatic bile ducts. *Arch Surg* 1957; 75: 450-61.

184. Klatskin G. Adenocarcinoma of the hepatic duct at its bifurcation within the porta hepatis. *Am J Med* 1965; 38: 141-56.

185. Brown G. Surgical removal of tumours of the hepatic ducts. *Postgrad Med* 1954; 16: 79.

186. Launois B, Campion JP, Brissot JP, Gosselin M. Carcinoma of the hepatic hilus: surgical management and the case for resection. *Ann Surg* 1979; 120: 151-7.

187. Blumgart LH, Benjamin IS, Hadjis NS, Beazley R. Surgical approaches of cholangiocarcinoma at the confluence of the hepatic ducts. *Lancet* 1984; 1: 66-70.

188. Launois B, Terblanche J, LakehaL M, Catheline JM, Bardaxoglou E, Landen S, *et al.* Proximal bile duct cancer: high resectability rate and 5-year survival. *Ann Surg* 1999; 230: 266-75.

189. Pichmayr R, Ringe B, Lauchart W, Bechstein WO, Gubernatis G, Wagner E. Radical resection and liver grafting as the two main components of surgical strategy in the treatment of proximal bile duct cancer. *World J Surg* 1988; 12: 99-101.

Chapter 8

Surgery of the pancreas

Jackie Y Tracey MD, Postdoctoral Fellow in Surgery

Abdool R Moossa MD FRCS (Eng & Edin) FACS

Professor of Surgery and Emeritus Chairman

Associate Dean and Special Counsel to the Vice Chancellor for Health Sciences

Director of Tertiary and Quarternary Referral Services

UCSD Thornton Hospital, San Diego, California, USA

Introduction

Surgery of the pancreas belongs to the 20th century and beyond. Part of this delayed surgical importance is due to its location and functions; surgeons have feared its manipulation because of its irritability. Its complex anatomical relationship has been summarised as follows: "The pancreas cuddles the left kidney, tickles the spleen, hugs the duodenum, cradles the aorta, opposes the inferior vena cava, dallies with the right renal pedicle, hides behind the posterior parietal peritoneum of the lesser sac and wraps itself around the superior mesenteric vessels." [1] In addition, it is largely hidden from view in the retroperitoneum. Thus, exposure of the anterior surface of the gland demands a major laparotomy, wide division of the gastrocolic omentum, elevation of the stomach, and downward retraction of the transverse colon and mesocolon. Palpation of the head of the gland can only be performed after a wide Kocher manoeuvre, elevating the pancreaticoduodenal segment off the posterior parietal structures, i.e. the right kidney, right renal vessels, inferior vena cava, left renal vein, and aorta. Full examination of the body and tail of the gland necessitates division of the lienorenal ligament, and mobilisation of the spleen and body and tail of the pancreas off the left kidney and other posterior parietal structures. Moreover, the intimate association of the pancreas with major vessels of the epigastrium limits the extirpative extent of any procedure and dictates what must be removed. The need to excise vessels and regional lymph nodes often makes removal of adjacent organs, such as the duodenum, common bile duct and, sometimes, the spleen and part of the stomach, necessary. It is for these reasons, that the pancreas is difficult to manage surgically when compared with other abdominal viscera. As a result pancreatic surgery had to await the advances in anaesthesia, antisepsis and haemostasis before it could develop.

Early history

The pancreas is thought to have been discovered by Herophilus of Chalkidon [2], a Greek anatomist and surgeon about 300 BC. He is also acknowledged to be the first to perform human dissections before an audience and was one of the founders of the ancient school of Medicine in Alexandria, Egypt.

Four hundred years later, the term 'pan-kreas' was coined by a famous anatomist and surgeon, Ruphos of Ephesus in 100 AD. Pancreas in Greek means: pan = all; kreas = flesh, or meat. Apparently, the Greeks recognised that the pancreas was a discrete organ, but failed to understand its function. Galen (130-200) (Figure 1, Chapter 1), born in Asia Minor (later became 'Physician to the Gladiators' in Rome as well as to Emperor Marcus Aurelius), described the pancreas as a secreting gland, yet he thought that the pancreas mainly served as a cushion or pad to protect and support the large blood vessels that were lying immediately behind.

Incredibly, he did not identify the pancreatic duct; yet, he described its arterial supply and venous drainage. Galen's word or 'law' was not to be challenged for well over a 1000 years until Vesalius, in the 16th century, received tremendous hostility from the establishment, as described in the first chapter. It remains unclear whether Hippocrates had much regard for the organ.

Andreas Vesalius (1514-1564), the great Professor of Anatomy at Padua (Figure 2, Chapter 1) and, later of Bologna and Pisa, and physician to Charles V and Philip II of Spain, described the organ as glandular and separate from the omentum [2]. His illustrations focused extensively on the vessels running through it, although he did not identify it by name (Figure 1). An English translation from that period supplies the synonym 'swete bread'. Later translations of Latin anatomy books indicate that the term 'sweet-bread' was in general usage at that time.

The real study of the pancreas began with Wirsung in 1642. Johann Georg Wirsung (1606-1643) was a German émigré at the San Francisco Monastery in Padua, Italy, where he worked as the prosector to Veslingus when he described the main duct of the human pancreas and recorded it on a copper plate (Figure 2) [2, 3]. Unfortunately, he was murdered a year later by a disgruntled student. At that time the function of the duct eluded him and he wondered if it was an "artery or a vein". As he had "never seen blood in it", a colleague named it "The Duct of Wirsung".

Later, in 1663, a 22-year-old student, Reinier de Graaf (1641-1673) in Leiden, Netherlands, used a goose quill to cannulate a dog's pancreatic duct. De Graaf began the task of using experimentation rather than dogma as a basis for medical understanding, but unfortunately, he died of bubonic plague at age 32. In 1720, Abraham Vater [2, 4] of Wittenberg (1684-1751), described the duodenal ampulla named after him and, in 1742, Santorini [2, 4] of Venice illustrated the accessory duct bearing his name.

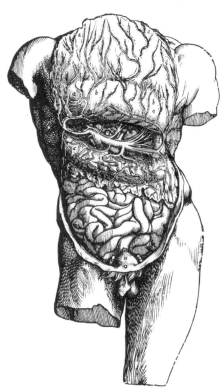

Figure 1. Anatomical drawing by Vesalius of the pancreatic region. *Reproduced with permission from the Classics of Surgery Library (Gryphon Editions), New York, USA.*

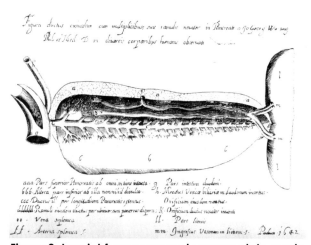

Figure 2. Imprint from engraved copper plate made by Wirsung in 1642. *Reproduced from Opie EL. Disease of the Pancreas: its cause and nature. Philadelphia and London: JB Lippincott Co., 1903: 17-45. Original source: Schirmer AM. Beitrag zur Geschichte und Anatomie des Pankreas. Basel, 1893: 11-9.*

History of endocrine function

Diabetes was recognised since the papyrus Ebers (about 1500 BC). Aretaeus of Cappadocia [2] (81-138 AD) first described the disease as "a melting down of the flesh and limbs into urine" and named the disease 'diabetes' from the Greek word for 'siphon'. It was later widely known as the 'Pissing Evil'. But, the association of diabetes and the pancreas was not made until 1889 when Oskar Minkowski (1849-1908) and Joseph von Mering [2] found that extirpation of the dog's pancreas resulted in urine which attracted flies whereas the urine of the non-pancreatectomised dogs attracted none. This observation led Minkowski [2] to analyze the urine and find glycosuria. Many further discoveries quickly followed: Paul Langerhans [4] (1847-1888), in his doctoral thesis described the islets of the pancreas; Laguesse [2] in 1893 suggested abnormalities of the islets might be the cause of diabetes; and, Eugene Opie [3] (1873-1971) found hyaline changes and destruction in the islets of the pancreas in diabetics and provided evidence towards the cause of the disease.

Frederic Banting (1891-1941), a surgeon, and Charles Best (1899-1878) (Figure 3), a medical student, showed that the extract of the pancreas, following previous ligation of its main duct, decreased the hyperglycaemia in diabetic dogs [5].

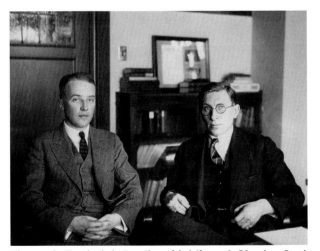

Figure 3. Frederick Banting (right) and Charles Best (left). *Reproduced with permission from the Thomas Fisher Rare Book Library, University of Toronto, Banting Papers.*

Insulin, was crystallised by J.J. Abel [6] (1857-1938) in 1926. One year later, a physician with severe hypoglycaemia was studied at the Mayo Clinic and explored by William Mayo [7], who found a tumour of the pancreas with metastasis to the liver. The biopsy showed a tumour of islet tissue. In 1929, Roscoe Graham of Toronto removed a functioning adenoma of islet cells of the pancreas from a woman. She was completely cured of her attacks for longer than 20 years of follow-up. In 1953, Whipple and Franz [8] reviewed 35 cases of insulin-secreting tumours and indicated the primary diagnostic criteria which became known as Whipple's triad:

- symptoms are reproduced by fasting and/or exercise;
- hypoglycaemia (blood sugar <50mg/dl) is confirmed with symptomatic episodes; and
- symptoms are relieved by glucose intake.

The amino acid sequence of insulin was determined in 1955 by Fred Sanger and colleagues and synthesis was attained in China, Germany and the US, with the secondary and tertiary structure determined in 1969. The next step in the evolution of pancreatic endocrinology is attributed to the brilliant work of Solomon A. Berson and Roslyn S. Yalow [9], who launched the era of radio-immunoassay with the famous measurement of endogenous plasma insulin in 1957. Further work was done by numerous workers, especially the University of Chicago group, led by Steiner and Rubenstein, which demonstrated that insulin is produced as a single chain precursor, pro-insulin, usually comprising 20% or less of the total serum immunoreactive insulin under ordinary circumstances. This pro-insulin is then split into C-peptide (connecting peptide) and insulin prior to storage in the beta cell granules. Thus, the modern diagnosis of hyperinsulinaemia now rests on the determination of glucose, insulin, pro-insulin, and C-peptide levels in the same serum specimen during fasting or during a symptomatic episode.

Numerous other peptides have now been identified as being secreted by the islet cells. Amylin or islet-amyloid associated polypeptide (IAPP) and pancreostatin have been identified, isolated and purified from the insulin-producing B-cells. Their physiological role has not been elucidated. Glucagon,

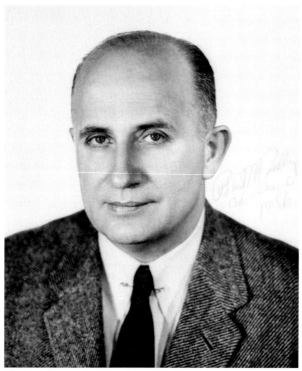

Figure 4. Robert M. Zollinger (1903-1992). *Reproduced with permission from the National Library of Medicine, Bethesda, Maryland, USA.*

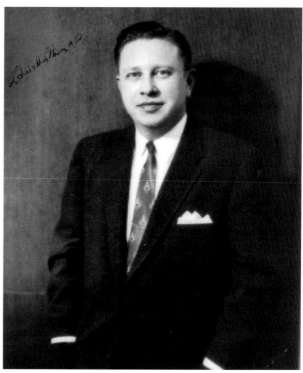

Figure 5. Edwin H. Ellison (1918-1970). *Reproduced with permission from the National Library of Medicine, Bethesda, Maryland, USA.*

the hormone antagonising the effects of insulin, is produced by the islet A-cells. Somatostatin is produced by the Delta or D-cells of the pancreatic islets, as well as D cells of the GI tract, as a 92-amino acid polypeptide prosomatostatin. Diazepam binding inhibitor (DBI) is an 86-amino acid polypeptide, also produced in the D cells of the acinar islets. Its physiological function is unknown.

The era of pancreatic endocrine surgery can be said to have been catapulted in 1955 when Robert M. Zollinger and Edwin H. Ellison [10] (Figures 4 and 5) presented two cases to the American Surgical Association, the proceedings of which were published later in the *Annals of Surgery*. Both patients died of multiple complications of intractable peptic ulcer disease. Drs. Zollinger and Ellison found metastatic non-B islet cell tumour in the abdomen and postulated that the tumour produces a secretagogue that simulated gastric hypersecretion.

Benjamin Eiseman of Denver first proposed that the clinical entity be named the Zollinger-Ellison (ZE)

syndrome. At about that time, Gregory in Liverpool, was busy isolating and purifying gastrin from the antral mucosa. At some point, a Zollinger-Ellison tumour was sent from UCLA by Morton Grossman to Gregory who extracted a high concentration of a gastrin-like substance from it. Gregory and his colleagues went on to isolate the pure peptide, gastrin, and identified its amino acid sequence.

The term 'gastrinoma' was first proposed by Morton Grossman [11] to describe the ZE tumour. Wilfred Circus of Liverpool and, later, of Edinburgh, defined the ZE syndrome as "recurrent ulcerators, persistent perforators, and bleeders unto death". Since the patients died of complications of the peptic ulcer diathesis and the tumours were metastatic or unidentified, the recommended treatment in the 1960s was removal of the end organ, namely, a total gastrectomy [12]. The 1970s witnessed the advent of H-2 receptor antagonists and later, proton pump inhibitors, all potent inhibitors of gastric acid secretion. This led to pharmacologic suppression of gastric hypersecretion, followed by evaluation of the patient to locate the gastrinoma. It soon became clear that there are two distinct types of patients with the ZE syndrome. One group, with metastatic disease as first described by Zollinger and Ellison, no longer need a total gastrectomy and is medically treated. The second group includes those who have a localised gastrinoma, usually in the 'gastrinoma triangle', which can be identified by modern imaging techniques and/or exploratory laparotomy. Such isolated tumours can now be resected with a high percentage of cure. Further refinement of radio-immunoassay and peptide chemistry led to the discovery of several other peptide hormones which are secreted by various islet cell tumours to produce well documented clinical syndromes. The term 'islet cell tumour' was replaced by apudoma (neoplasms that arise from pancreatic amine precursor uptake decarboxylase [APUD] cells). This was later changed to the current nomenclature of neuroendocrine tumour [13, 14]. Non-functioning neuroendocrine tumours do not produce any clinical syndrome, but may secrete chromogranin A and/or human pancreatic polypeptide. Serial radio-immunoassay of either of these peptides is now routinely used for diagnosis and monitoring response to therapy. The era of pancreatic endocrinology was further expanded when the hereditary syndromes of multiple endocrine neoplasias were documented in the 1980s. The genetic profile of many of these tumours has now been elucidated and further progress is on the way with the evolution of molecular genetics.

History of exocrine function

Ernest study of the pancreas' exocrine function began with Reinier de Graaf [2], a Dutch anatomist and physiologist (1641-1673). One of the dogs is shown in Figure 6. He inserted a duck's quill in the duct and tasted the juice, wrongly deciding that it was acidic; he then postulated that the juice played a role in digestion.

Claude Bernard [15] (Figure 8, Chapter 7) studied pancreatic juice from 1849 to 1856 and showed that it emulsified fats, splitting them into fatty acids and glycerol and that it converted starch to sugar. Thus, he showed that all digestion did not occur in the stomach and that pancreatic juice further aided in digestion of proteins which began in the stomach. The control of pancreatic exocrine secretion was first studied by Pavlov [2] and his pupils in 1888, using methods similar to those they used for gastric secretion. They stimulated the cervical vagus nerve in an acute experiment in which the pyloric canal was occluded in such a manner as to prevent entry of gastric acid into the duodenum but, not damage the vagal nerve fibres. This stimulation caused a slow flow of pancreatic juice enriched with enzymes. This conclusively proved that the vagus is a true secretory nerve to the pancreas and that it is responsible for the stimulation of enzyme secretion, but not water and salts.

In 1902, Bayliss and Starling [16] showed that introduction of a dilute HCL solution into the duodenum or an isolated loop of jejunum produced marked secretion of pancreatic juice. Extract of jejunal mucous membrane in a dilute HCL solution produced pancreatic secretion when injected into the jugular vein. They deduced that in the upper small intestine resides a humoral agent (secretin) which stimulated pancreatic secretion. The existence of the hormone, secretin, was soon confirmed by further physiological evidence. Nearly half a century later, the discovery of pancreozymin (cholecystokinin, CCK) by Harper and Raper in 1943 [17], became the third major advance in

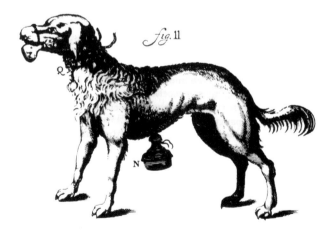

Figure 6. Reinier de Graaf's dog with collections of salivary and pancreatic juices taking place. *Reproduced from de Graaf R. Tractatus anatomico-medicus de succi pancreatici natura & usu. Lugd. Batavorum: Ex Officina Hackiana, 1671.*

our knowledge of the mechanism concerned in the stimulation of pancreatic secretion, those preceding it being the demonstration of the effect of the vagus nerve and the discovery of secretin. The hormonal status of pancreozymin (CCK) clarified a great many previous observations lacking satisfactory explanation since the time of Pavlov. The action of pancreozymin (CCK) is identical to that of the vagus on the secretion of enzymes with little or no significant flow of water, salts and alkali, but the pancreozymin (CCK) effect differs from that of the vagus in that it is resistant to atropine. Thus, a complete explanation of facts observed over 40 years, namely the varying power of different crude secretin preparations to excite enzyme production in addition to water and alkali, is the presence of varying amounts of secretin and pancreozymin (CCK) in different extracts. The eventual availability of pure secretin and pancreozymin (CCK) led to the development of multiple pancreatic function tests and pain reproduction tests over the end of the last century. These have now been largely abandoned because of poor accuracy or correlation with clinical symptoms and lack of patient acceptance.

Pancreatic imaging

The last 30 years can be labelled 'the age of imaging' and have witnessed the rapid evolution of diagnostic imaging techniques with complementary guided interventional procedures on the pancreas and other organs. In the 1950s and 1960s, the pancreas was indirectly visualised using contrast studies of the upper gastrointestinal (UGI) tract, namely, barium swallow and hypotonic duodenography. Reliance was placed on extrinsic compression and indentation, and rugal and mucosal abnormalities of the UGI tract. A pancreatic neoplasm had to be large or extensive to be diagnosed by these methods, which are now obsolete. In the 1960s, radionucleotide scintigraphy using ^{75}Se-L-selenomethionine became temporarily popular. Dilemmas in interpretation and faint or, partial, visualisation of the pancreas was such that this technique was also abandoned. The 1970s saw the emergence of non-invasive imaging using ultrasound and computed tomography. At the same time, the development of fiberoptic endoscopes in Japan led to the use of the invasive endoscopic retrograde cholangiopancreatography (ERCP).

General factors that handicap study of the pancreas by ultrasonography are gas in the GI tract, alteration of anatomy by previous abdominal operations, barium in the colon, and obesity. These factors may be partially overcome by transducer compression of the abdominal wall, changing the patient's position, and the use of the spleen, kidney and distended stomach (with water) as an acoustic window. The evolution of CT scans has largely replaced ultrasound as a method of visualising the pancreas. However, endoscopic ultrasound continues to be useful, but it is invasive and mandates the availability of an experienced endoscopist/ ultrasonographer.

Spiral CT scans with intravenous contrast and oral water (pancreatic protocol) is now the diagnostic modality of choice for pancreatic disorders. The size, contour and shape of the gland, the presence of any mass or ductal dilatation, its relationship to adjacent structures, such as the duodenum, common bile duct, and major vessels, can all be assessed. Modern CT scanning has virtually rendered diagnostic visceral angiography obsolete.

The rapid evolution of magnetic resonance imaging (MRI) has added a new dimension to diagnosing pancreatic disease. The addition of gadolinium contrast agents allows the identification of differences in enhancement patterns between the normal pancreas, pancreatitis, and carcinomas. MRIs have several disadvantages including a long imaging time, high cost, limited availability, and a high level of experience and expertise requirement for accurate interpretation. At present, MRI should be reserved for difficult cases when the CT scan is inconclusive or confusing, and when allergies to contrast or, renal impairment, prevents the use of a CT scan. As MRI technology improves, magnetic resonance imaging pancreatography (MRCP), may well emerge as the single best test for visualising the hepatobiliary system and the pancreas.

Since the 1970s, the development of and refinement in fiberoptic endoscopy, pioneered by the Japanese and Americans, led the impetus to cannulate the ampulla and perform both retrograde cholangiogram and pancreatogram (ERCP) for diagnostic purposes. Because of its invasiveness and the risk of developing pancreatitis and cholangitis, ERCP is now reserved for therapeutic purposes only, such as common bile duct stone retrieval or stent placement.

Early beginnings of direct operations on the pancreas

Chronologically, operations in the peri-ampullary area started with biliary-enteric anastomoses, followed by direct attack on the ampulla of Vater, before confronting the feared pancreaticoduodenal resection.

Biliary-enteric anastomosis

Early on it was recognised that pancreatic cancer gave rise to obstructive jaundice resulting in unbearable itching and bleeding, and quite often, terrible pain. The understanding that the absence of bile in the digestive tract and coagulopathy were related, led to the early operations to restore the flow of bile and correct bleeding. Bile peritonitis was also appreciated and was a feared sequel of any operation involving the biliary tract. In 1882, Alexander von Winiwarter [7] (1848-1917), a disciple of Billroth, created the first successful cholecystojejunostomy for a patient with a mass in the head of the pancreas. He came about this rather circuitously having first created a cholecystostomy and colostomy, believing the two fistulas would communicate. This, however, did not occur and at the fifth attempt the definitive cholecysto-jejunostomy endured and the patient survived. In 1887, Ruggiero Oddi successfully anastomosed the gallbladder to the stomach in three dogs after ligation of the common bile duct.

In 1888, Monastyrski [7] in Russia performed the first cholecystoduodenostomy in a patient suffering from pancreatic cancer. A year later, the French surgeon, Terrier [7], described a patient with pancreatic cancer and an enlarged gallbladder, in which he successfully performed a cholecystoduodenostomy.

Shortly thereafter in 1890, Ludwig Courvoisier (Figure 7), the Swiss surgeon, described his autopsy experience with jaundiced patients who died [7]. Courvoisier presented it as a description or 'sign', 'Courvoisier-Zeichen' (Courvoisier's sign) or 'Courvoisier-Regel' (Courvoisier's rule). He would no doubt disapprove of his observation being a 'law' as it is in English medical literature. He actually wrote: "Bei Steinobstruction des Choledochus ist Ectasie der Gallenblase selten; das organ ist vorher schon gewöhnlich geschrumpft. Bei Obstruction andrer Art ist dagegen ectasie das Gewöhnlich; Atrophie besteht nur 1/12 diese Fälle." When translated this means: "Thus with stone obstruction of the duct, dilation of the gallbladder is rarely observed; the organ has already undergone contraction; with obstruction from other causes, dilation is to be expected; atrophy exists in only 1/12 of these cases." [18]

In France it is often referred to as the 'Courvoisier-Terrier' Law. A possible exception to this rule is the simultaneous impaction of a stone in the cystic duct and another at the lower end of the common bile duct. In 1892, Murphy [7] in Chicago (Figures 7 and 8, Chapter 10), developed a metallic button to aid in the formation of the anastomosis and successfully performed three cholecystoduodenostomies. In 1882, Robert Gersuny [7], another Billroth protégé, performed a cholecystogastrostomy, as the duodenum and jejunum were blocked by cancer. The patient survived with resolution of her jaundice and this operation sustained itself due to its simplicity for the following four decades. These early biliary enteric operations were generally performed alongside a

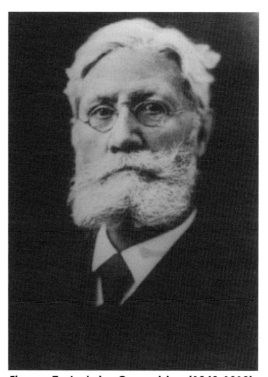

Figure 7. Ludwig Courvoisier (1843-1918).
Reproduced with permission from The Royal Society of Medicine, London, UK.

gastroenterostomy to decrease the likelihood of food refluxing into the gallbladder and to allow food to bypass the obstructed duodenum. Monprofit in 1904 [7] employed a Roux loop for cholecystojejunostomy; in 1908 [7] he proposed in a contribution to the French Congress of Surgery that it be used for hepatico-jejunostomy. Dahl was the first to successfully use a Roux loop in biliary surgery in 1909. Cholangitis had previously plagued many biliary-enteric anastomoses. This arrangement prevented the reflux of digestive tract contents into the biliary tree and decreased the likelihood of cholangitis.

Papillary operations

Before the turn of the 20th century, surgeons were removing biliary tract calculi by creating a duodenotomy and performing papillotomies for impacted calculi. The most famous was by Charles McBurney (Figure 8, Chapter 12), who had performed elective duodenotomy and papillotomy for embedded calculi in 1878. Kocher [7] (Figure 14, Chapter 12) popularised the choledochoduodenostomy following the removal of choledochal calculi, having performed some 20 of these by 1899. In the 1890s, attempts by surgeons in Germany and France to excise tumours in the ampullary area were unsuccessful. William Halsted of Baltimore (Figure 6, Chapter 10) was the first to remove a carcinoma of the ampulla by the duodenal route. Next came the report of William Mayo in 1900 of the successful resection of a peri-ampullary tumour [7]. This beckoned the quick technically feasible 'ampullectomy', or removal of the papilla, in the jaundiced, hypocoagulable patient with a peri-ampullary tumour. Vitamin K was yet to be discovered, so that patients with long-standing jaundice tended to bleed uncontrollably.

Direct operations on the pancreas

The earliest record of a direct surgical procedure involving the pancreas was the excision of part and, at times all, of the dog's gland by Johann Brunner [2] (1653-1727). Although his dogs were extremely thirsty postoperatively, he did not make the connection of polydipsia and diabetes. However, in humans, direct pancreatic surgery initially involved the drainage or resection of large cysts with the resulting formation of external fistulas. In 1883, Gussenbauer [7], another pupil of Billroth, marsupialised a pancreatic pseudocyst with survival; others soon followed. Antoni T. Jurasz (1882-1961) was the first to perform marsupialisation of the pancreatic cyst into the stomach. Subsequent attempts included the first cyst-enteric anastomosis in 1909 when Coffey [7] anastomosed the tail of the pancreas to a loop of small bowel. In 1911, the duodenum was used by Ombredanne [7]. The gallbladder was also employed for cyst drainage and although the patients survived and the procedure was technically feasible, it was rapidly abandoned. The development of the cyst-jejunostomy in 1943 by Chesterman [7] was met with more durability and the procedure persists to this day.

Pancreaticoduodenectomy

In 1898, Alessandro Codivilla [7], an Italian surgeon, performed the first pancreaticoduodenectomy for a mass in the head of the pancreas in a jaundiced patient. He resected the head of the pancreas, duodenum and pylorus and closed the duodenal stump, ligated the common bile duct above the pancreas and performed a cholecystojejunostomy with a Murphy's button, and a Roux-en-Y gastro-enterostomy. Unfortunately, the patient died 24 days later. But, this led other surgeons to follow his lead. It would be Walter Krausch [7] (1909-1967), the disciple of Mikulicz, who would be credited with the first successful two-staged pancreaticoduodenectomy while working in Berlin. At the first operation he performed a cholecystojejunostomy and six weeks later he completed a side-to-side gastroenterostomy in four hours, resected the head of the pancreas, pylorus and first and second parts of the duodenum and created a pancreaticojejunal anastomosis. The patient survived for nine months.

In 1935, Allen Oldfather Whipple performed an excision of a carcinoma of the ampulla of Vater and part of the head of the pancreas, using catgut sutures and ligatures. The patient died two days later. Autopsy showed digestion of the catgut with subsequent duodenal leakage. Whipple had previously used silk sutures on several patients with islet cell tumours without adverse effect. He was now convinced of the importance of non-absorbable suture material and the need for a more radical operation.

Lester Dragstedt of Chicago, in 1918, had successfully removed the duodenum from a dog with no ill effect. Hence, Whipple [7] (Figure 8) decided to resect the head of the pancreas with a complete duodenectomy, the distal common bile duct and terminal stomach, making an anastomosis between the end of the common duct and a limb of jejunum with a distal gastrojejunostomy. He performed the operation at first in two stages, but changed to one

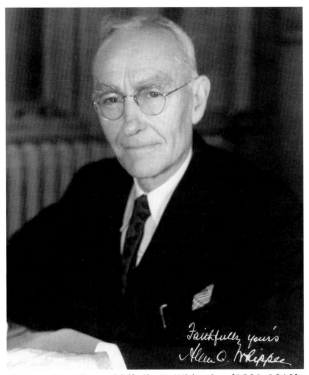

Figure 8. Allen Oldfather Whipple (1881-1963).
Reproduced with permission from the family of Dr. Whipple.

stage on March 8th, 1940 [7], after the discovery of Vitamin K by Dam. At first, the operative mortality of the operation was approximately 30-40%. This has gradually decreased and is currently under 2% in expert hands.

The three decades following Whipple's contributions can be labelled 'the age of surgical experimentation and technical development'. Dissatisfaction with the high morbidity coupled with the poor survival after the Whipple operation for cancer led many surgeons to try total pancreatectomy as an alternative.

The first successful total pancreatectomy was done for an unlocated functioning islet cell adenoma by Priestley in 1944 [19] at the Mayo Clinic. Total pancreatectomy was soon advocated in the 1960s for cancer in the head of the pancreas to eliminate the possibility of multicentric disease. An added attraction was the elimination of the pancreaticojejunal anastomosis and its inherent leak rate which was often fatal. This premise did not survive critical appraisal, especially as the long-term survival did not improve and the complications of the ensuing diabetic state became a major impediment. In 1973, Fortner proposed extension of the Whipple operation into the concept of a 'regional pancreatectomy'. This entails removal of a major portion of the head and neck of the gland together with resection of the confluence of the portal and superior mesenteric veins, subtotal gastrectomy and regional lymph node excision. The operation was extended further to include partial resection with graft reconstruction of the hepatic and superior mesenteric arteries. It was soon realised that excision of major arteries did not improve survival and carried a prohibitive mortality and morbidity. On the other hand, excision of a short segment of vein with reconstruction is still recommended if it helps the surgeon to achieve gross negative surgical margins. Many variations of the Krausch-Whipple operations have been and are still being proposed. Many surgeons favour preserving the entire stomach and first part of duodenum if at all possible.

The 1970s witnessed the beginning of major advances in anaesthesia, critical care, interventional radiology, and imaging techniques. These disciplines, coupled with better patient selection, better surgical expertise, and the trend towards centralisation of complex procedures, are responsible for the appreciable improvement in our surgical results.

Surgeons operating on pancreatic cancer today can be classified into three groups:

♦ the 'aggressive-radical' surgeon who will always attempt major extirpative procedures with resection of major vessels and vascular reconstruction. Such 'tour de force' is still popular in Japan;

- the 'nihilist-timid' surgeon who avoids getting involved in complex time-consuming risky procedures; and
- the 'rational' surgeon who will tailor the operation to the stage of the disease, and the patient's general condition and ability to tolerate the operation.

Acute pancreatitis

Reginald Fitz (Figure 7, Chapter 12), a pathologist at the Massachusetts General Hospital in Boston, gave the first clear description of acute pancreatitis in 1889. In the majority of patients the disease has a mild self-limiting form which may be treated successfully with simple conservative measures. In approximately 15-20% of patients, the disease is severe and is associated with widespread pancreatic and peri-pancreatic necrosis, serious local infective and systemic complications, and finally, multi-organ system failure. Because the natural history of the mild form of the disease is so different from that of necrotising pancreatitis, early identification of patients who will develop severe disease is crucial.

Clinical assessment is notoriously difficult and even experienced clinicians can predict prognosis in only about 39% of cases. This led to the development of multi-factorial scoring systems to predict the natural history of acute pancreatitis. The first such system was developed in New York by Ranson [20] in 1974. Five laboratory and clinical parameters are measured at admission, and six more are assessed at the end of the first 48 hours of hospitalisation to estimate a likelihood of ultimate mortality. Unfortunately, the criteria required a full 48 hours to establish and were not helpful in the crucial early hours. Imrie [21] modified Ranson's criteria, including only nine factors (the Glasgow criteria) which could be used on admission. Several other predicting factors and systems have since come and gone. Probably the most popular system at present is the Acute Physiological and Chronic Health Evaluation (APACHE II) scores. The APACHE scoring system may be applied to any critical illness and correlates with the severity of disease and associated risk of in-hospital death. It allocates points to each physiological variable and takes into account age, severe previously diagnosed medical condition and surgical status. It must be

emphasised that these prognostic factors or scoring systems are useful to compare populations and treatment regimens, but they do not help in the management of the individual patient.

Because of the cumbersome nature of these multifactoral systems, and the difficulty of memorising the factors, attempts have been made to estimate prognosis using a single indicator. The use of CT scanning is probably the best at present; it documents the degree of pancreatic and peripancreatic inflammation, the presence of associated fluid collections, and the degree of pancreatic and peri-pancreatic necrosis. The Balthazar CT severity index [22] measured by CT scanning, was found to be more reliable to predict severe disease.

The high probability of death for patients with severe pancreatitis prompted surgeons in the 1960s to approach the disease in the same way that they treat acute appendicitis or acute cholecystitis, namely, removal of the entire affected organ. Watts, in 1963, performed the first total pancreatectomy in the UK. The wave of enthusiasm for the procedure, especially in France, was short-lived because of the prohibitive mortality and morbidity in these very ill patients. By trial and error over the years, it is now widely accepted that the early management of severe acute pancreatitis is non-operative. Operation is reserved for infected pancreatic necrosis, extensive non-infected necrosis causing toxic symptoms, and other rare complications, such as rupture into adjacent viscera. Largely as a result of the German workers led by Hans Beger [23] from Ulm, when operative intervention is needed, the principle of debridement, removal of necrotic and infected material in the lesser sac and postoperative irrigation of the lesser sac combined with antibiotics and other supportive therapy in the ICU, has become the standard of care and has reduced the mortality from around 60% to less than 10%.

Chronic pancreatitis

The surgical treatment of this disease does not have an impressive record. Chronic pancreatitis implies the progressive irreversible destruction of the entire gland with eventual development of both exocrine and endocrine insufficiency. By definition, it is not primarily a surgical disease and, therefore, no surgical procedure can restore either the endocrine or the exocrine function of the pancreas; nor is it likely to prevent further loss of glandular function.

Alcoholism is the aetiologic factor in the Western world and most patients are also addicted to narcotic drugs by the time they seek surgical intervention for pain relief. We have learned, the long, hard way, that avoidance of alcohol is a more important determinant of outcome after operation than the type of procedure.

The results of operation for pain are still neither consistent nor impressive. First reported in 1943 by Mallet-Guy [24] and other French surgeons, splanchnicectomy and coeliac plexus ablation for the management of intractable pancreatic pain gave, at best, inconsistent results and was quickly abandoned. It is currently being re-advocated using minimal access (laparoscopic and thoracoscopic) approaches but long-term follow-up is lacking [25]. Doubilet and Mulholand in New York proposed in 1948 intra-operative pancreatography and sphincterotomy to drain the duct of Wirsung. This was first accomplished transcholedochally and later, transduodenally. The results were disappointing. In the 1950s, DuVal, Zollinger and Longmire [26-28] independently proposed amputating the tail of the pancreas and draining the duct of Wirsung retrogradely into a loop of jejunum. This, too, was unsuccessful.

Cattell [29] (Figure 2, Chapter 13), at the Lahey Clinic, used for the first time, in 1947, a side-to-side anastomosis between a loop of jejunum and a distended duct of Wirsung to relieve pain in patients with cancer in the head of pancreas. Eventually, the 'chain of lakes' description of Wirsung's duct in some patients with chronic pancreatitis, led Puestow and Gillesby [30] (1958) of Chicago to propose un-roofing the pancreatic duct and its anastomosis to the jejunum in a side-to-side fashion. Numerous modifications of the technique still abound today.

The past 30 years have witnessed multiple techniques of partial or total pancreatic resection with variable results. Various combinations of partial head resection with duct drainage ensued but none has been uniformly successful for pain relief. The multiplicity of surgical procedures recommended for chronic pancreatitis attests to the fact that not one single procedure has the answer to this disease.

Pancreatic transplantation

Pancreatic transplantation is the last surgical frontier to be tackled over the past 50 years. As early as 1959, Brooks and Gifford in Boston attempted homografting of pancreatic tissue in man by implanting fragments of pancreas from still-born infants into the quadriceps muscles of their diabetic mothers. Their lack of success in achieving glucose homeostasis led to the subsequent use of diffusion chambers containing insulinoma tissue. They reported a transient reduction of insulin requirement in two diabetic patients.

Vascularised whole organ (pancreatoduodenal) allotransplantation was first undertaken by Lillehei's group at the University of Minnesota in 1966 [31]. Technical refinements and development of immunosuppressive drugs have ensued over the past 40 years. The number of pancreas transplants performed in the US increased from 79 in 1988 to 1221 in 1998, according to a United Network for Organ Sharing (UNOS) report [32]. Simultaneous kidney-pancreas transplant has generally been preferred, but the number of isolated pancreas transplants continues to increase. Several techniques have evolved to deal with the exocrine secretion - ligation of the pancreatic duct or neoprene injection into the duct have been largely abandoned. The previously popular drainage of the duodenal stump into the urinary bladder has now been largely supplanted by enteric drainage. Most surgeons still drain the splenic vein of the graft into the iliac vein, but there is a trend towards draining the splenic vein into the portal venous system.

The concept of isolating islets from the pancreatic exocrine tissue has occupied scientists for over 35 years. Isolation of islets from the human pancreas by the collagenase technique is feasible but yields relatively few islets. Numerous laboratories are still attempting to improve the yield, because a large number of islets is required for successful reversal of Type I diabetes mellitus.

Intraperitoneal, intramuscular and intrasplenic implantation of islets in animals have been shown to transiently improve the hyperglycaemic state. In 1976, Sutherland and his colleagues [33] reported ten transplants of islet tissue into seven diabetic patients who had previously undergone renal transplantation for end-stage diabetic nephropathy. The islet tissue from fresh cadavers were transplanted intraperitoneally in five patients, into a muscle pocket in one, and in the portal vein in four cases. These transplants had no impact on the diabetic status of the patients, probably due to the small amount of islet tissue isolated and transplanted as well as to immune rejection.

Over the past 20 years, work at the University of Edmonton in Canada [34] has reactivated this line of research by providing significantly better results with islet cell transplantation. Encouraging results have been achieved by improved technique of islet cell extraction, better combination of immunosuppressive drugs, and direct infusion of the islets into the liver via the transjugular route via the vena cava into the hepatic veins by the interventional radiologist.

The future at present appears to reside in stem cell research. Preliminary experiments suggest that undifferentiated stem cells can be stimulated in tissue culture to differentiate into insulin-secreting cells.

Dedication

This chapter is dedicated to the memory of Dr. Robert M. Zollinger and his colleague, Edwin H. Ellison. Their seminal contribution was based on a report of two cases. They were able to find previous reports of four similar cases with extremely high gastric acid output, peptic ulceration, and non-insulin-secreting islet cell adenomas of the pancreas. Their deduction that a gastric acid secretagogue was produced by the tumours revolutionised gastro-intestinal and endocrine pathophysiology and surgery. Dr. Zollinger was Chairman of the Department of Surgery at The Ohio State University for over a quarter of a century. Apart from his surgical contributions, he was an outstanding teacher of students and residents. His sharp wit was often at the expense of other surgeons who largely deserved it. One of his famous aphorisms, "every surgeon should dilate the lower end of the common bile duct with the same temerity as he would his own urethra", is still widely quoted today.

Dr. Ellison left The Ohio State University and became Chairman of the Department of Surgery at Marquette University School of Medicine, which later became the Medical College of Wisconsin. Both Dr. Zollinger and Dr. Ellison were instrumental in the training of Dr. Larry C. Carey, who, upon Dr. Zollinger's retirement, became the first Zollinger Professor of Surgery and Chairman of the Department. Ironically, Dr. Zollinger died of pancreatic cancer and Dr. Ellison died of complications of diabetes mellitus. The current holder of the Zollinger Chair at The Ohio University is Christopher Ellison, who is the son of the late Edwin Ellison. He was trained by Dr. Larry Carey and was the surgeon who operated on Dr. Zollinger during his terminal illness.

References

1. Derman H. *Measurement of exocrine and endocrine functions of the pancreas.* Sutherland FW, Sutherland FW Jr., Eds. Philadelphia: Lippincott Co, 1961.

2. de Graaf R. *Tractatus anatomico-medicus de succi pancreatici natura & usu.* Lugd. Batavorum: Ex Officina Hackiana, 1671.

3. Opie EL. *Disease of the pancreas: its cause and nature.* Philadelphia: JB Lippincott, 1903.

4. Brooks JR. *Surgery of the pancreas.* Philadelphia: Saunders, 1983.

5. Banting FG, Best CH. The internal secretion of the pancreas. *J Lab Clin Med* 1922; 7: 251.

6. Abel JJ. Crystalline insulin. *Proc Natl Acad Sci USA* 1926; 12: 132-6.

7. Trede M, Carter Sir David C, Eds. *Surgery of the pancreas.* Foreword By William P Longmire, Jr. New York: Churchill Livingstone, 1997.

8. Whipple, AO, Franz VK. Adenoma of the islet cells with hyperinsulinism. *Ann Surg* 1935; 101: 1299.

9. Yalow RS, Berson SA. Assay of plasma insulin in human subjects by immunologic methods. *Nature* 1959; 183: 1648.

10. Zollinger RM, Ellison E. Primary peptic ulceration of the jejunum associated with islet cell tumors of the pancreas. *Ann Surg* 1955; 142: 709.

11. Grossman M. Personal communication quoted by Isenberg J, 1980.

12. Ellison EC, Carey LC, Sparks J, *et al.* Early surgical treatment of gastrinoma. *Am J Med* 1987; 82(5B): 17-24.

13. Pearse AGE, Polak JM. Neural crest origin of the endocrine polypeptide (APUD) cells of the gastrointestinal tract and pancreas. *Gut* 1971; 12: 783-8.

14. Fontaine J, LeDouarin N. Analysis of endoderm formation in the avian blastoderm by the use of quail-chick chimeras. The problem of the neuroectodermal origin of the cells of the APUD series. *J Embryol Exp Morphol* 1977; 41: 209-22.

15. Bernard C. *Memoir on the pancreas and on the role of pancreatic juice in digestive processes: particularly in the digestion of neutral fat.* London; Orlando, Fla.: Academic Press,1985.

16. Bayliss WM, Starling EH. The mechanism of pancreatic secretion. *J Physiol* 1902; 28: 325.

17. Harper AA, Raper HS. Pancreozymin, stimulant of secretion of pancreatic enzymes and extracts of small intestine. *J Physiol* 1943; 102: 115-25.

18. Courvoisier LG. *Casuistisch-statistische Beiträge zur Pathologie und Chirurgie der Gallenwege.* Leipzig: Verlag von FCW Vogel, 1890: 57-8.

19. Priestley JT, Comfort MW, Radcliff JJ. Total pancreatectomy for hyperinsulinism due to islet cell adenoma: survivial and cure at 16 months after operation; presentation of metabolic studies. *Ann Surg* 1944; 119: 221.

20. Ranson JHC, Rifkind KM, Roses DF, *et al.* Objective early identification of severe acute pancreatitis. *Am J Gastroenterol* 1974; 61: 443-51.

21. Blamey SL, Imrie CW, O'Neill J, *et al.* Prognostic factors in acute pancreatitis. *Gut* 1974; 25: 1340-60.

22. Balthazar EJ, Robinson DL, Megibow AJ, Ranson JHC. Acute pancreatitis: value of CT in establishing prognosis. *Radiology* 1990; 174: 331-6.

23. Opie EL. The relation of diabetes mellitus to lesions of the pancreas. Hyaline degeneration of the islands of langerhans. *J Exp Med* 1901; 5: 527-40.

24. Mallet-Guy PA. Late and very late results of resections of the nervous system in the treatment of chronic relapsing pancreatitis. *Am J Surg* 1983; 14: 234-8.

25. Stone H, Chauvin E. Pancreatic denervation for pain relief in chronic alcohol-associated pancreatitis. *Br J Surg* 1990; 77: 303-5.

26. DuVal MK. Caudal pancreaticojejunostomy for chronic pancreatitis. *Ann Surg* 1954; 140: 775.

27. Zollinger RM, Keith LM, Ellison EH. Pancreatitis. *New Engl J Med* 1954; 251: 497-502.

28. Longmire WP, Jordan PH, Briggs JD. Experience with resection of the pancreas in the treatment of chronic relapsing pancreatitis. *Ann Surg* 1956; 144: 681.

29. Cattell RB. Anastomosis of the duct of Wirsung; its use in palliative operations for cancer of the head of the pancreas. *Surg Clin N Am* 1947; 27: 636-43.

30. Puestow CB, Gillesby WJ. Retrograde surgical drainage of pancreas for chronic relapsing pancreatitis. *AMA Surg* 1958; 76(6): 898-907.

31. Kelly WD, Lillehei RC, Merkel FK, *et al.* Allotransplantation of the pancreas and duodenum along with the kidney in diabetic nephropathy. *Surgery* 1967; 61(6): 827-37.

32. Sutherland DE, Cecka M, Gruessner AC. Report from the International Pancreas Transplant Registry - 1998. *Transplantation Proceedings* 1999; 31: 597-601.

33. Sutherland DE, Matas AJ, Goetz FC, Najarian JS. Transplantation of dispersed pancreatic islet tissue in humans: autografts and allografts. *Diabetes* 1980; 29(11): 31-43.

34. Shapiro AM, Lakey JR, Ryan EA, Korbutt GS, Toth E, Warnock GL, *et al.* Islet transplantation in seven patients with type 1 diabetes mellitus using a glucocorticoid-free immunosuppressive regime. *New Engl J Med* 2000; 343(4): 230-8.

Chapter 9

The challenge of intestinal obstruction

David FL Watkin MChir FRCS

Emeritus Consultant Surgeon, Leicester Royal Infirmary, Leicester, UK

Introduction

Mechanical intestinal obstruction is a condition clearly demanding surgical treatment. The typical clinical features were graphically described in the 14th century by John of Arderne: "[Passio iliaca] cometh with constipation of the belly and busy costing [vomiting] and with huge acheing and sorrow, as though the guts were bored with a wymball [gimlet] ... and the matter that should pass out beneathenforth cometh out of the mouth." [1]

Obstructions due to strangulated external hernias were recognised in antiquity but understanding of the intra-abdominal causes had to await autopsy evidence in the 16th and 17th centuries. Thus, strangulated hernias account for almost all the early operations for obstruction, while the intra-abdominal conditions were looked after by physicians. Some distal large bowel obstructions were identified clinically in the 19th century and treated by the creation of an artificial anus. Then, following the introduction of anaesthesia and antisepsis, surgical treatment of intra-abdominal causes of obstruction became feasible, although mortality rates remained high until the 1930s, when the value of gastric aspiration and intravenous fluid replacement was appreciated. Improved anaesthesia and the development of antibiotics contributed to further reductions in mortality.

This complex story will be unravelled thematically, in approximately chronological order. In the evolution of surgical treatment the focus will move from country to country, with a bias towards reports in the English language. Many of the early writings described operations without any evidence that the author (or indeed anyone else) had performed them. Actual reports of surgery, with data, take precedence, but expressions of opinion are also useful, particularly to indicate that a procedure was not yet in general use. Developments since 1950 are described only in outline, as references to these are readily available.

Terminology

Hippocrates used 'ιλeus' for a severe abdominal pain which will usually prove fatal [2]. Later, ileus was limited to cases of intestinal obstruction and then, when it was recognised that not all obstruction is due to a blockage, it was divided into mechanical and paralytic ileus. The latter continues in use (though 'paralytic' is often omitted) but the former survives only as gallstone ileus.

The surgical vocabulary was different in the 19th century: 'abrogation of ingesta' would now be 'nil by mouth'; 'alvine dejections' were faeces; 'injection', without further qualification, meant administration of an enema. 'Gastrotomy' indicated opening of the peritoneal cavity, gradually being replaced by abdominal section. Similarly, 'gastroenterotomy' meant jejunostomy. 'Laparotomy' had been used in Europe but was not established in the American literature until Ashhurst[3] drew attention to the confusion caused by the dual meaning of 'gastrotomy' in 1874. For clarity, the modern equivalents will be used, other than as direct quotations.

Strangulated hernia

The early history of the operative treatment of strangulated hernia was reviewed by Wangensteen and Wangensteen[4]. Aurelianus in the 5th century referred to an operation by Praxagoras in the 4th century BC, in which he "made an incision over the swelling of a strangulated groin hernia, freed the gut and cut into the bowel to establish an artificial anus". In the 13th century, Saliceto, and then Lanfranc, resected the involved intestine and made anastomoses using animal gut and trachea as stents. In 1561, Pierre Franco, from Lyons, described approximately 200 hernia operations, advocating an incision at the neck of the scrotum. For strangulation he first tried venesection and rectal insufflation of tobacco smoke; if unsuccessful he operated using a goose quill to decompress the bowel and then incising the constriction. The aim was reduction, not repair.

In 1615, Pierre Pigray, from Rouen, published a similar description of the operation. Having opened the sac, he introduced a finger lubricated with butter; if the hernia could not then easily be reduced he deflated the bowel with a needle. Elsewhere, progress was delayed. Heister reported that his senior, Rau, encountered dead bowel when operating for strangulated hernia; he informed the patient that he would die, gathered up his instruments and left!

In the early 18th century, members of the newly formed Royal Academy of Surgery in Paris resected gangrenous bowel, with formation of an artificial anus. In 1701, Mery's patient recovered. La Peyronie (Figure 1) excised devitalised bowel and, by traction on a suture placed through the mesentery of the adjacent ends, was able to hasten closure of the fistula. By 1790, Petit (Figure 9, Chapter 15) had a series of 11 cases of strangulated hernia with seven known survivors, although only one had gangrenous gut[5]. This flowering of surgery in France suffered a setback in the next century, Maunoury[6] bemoaning the timidity of contemporary surgeons, such as Dupuytren, who delayed operation and failed to deal appropriately with devitalised bowel.

Meanwhile, in the UK, successful resections were carried out by William Cookesley, a country surgeon from Crediton in Devon in 1731, and by de Ronsil[7] in London, in 1732. Cheselden removed 26 inches of 'mortified gut' after a strangulated umbilical hernia had burst, and the patient survived for some years with a faecal fistula[8]. Less successful was the case of Queen Caroline (wife of George II) who suffered strangulation of an umbilical hernia in 1737. After four days of alternative remedies, she finally permitted examination of the abdomen. The swelling was lanced and she developed a faecal fistula, but died five days later.

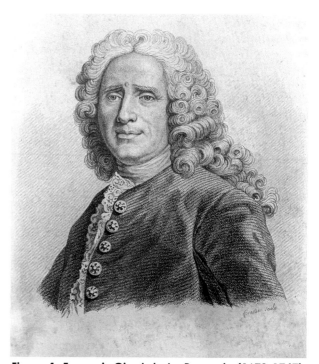

Figure 1. François Gigot de La Peyronie (1678-1747). *Reproduced with permission from the Wellcome Library, London.*

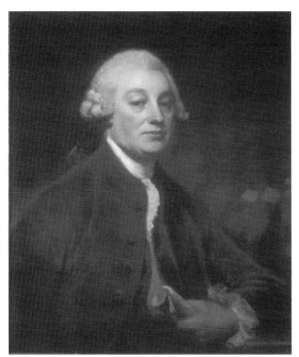

Figure 2. Percival Pott (1714-1788). *Reproduced with permission from The Royal College of Surgeons of England.*

Percival Pott (Figure 2), in a treatise on hernia in 1756, advised early operation for strangulation, acknowledging that often it will not cure the hernia [9]. He described incising the constriction ring to permit reduction of viable bowel, but "no altered or mortified part should be returned loose to the belly". When gangrene required excision, he advised that one end should be invaginated into the other and the portions sutured together and to the peritoneum, "so that if union does not take place the faeces may be delivered from the wound". Despite these clear practical instructions, there is no indication of his results.

Nevertheless, surgeons were reluctant. Lawrence advocated taxis, bloodletting (faintness facilitating reduction), purgatives to excite the bowel (and so extract it from the hernia) and a tobacco enema, with operation as a last resort [10]. Astley Cooper (Figure 3), in 1821, was reported to have said: "It is a most unpardonable neglect in the practitioner not to use tobacco in strangulated hernia, which ought to be impressed on every surgeon." [11]

Cooper emphasised the risks of operation to his students but his results, 19 survivors from 33 operations for strangulated hernia, were creditable. It is not clear how many had gangrenous bowel, for which he favoured incision rather than resection.

By 1883, Browne was able to report 44 personal cases in seven years, with a mortality of 25% in hospital and 18% in private practice [12]. He advised immediate operation and aimed for a radical cure. Thereafter, results were usually published in the context of intestinal obstruction in general, but in 1931, Frankau surveyed 1480 operations for strangulated hernia in the UK and Ireland [13]. Mortality was 13% for inguinal and femoral hernias and 41% for umbilical hernias; if a bowel resection was necessary, the mortality averaged 43%.

Treatments used by physicians

Prior to the advent of anaesthesia, the treatment of intestinal obstruction, except for strangulated hernias, was generally in the hands of physicians. Sydenham,

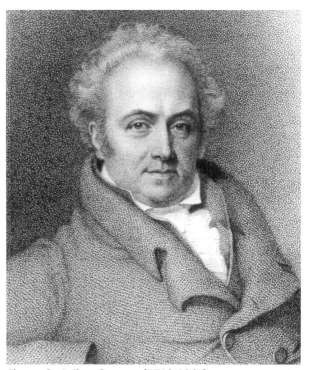

Figure 3. Astley Cooper (1768-1841). *Reproduced with permission from The Royal Society of Medicine, London, UK.*

in the 17th century, recommended opium, rest, horse-riding or a warm kitten placed on the abdomen [14]. By the 19th century there was an amazing variety of treatments [4], including purgatives, enemata and leeches (applied to the abdomen or anus). Opium and belladonna were popular drugs, the latter being rubbed on the abdomen or given rectally. Tuckwell described a patient, obstructed for ten days, who recovered after administration of belladonna. Up to seven pounds of metallic mercury, administered orally, was designed to force a passage past an obstruction [15]. When it became available, electricity was applied to the abdomen or via the pneumogastric (vagus) nerve in the neck. Surgeons applied abdominal taxis: the patient was shaken while suspended by the feet, had the abdomen kneaded and finally was placed prone, with the pelvis supported on a pillow [16]. More logical was the practice of puncturing the distended intestine to provide symptomatic relief. Some patients were cured by these manoeuvres; presumably their disorders were capable of spontaneous resolution.

Brinton (Figure 4) in 1867 gave a clear account of the clinical features, distinguishing mechanical and paralytic obstructions, and pointed out that the nearer an obstruction is to the stomach the smaller is the amount of urine passed [17]. He allowed that colostomy was indicated for stricture of the large intestine and laparotomy was appropriate for obstruction due to bands or a (Meckel's) diverticulum, but only after a full trial of medical measures. Of 600 collected cases of obstruction, 43% were due to intussusception, for which he opposed operation because the success rate was lower than the alleged 30-50% chance of recovery by sloughing of the inner layers. He considered that opium should be administered freely: "Certainly nothing in the whole action of remedies can surpass the comparative painlessness into which I have seen an agonising intussusception converted [by belladonna and opium] during the many days that have intervened before its unavoidable termination in death." [17]

Pathology of intestinal obstruction

The main types of intraperitoneal obstruction were recognised during the 19th century. Indeed, discussion of the lesions responsible formed the greater part of treatises on obstruction [17]. The fundamental concepts discussed were strangulation, paralytic ileus and the distinction between small and large bowel obstruction.

Strangulation

Although strangulation had been well recognised in hernias for hundreds of years, the changes were attributed to inflammation until Bryant [18] described the mechanism of venous obstruction, due to bands, hernias, intussusception or volvulus. He pointed out that the effects of strangulation precede the effects of obstruction and that patients with simple obstruction survived far longer. Treves included obstruction due to mesenteric thrombosis and referred to one successful case of resection for this [19]. However, until the 1920s the effects of gangrenous bowel were submerged in the more general theory of toxaemia (see later section); for example, McGlannan attributed 75% of 127 deaths to toxaemia, although only 20 had gangrenous bowel [20].

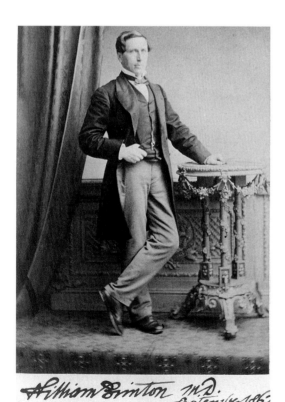

Figure 4. William Brinton (1823-1867). *Reproduced with permission from the Wellcome Library, London.*

Hausler and Foster, in 1924, drew a clear pathological distinction between simple and strangulating obstructions, exemplified by animal experiments and typical clinical cases [21]. Scott and Wangensteen [22] demonstrated that in strangulation, blood volume was lost, proportionate to the length of bowel involved. Experiments showed that increased intraluminal pressure, proximal to an obstruction, interfered with blood flow in the bowel [23], especially in a closed loop [24] or in the caecum with a competent ileocaecal valve [25]. In 1962, Cohn comprehensively reviewed the experimental evidence, concluding that bacteria, ischaemia and intraluminal pressure all contribute to the release of a toxin [26].

Paralytic ileus and early postoperative obstruction

The distinction between paralytic and mechanical obstruction in the postoperative period is difficult. Treves [27], in 1884, mentioned 'ileus paralyticus', but by 1901 was dismissive [28], stating that "paralysis following operations for strangulated hernia or volvulus can be explained by peritonitis". Then Murphy

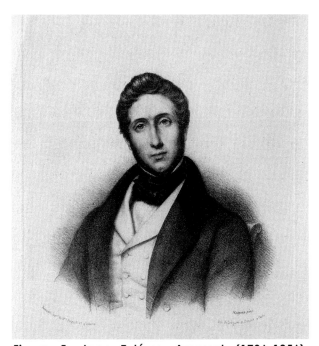

Figure 5. Jean Zuléma Amussat (1796-1856).
Reproduced with permission from the Wellcome Library, London.

in 1896, gave a comprehensive account of adynamic ileus due to abdominal operations, spinal injury, peritonitis, uraemia or renal or biliary calculus [29]. Richardson, in 1920, distinguished between early and late postoperative obstruction, separating these at four weeks [30]. Most early obstructions occurred within two weeks; they could be paralytic or mechanical [31], while late postoperative obstruction was due to adhesions.

Small and large bowel obstruction

Brinton [17] recognised the clinical features of small and large bowel obstructions and appreciated that most of the latter were due to strictures and of less acute onset. Some early authors excluded large bowel obstruction due to carcinoma from their acute series, regarding it as chronic.

Early operations for large bowel obstruction

Apart from hernias, the only obstructions that could be accurately diagnosed in the 18th century were imperforate anus or a palpable rectal stricture. Cope reviewed the early history of colostomy for the relief of these conditions [32]. Littré, in 1710, suggested that infants with imperforate anus might survive if the colon was opened in the left iliac fossa and Duret did this successfully in Brest in 1793, but without follow-up. Over the next 23 years, 11 more cases were reported, with three survivors.

During this period a few colostomies were performed in adults. Fine had the first success in 1797, the patient living for three and a half years, and Pring had a further long-term survivor in 1819, stating: "It may be worthwhile to observe that the inconveniences of an anus in this situation are not such as to have caused her any regret .... on the contrary .... it has afforded her moral as well as physical advantage, for she is now at no loss for an interest and is provided with something to think about for the rest of her life." [32]

However, surgeons were concerned about the risk of peritonitis after opening the abdomen. In an early example of experimental surgery, Amussat (Figures 5 and 6), in 1839, inflated the large bowel of a cadaver and showed that it was possible to reach the descending colon extraperitoneally, via an incision in the loin [33]. He then performed a successful lumbar colostomy in one patient, and six weeks later in another, after this patient had talked to the previous one - an early example of pre-operative counselling.

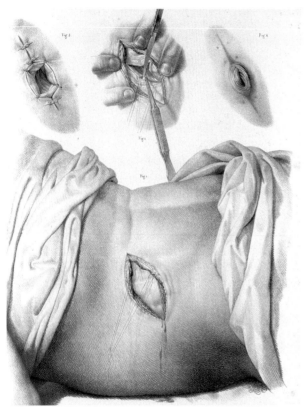

Figure 6. Amussat's lumbar colostomy. *Reproduced with permission from the Wellcome Library, London.*

By 1852, Caesar Hawkins was able to collect 44 cases of colostomy, the majority by the lumbar route, although this was difficult in the obese and often the peritoneum was opened inadvertently [34]. Hilton, in 1853, performed a lumbar colostomy on a surgical colleague who returned to work, seeing 30 to 40 patients per day [35]! Others were doubtful, as indicated by Brown: "But I much question the propriety of such an operation ... since if the patient survives he must become ... loathsome to himself and to those around him." [15]

The development of antisepsis prompted a return to transperitoneal colostomy, with some surgeons

advocating caecostomy. In the late 19th century, the mortality for colostomy was generally lower than after operations for small bowel obstruction.

Surgery for intraperitoneal obstructions

In about 1672, Paul Barbette in Amsterdam suggested surgery for intussusception, although there is no indication that he followed this advice: "Would it not be better to make an incision and draw out the strangulated intestine with fingers, than leave the patient in danger of his life!" [36]

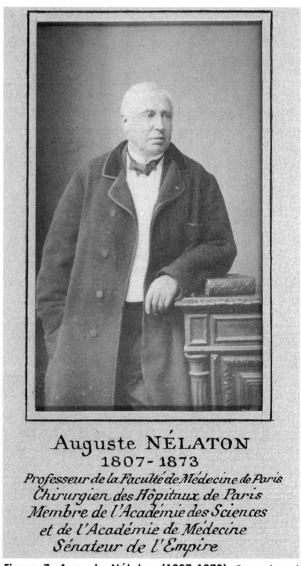

Auguste NÉLATON
1807-1873
*Professeur de la Faculté de Médecine de Paris
Chirurgien des Hôpitaux de Paris
Membre de l'Académie des Sciences
et de l'Académie de Médecine
Sénateur de l'Empire*

Figure 7. Auguste Nélaton (1807-1873). *Reproduced with permission from the Wellcome Library, London.*

Later in the 17th century, there were isolated second-hand accounts of Theophilus Bonet reporting and of Antonj Nuck supervising successful operations for volvulus. In 1853, Brown, a practitioner from the Leicestershire village of Wymeswold, envisaged the possibility of operation for intra-abdominal obstructions, but stated that: "Of course no one would be bold or mad enough to attempt an operation of this kind without a consultation." [15]

Gay, in 1861, collected 54 autopsy cases of obstruction by a band, for which surgical treatment might have been possible [37]. Then in 1867, Brinton [17], a physician, acknowledged that colostomy for a large

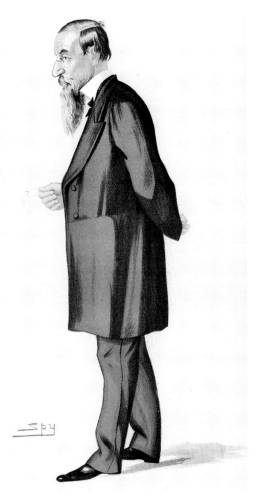

Figure 8. Caricature of Jonathan Hutchinson (1828-1913) by Spy. *Reproduced with permission from the Wellcome Library, London.*

bowel stricture or laparotomy for intussusception or band obstruction might be justified. With anaesthesia, surgical relief of intra-abdominal obstruction became feasible, but there was great anxiety about the danger of opening the peritoneum and the difficulty of replacing protruding intestines. In 1874, Ashhurst collected from the literature since 1819 a total of 57 laparotomies for intestinal obstruction, with 18 survivors [3].

The early abdominal operations, done via a two-finger incision, were usually enterotomies, draining a distended loop of small intestine as originally described by Nélaton [38] (Figure 7). This gave relief of distension and vomiting but not a cure unless the cause resolved. On that basis traditional non-operative treatments could easily be justified. In the later decades of the 19th century the controversy over the treatment of intestinal obstruction was documented in reports from two meetings of the British Medical Association (BMA). In 1878, Hutchinson (Figure 8), who in 1874 had performed the first successful operation for intussusception in a child [39], gave a comprehensive lecture on intestinal obstruction [16]. Except for children, in whom the diagnosis was likely to be intussusception, and for incurable disease of the lower bowel for which colostomy was appropriate, he favoured conservative measures: "Exploratory operations for intestinal obstruction, the cause of which is not known, are not warrantable."

Nevertheless, he did suggest that patients with obstruction should be under the care of surgeons, at that time a revolutionary idea! In the discussion, Allbutt (Figure 9), a physician, supported operation for patients with 'twists or internal herniae', referring to Teale's results [40]. These comprised six cases of abdominal section; there was only one survivor, but it was thought that earlier operation would have benefited others.

In the same year, Bryant (Figure 10) made a well argued plea for laparotomy as soon as strangulation was diagnosed: "In cases of intestinal obstruction, when the physician's art has failed to give relief, the surgeon's aid is occasionally requested and it would be well for the medical mind to recognise that in a

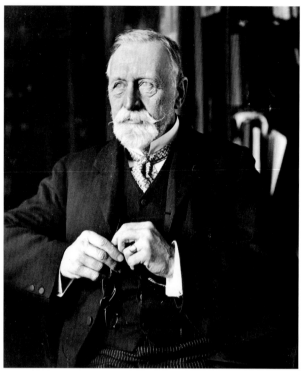

Figure 9. Thomas Clifford Allbutt (1836-1925). *Reproduced with permission from the Wellcome Library, London.*

large proportion of cases this aid is sought at too late a period." [41]

At that time he had but one survivor from such an operation. In 1884, he published 17 years' experience, describing the pathological features of strangulation [18]. Of 12 patients with band obstruction and 20 with intussusception (all proven at autopsy), only four had laparotomy and none survived. He concluded that laparotomy was indicated as soon as strangulation was diagnosed. Gangrenous bowel should be exteriorised and then resected, leaving an artificial anus. Enterotomy was reserved for situations where laparotomy was rejected or inappropriate.

The crucial questions of whether and when operation was indicated were discussed at another session of the BMA in 1883. Except for strangulated hernia, Parker, Professor of Surgery in Liverpool, advocated "proper expectant treatment" [42]. This policy would give some survivors, "while it is decidedly less frequently fatal than abdominal

section". Only when the patient was "passing into the commencement of collapse" would he consider enterotomy. In discussion Tait responded vigorously: "It is wholly unnecessary, and dangerous, to wait for an accurate diagnosis. This can be done only by abdominal section, and this had better be done before death than after it."

Then in 1884, Treves (Figure 11) gave a comprehensive account of intestinal obstruction [27]. He attributed shock to sudden stretching of the visceral peritoneum, but by the second edition he was invoking a toxin: "Subjects with acute intestinal obstruction die from the phenomena of septic

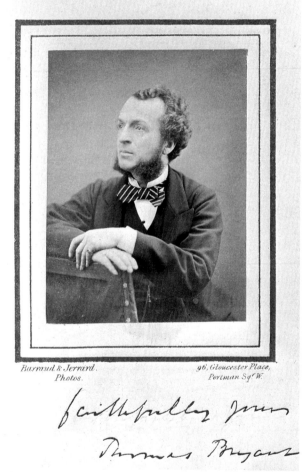

Barraud & Jerrard.   96, Gloucester Place,
Photos.   Portman Sqʳ W.

Figure 10. Thomas Bryant (1828-1914). *Reproduced with permission from the Wellcome Library, London.*

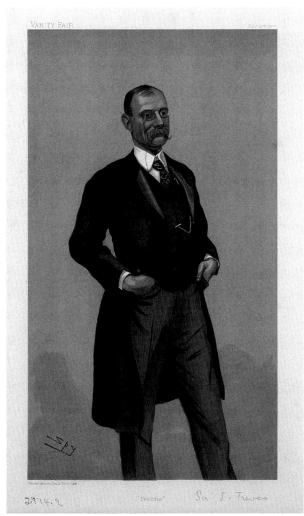

Figure 11. Caricature of Frederick Treves (1853-1923) by Spy. *Reproduced with permission from the Wellcome Library, London.*

poisoning." [28] Discussing treatment he felt bound to cover the full range of traditional non-operative measures, emphasising the value of opium and enemata and condemning aperients, before considering operation. Reviewing the alternatives, from percutaneous puncture to laparotomy he wrote: "This [laparotomy] is one of the most important operations concerned in the treatment of intestinal obstruction, and is a procedure likely in the future to occupy a still more conspicuous position." [27]

The peritoneum was to be opened with great care to avoid protrusion of viscera. By 1899 he had moved on: a two-finger incision might suffice for division of a band or for enterostomy, but enlargement to four fingers' breadth might be needed for diagnosis and if necessary the bowel could be allowed to protrude [28]. In advanced cases, after relief of the obstruction, enterostomy (using Paul's tube) was advised. Gangrenous bowel was to be exteriorised and incised, or, if the patient was not too ill, 'suspect' bowel might be resected, with anastomosis. Treves estimated the mortality of such operations as 50%. To counteract patients' reluctance he wrote: "It is less dangerous to jump from Clifton Suspension Bridge than to suffer from an acute intestinal obstruction and decline an operation." [28] *

Meanwhile in Boston, Fitz (better known for understanding the nature of appendicitis) collected 295 cases of intestinal obstruction, excluding herniae, from the literature of the previous eight years, with 70% mortality [43]. He advocated a warm water enema, to assess whether the large bowel was the site of obstruction and for the possible reduction of intussusception. He concluded: "Acute intestinal obstruction is diagnosticated by exclusion (e.g. of peritonitis). Its seat [large or small bowel] is fixed by injection [i.e. enema]. Its variety is determined by its seat and the age, antecedents and symptoms of the patient. Its treatment is surgical on or after the third day, if the symptoms are urgent and forced injections fail."

Senn, in 1889, gave a surgical mortality of 69% [44], writing that operation for intestinal obstruction was still in its infancy. Kocher described his experience of 77 cases in Berne, emphasising drainage of the toxic material from the bowel proximal to the obstruction (as did Treves [45]) and, if the patient was in good condition, correction of the obstruction [46]. His overall mortality was 36% - remarkably low for the time. Elliott recommended a two-stage procedure for bowel resection, forming a double-barrelled stoma and later crushing the spur [47]. In 1895, Holmes published a consecutive series, comprising seven years' experience of laparotomy at St. George's Hospital, London, including 31 operations for intestinal obstruction, with only six survivors [48].

---

* The Clifton Suspension Bridge was completed in 1885, 245 feet above the high water level in the Avon Gorge. In 1885 Sarah Ann Hanley, following an argument with her boyfriend, threw herself from the bridge; crinoline petticoats slowed her fall and she survived and lived to the age of 84.

Management 1900-1930: 'toxaemia'

The management of intestinal obstruction in the early 20th century was dominated by the concept of toxaemia. Whereas mortality rates for many other elective and emergency procedures fell dramatically to around 10% [49], those for intestinal obstruction remained stubbornly in the range of 30%-60% (Table 1). There are many descriptions of the patients becoming increasingly unwell, with a dry mouth, sunken eyes and reduced urine output. Tuttle reviewed 128 operations for obstruction, with zero mortality for those operated upon within six hours of onset, rising to 15% at 24 hours and 37% at six days, so demonstrating the benefit of early operation [50], and others concurred [20, 30, 51, 52]. This was all attributed to increasing absorption of a toxin, as originally suggested by Amussat [33].

Experiments showed that intravenous injection of the contents of the obstructed upper small bowel resulted in the death of the animal within 12-24 hours [53, 54]. Some believed that the toxin was the result of bacterial action within the lumen; Williams suggested *Cl. Welchii* [55], while others hypothesised that it was the product of deranged mucosal secretions [56]. No one demonstrated how the toxin reached the systemic circulation. The practical application of this theory was to urge doctors to recognise obstruction and refer promptly and surgeons to operate early, using enterostomy to remove the toxin from the distended bowel [57, 58]. Saline solutions, often hypertonic up to 15% [59], but in relatively small volumes, were given subcutaneously, in the belief that chloride could neutralise the toxin.

By the 1920s treatment was adapted to three stages of obstruction [60]. Early cases would have the cause removed at laparotomy under general anaesthetic. Those with a two to four-day history, but in good condition, would have in addition a jejunostomy tube to allow toxins to be washed out with bicarbonate solution. Late cases, in poor condition, "presenting the appearance of being poisoned by toxins", would have a jejunostomy under local anaesthetic; if they survived, a laparotomy might be carried out a week later.

But the results did not improve. In 1925, Souttar, in a survey of 3064 operations among British teaching hospitals, found mortalities of 32% for intraperitoneal obstruction and 19% for strangulated hernias [61]. Seven years later the figures were no better, with mortalities of 39% and 18% respectively [62]. Fifty-three percent of operations for intraperitoneal obstruction involved reduction of intussusception or simple division of adhesions. More than half of the remainder had enterostomy alone, though van Beuren and Smith began to question the value of this [63]. Although some personal series had produced lower rates [64, 65], the mortality for hospital series remained stubbornly in the range 40-65% (Table 1).

All these authors regarded toxaemia as the major factor in mortality, but some also gave "large quantities of isotonic saline" [66]. Then, during the 1930s in the US, three important developments occurred in parallel: intravenous fluids, suction decompression and plain film radiology.

Fluid therapy

Intravenous fluids are essential in the management of intestinal obstruction, but the early history is difficult to establish. Saline was used by O'Shaughnessy [67] in the treatment of cholera in the 1820s, after he found that the concentration of salts in the serum was reduced. He believed that chloride neutralised a toxin and gave saline to support this process, but only a surprisingly small amount: "In severe cases I would not hesitate to inject some ounces of warm water into the veins. I would also, without apprehension, dissolve in that water the mild innocuous salts which nature herself is accustomed to combine with the human blood."

In intestinal obstruction, oligurea and the disappearance of chloride from the urine were noted by Brinton [17], who attributed this to fluid loss and suggested that this might be replaced rectally. Treves followed this policy [27] and later wrote: "No evidence has been adduced in favour of intravenous injection as a means of allaying intense thirst." [28] Matas [68], in New Orleans in 1891, described giving one to four pints of intravenous saline, but the indication in the 19 traumatic or postoperative cases was blood loss.

Table 1. Mortality figures for intra-abdominal obstruction (1888-1986).

First author	Years of data collection	Centre / Country	No. of cases	Case mortality %
Gibson [150]	1888-1898	Collected from literature	646*	47
Scudder [30]	1898-1907	Boston	121	60.4
McGlannan [20]	Pre-1915	Baltimore	276	45.7
Deaver [51]	1903-1913	Philadelphia	120	61.7
Richardson [30]	1908-1917	Boston	118	41.5
Burgess [104]	1913-1922	Manchester	445	39.6
Souttar [61]	1920-1924	UK	1655	32
McIver [111]	1918-1927	Boston	156	44
Brill [66]	1922-1928	Philadelphia	80	49
Miller [52]	1924-1929	New Orleans	246	74
Vick [62]	1925-1930	UK	3625	39
McKittrick [109]	1928-1937	Boston	136	20
Hudson [156]	Pre-1941	London	370	32
Eliason [157]	1934-1943	Philadelphia	230	11
Becker [125]	1940-1949	New Orleans	702	21.5
Nemir [158]	1940-1950	Philadelphia	340	11
Smith [121]	1942-1953	Minneapolis	1122	13
Barling [159]	1950-1953	Sydney	245	21
Savage [98]	Pre-1959	London	179	15
Waldron [160]	1944-1956	Houston	435	14.7
Silen et al [123]	1944-1959	San Francisco	480+	10.5
Davis [161]	1956-1966	Los Angeles	185+	4
Laws [162]	1963-1972	B'ham Al.	465+	8
Stewardson [120]	1967-1976	Chicago	181+	6.6
Fevang [163]	1960-1995	Bergen	714+	4.5
McEntee [127]	1985-1986	Darlington etc	177	13

Reports are sequenced by the midpoint of data collection

* Gibson's was a collected series; all others were from single hospitals

The multiple reports from Boston, Philadelphia and New Orleans were from the same hospital in each case

Some series have been re-calculated to exclude external hernias

+ Small bowel obstruction only

Others recommended saline, generally in high concentration and as a bolus injection, for the treatment of traumatic shock [69] and to neutralise the 'toxin' in obstruction.

Between 1912 and 1930, both animal experiments and the biochemical analysis of plasma identified fluid depletion as an explanation for the poor condition of patients with obstruction. Hartwell, Hoguet and Beekman showed that in high small bowel obstruction in dogs, subcutaneous saline, in a volume matched to the measured losses, prolonged survival [70]. Others produced similar results [71, 72], while still paying lip service to the toxin theory, but gradually the latter was abandoned [73, 74]. Gamble (Figure 12) and Ross emphasised the importance of sodium in the deficit resulting from pyloric obstruction and demonstrated that the rise in blood urea was a consequence of reduced blood volume [75]. They were the first to integrate electrolyte and water depletion: "It has been shown that in the presence of considerable reductions of the volume of body water the total concentration of dissolved electrolytes tends to remain stationary."

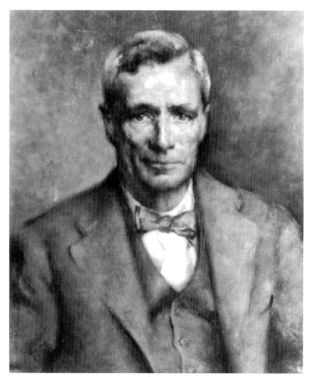

Figure 12. J.L. Gamble (1883-1959). *Reproduced with permission from the National Library of Medicine, Bethesda, Maryland, USA.*

These policies slowly came into use clinically [21, 30, 52, 72], while at a technical level Penfield and Teplitsky [76] described a system for controlling the flow of fluid with a needle valve and a water manometer. Their 'prolonged' infusions administered about three litres in two to four hours! This method was superseded by the introduction by Mattas of a glass chamber and the term 'drip' [77]. But intravenous fluids were not yet widely used. At a meeting of the BMA in 1932, Newland [78], giving the opening paper on intestinal obstruction, emphasised early diagnosis but did not mention saline, although others did [79]. However, in 1935, Gatch and Culbertson were able to write: "[It is] now accepted by everyone that the chief cause of death in simple obstruction of the small bowel... is circulatory failure due to loss of water and electrolytes." [80]

In 1933, Wangensteen and Paine [81], reporting on 32 patients with adhesive obstruction, administered intravenous fluid in sufficient amounts to give a urine output of 800 to 1000ml per 24 hours. Coller *et al* [82] published studies of the electrolyte levels in postoperative patients given saline replacement for their measured losses and offered formulae for the volume to be administered. Gradually the idea of fluid balance developed; in 1939, Wangensteen and colleagues asked: "When will these items [gastric aspirate and urinary output] be recorded on the face sheet of all hospital records for the orientation of the surgeon?" [83]

There was also concern about the risk of fluid overload, ultimately resolved by CVP monitoring [84]. The need for potassium replacement was recognised in the 1940s [85].

Intravenous fluid replacement could have been introduced earlier, but was delayed by adherence to the toxaemia theory and the lack of facilities for sodium estimations. Only gradually was it appreciated that the requirement was for a balanced prescription of salt and water to replenish the extra-cellular compartment. Nevertheless, intestinal obstruction provided the lead for intravenous fluid therapy in other fields of medicine.

Bowel decompression

The history of gastric and duodenal intubation was comprehensively reviewed by Paine [86]. Initially, gastric tubes, passed orally, were used for the treatment of poisoning and then for physiological research. With the introduction of the Levin tube [87] inserted via the nose, surgeons in the late 1920s began to apply syphonage for postoperative distension. Then, Wangensteen (Figure 15) developed continuous suction for effective decompression of the small bowel.

Gastric lavage was used by Fitz [43] and Treves [28] for symptomatic relief in intestinal obstruction. Later, the risk of aspiration during anaesthesia was recognised as an indication [58] and forcefully described by Grey Turner who "most vividly remembered cases in which, at necropsy, the faecal matter could be squeezed from the lungs like a wet sponge". [88]

In 1910, Westermann [89] used a duodenal tube for postoperative distension, but it was not adopted widely. It was known that some obstructions resolved completely after enterostomy and in 1932, Wangensteen tried gastroduodenal suction via a Levin tube in three patients, resulting in resolution of the obstruction [25]. The following year he described its use in 38 patients [81], mostly with adhesion obstruction, 20 of whom were decompressed, with one death plus two other unrelated deaths, while 18 patients came to operation. Wangensteen and Rea demonstrated that the avoidance of swallowed air enabled dogs with low small bowel obstruction to survive much longer, confirming that distension is a lethal factor [90], while Gatch and Culbertson showed experimentally that intestinal distension impaired mucosal blood flow [80].

Abbott and Johnston used the longer Miller-Abbott tube, which could reach the ileum, to achieve more complete decompression of the small bowel [91], enthusiastically supported by Smith in a series of 1000 cases [92]. Long naso-intestinal aspiration tubes never became popular in Britain and have perhaps been less used in the US since Bizer *et al* [93] found no significant difference in the rate of successful decompression between short and long tubes. A randomised trial showed no benefit from the long tube [94] and a recent major Anglo-American textbook mentions only nasogastric decompression [95].

Methods of operative decompression also need to be considered. Aspiration of the bowel started in the 16th century with Franco's use of a goose quill in strangulated hernia, later superceded by a needle or a trocar and cannula. In 1905 Monks demonstrated, in the cadaver, that four feet of small bowel could be telescoped over a glass tube [96]. Holden attached a rubber hose and milked the bowel contents out through it, "leaving the bowel empty and ribbon like" [65]. Wangensteen described the use of a catheter passed via a trocar, to achieve "aseptic decompressive suction" [97]. This concept was not brought into general use in Britain until 1958 when Savage [98] presented a 14-inch metal tube for suction decompression via a small enterotomy. A year later, Baker described a 40-inch catheter which could be retained postoperatively [99].

Diagnostic methods

Rectal examination

Rectal examination had been practised from at least the 17th century, but clearly many were reluctant about it, as indicated by Codman in 1920: "Rectal examination must not be neglected in diagnosis … I do not mean instrumental but digital examination. This procedure is so repulsive to both physician and patient that it is readily passed by … [To omit it] is criminal where the suspicion of obstruction has arisen." [64]

Examination with a rectal sound was suggested, but it was abandoned because it could never be passed beyond mid sigmoid [27] and risked perforation [43]. Mayo described insertion of the whole hand, under chloroform, to identify a constriction at eight inches [100]. In 1929, sigmoidoscopy was first recommended in suspected large bowel obstruction, "where it is valuable to be able to say that the distal 8 to 11 inches is clear" [49].

Enemas, originally employed as treatment, were used to exclude an obstructing lesion in the colon; if the volume accepted was less than six quarts, the obstruction was colonic and a blind colostomy was appropriate [43]. Treves added the refinement of applying the stethoscope over the caecum to detect the arrival of the enema fluid there [27]. The lack of a faecal result from a second enema as diagnostic of obstruction remained orthodox teaching in the mid-20th century [101].

Auscultation

The application of the stethoscope in intestinal obstruction was rarely mentioned in articles or textbooks until Burgess, in 1929, wrote: "Auscultation is a much neglected method of investigation and one to which I attach great value. After a little experience one gets to recognise certain sounds associated with distended intestines, and the contrast between the turbulent gurgling sounds of mechanical obstruction and the deathlike silence of paralytic ileus is very marked." [49]

These views were supported by Wangensteen [25] and auscultation became routine.

Radiology

Schwarz [102], in Vienna in 1911, first described the use of radiology in obstruction. He gave a small quantity of barium by mouth to identify levels in fluid-laden loops of small bowel and noted that fluid levels could be seen before the barium was given. Several publications followed in the German and French literature, and then in 1915 by Case in English, but he concentrated on radiology for postoperative obstruction [103]. Although mentioned occasionally [104], plain films were slow to catch on in the US and the UK, being subject to the objections that they were of little value [52] and would delay the urgent operation. At a meeting of the BMA as late as 1932, Newland [78] failed to mention radiology, Burgess [79] gave tentative support, but Paterson wrote: "The suggestion that radiography should be employed in the diagnosis of intestinal obstruction is one which should be condemned whole-heartedly ... I prefer the seeing eye of a living clinician to the scientific eye of a dead machine." [105]

In 1930, Ochsner (Figure 13) and Granger reported the use of plain films in 32 patients during the previous three years; in 20, a confident clinical diagnosis of obstruction was confirmed and in 12, when the clinical evidence was not diagnostic, they were of real value [106]. (Incidentally, this paper was not selected for presentation at the American Surgical Association!). Rabwin and Carter agreed, and noted a reduction in mortality during the preceding 18 months, as plain films led to earlier operation [107]. In 1940, Wangensteen was emphasising their value to establish whether obstruction was present, its level and whether it was complete [108] and McKittrick and Saris stated: "The so called scout film … is the most important objective finding in the patient with small bowel obstruction." [109] Radiology gave a positive result in 92% of their cases and was 'suggestive' in the remainder. However, as late as 1948 Samuel wrote: "When it is generally realised that most of these patients are well enough to be examined in the X-ray department ... the method will come into more general use." [110]

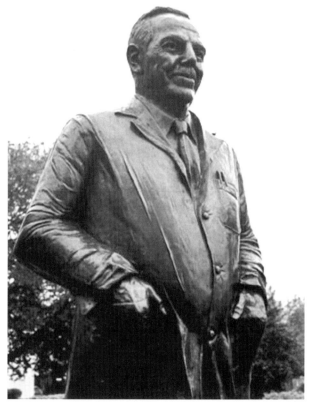

Figure 13. A statue of Alton Ochsner (1896-1981), which is sited in front of the Ochsner Clinic.

Other developments in the 1930s

Anaesthesia

Some had claimed lower mortality using spinal [31] or local anaesthesia [111] (mainly for blind enterostomy in late cases), but others had found the converse [52]. The appointment of specialist anaesthetists was doubtless a crucial factor in reducing risk [112]. Then the introduction of the cuffed endotracheal tube provided protection against aspiration and muscle relaxants facilitated access and closure.

Observation in hospital

It appears that until about 1930 patients with intestinal obstruction were not admitted to a surgical ward unless an operation was planned. In 1925, Vick suggested that the provision of an observation ward for patients suspected of obstruction might result in more timely operations [113]. Similarly, Wangensteen stated that "a patient suspected of having bowel obstruction should be under scrutiny and preferably in a hospital" [25] These were revolutionary ideas, paving the way for modern assessment.

Experience of the surgeon

Codman [64] attributed the high hospital mortality to leaving emergency operations to inexperienced juniors; there were 23 different operators for Richardson's 118 cases [30]. Miller concurred: "All these operations are of the gravest type and yet too often, chiefly because of the seniority system in our hospitals, they are undertaken by young and inexperienced men." [52] These comments were still relevant at the time of the CEPOD Report in 1987 [114].

The enlightenment

The major advances in the 1930s were creeping developments, occurring in parallel, so it is impossible to establish their individual contributions, but results certainly improved. In 1937, Orr, in a balanced review [115], summarised the important elements of treatment as operative relief of the obstruction, after first allowing a few hours for fluid replacement and relief of bowel distension.

Intravenous fluids and nasogastric suction were supported by Aird [116], and Smith agreed, adding radiological help in diagnosis, improved anaesthesia and the availability of antibiotics [117]. By 1958, Shires and Adwan proposed delaying operation, when strangulation was not thought to be present, to allow full fluid resuscitation: "It is obvious from the physiological consequences that if all patients with mechanical obstruction are operated upon as soon as the diagnosis is made, the operative mortality will be high. If there are signs of ischaemia immediate operation is indicated, otherwise allow time to replenish water and electrolyte deficits." [118]

Wangensteen and colleagues expanded their series to 190 cases, of which 126 were treated by suction, using nasoduodenal or Miller-Abbott tubes [83]. Decompression was achieved in 83 (6% mortality) and for 66 this was the only treatment needed. The most frequent operative procedure was still enterostomy (gradually to be replaced by suction and operative decompression). The overall mortality for treated cases was 15%. Using the Miller-Abbott tube as initial treatment, Leigh and Diefendorf achieved a mortality of 5% in 132 obstructed patients, of whom 29 avoided operation [119].

Tendler and Cartwright reviewed their results in a total of 2508 cases over 31 years [112]. The mortality fell from 51% in 1923-32 to 26% in 1933-46 and then 8.5% in 1947-53, and this trend is evident in other series (Table 1). They related the first stage of improvement to the 'enlightenment' of the use of X-rays, intravenous fluids and suction decompression. Subsequent progress was attributed to avoidance of prolonged suction, the use of a blood bank, antibiotics, availability of more appropriate fluids for intravenous use and the appointment of their first full-time anaesthetist.

When all obstructions were treated by immediate operation the detection of strangulation was unimportant. But when selecting patients for the alternative conservative management, it became vital not to miss strangulation and incur a mortality of 20-40% [120]. Strangulation predominantly affects the small bowel, while large bowel obstructions are chiefly due to carcinoma, so these two categories have increasingly been reported separately. Early postoperative obstruction merits independent consideration.

Small bowel obstruction

Wangensteen's group maintained that the incidence of missed strangulation was low enough to be offset by the gain from the avoidance of operation in a substantial proportion of patients [121]. Many others found that strangulation could not reliably be excluded and so called for early operation, delayed only by a few hours for fluid replacement and suction [109, 122-124] and Becker referred to "abuse of tube decompression" [125]. However, series involving a trial of aspiration in presumed adhesive obstruction, with no clinical evidence of strangulation, produced good results [93, 126, 127]. The consensus was that initial conservative treatment was indicated for recurrent adhesive obstruction or incomplete obstruction, subject to repeated reassessment and a time limit. Otherwise, particularly if there were any indicators of strangulation, early laparotomy was advised.

Diagnostically, a water-soluble contrast meal has been used to distinguish functional from mechanical small bowel obstruction or to indicate whether obstruction due to adhesions is likely to resolve on

conservative treatment [128]. Computed tomography may detect strangulation [129] and so clarify the decision.

Laparoscopy can identify the site of obstruction and treat many cases [130]. It can shorten hospital stay, but carries an increased incidence of early re-operation [131]. In adhesive obstruction it may have the specific benefit of a lower recurrence rate [132, 133].

There has also been recent discussion of the management of patients with obstruction due to extensive peritoneal metastases, for whom operation would be futile and whose management lies in the field of palliative care [134, 135].

Large bowel obstruction

Blind colostomy or caecostomy for left colon obstruction was discussed in an earlier section. The primary might then be resected as a second stage with later closure of the colostomy, but the mortality was high. Paul in 1895 adopted Mikulicz's exteriorisation/resection for obstruction (Figure 14), leaving only a minor second stage to close the double-barrelled colostomy [136]. At that time, obstruction in the right colon would have been treated initially by ileostomy or ileotransverse anastomosis.

Then it was shown that emergency primary anastomosis after right hemicolectomy was safe [137]. Staged management remained the norm for left-sided obstructions, although some advocated Hartmann's procedure [138] or subtotal colectomy [139]. Adventurous surgeons carried out primary resection and anastomosis [140, 141], but this did not become popular until the technique of on-table prograde lavage was described [142]. From then on primary resection and anastomosis were preferred, provided the patient's condition warranted it and the surgeon had the necessary skill [143]. A water-soluble contrast enema became standard practice, before operation for distal large bowel obstruction, to exclude pseudo-obstruction and avoid an unnecessary operation [144]. Recently, expanding metal stents, inserted endoscopically, have been used to defer operation or for palliation [145].

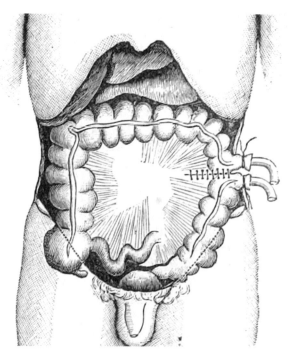

Figure 14. Paul-Mikulicz exteriorisation resection for colonic obstruction. *Reproduced with permission from the British Medical Publishing Group* [136].

The management of sigmoid volvulus was revolutionised by the realisation that it could be relieved in 90% of cases by sigmoidoscopic deflation [146], but an elective resection is necessary to prevent recurrence.

Early postoperative obstruction and paralytic ileus

Between 1900 and 1930, paralytic ileus, mainly due to peritonitis, was treated by enterostomy [57] or Handley's combination of jejunocolic anastomosis and caecostomy, with the objective of draining the small bowel [147]. Early postoperative obstructions were assumed to be mechanical; McIver [111] reported 84 operations (mostly within two weeks) accounting for 21% of all operations for acute obstruction, with a 44% mortality. Others suggested that many such cases would recover with suction decompression [93, 148], and

Leigh and Diefendorf treated 77 patients with paralytic ileus, of whom only five required operation [119]. In 1962, Miller and colleagues [149] concluded that the indications for operation in paralytic ileus were few, and this remains the modern view.

Changing causes of obstruction

Early collected series comprised only those conditions then considered suitable for operation [3] or combined these with autopsy reports [43] and so were subject to publication bias. The causes of obstruction in Gibson's collected series from 1900 [150] and subsequent large, single hospital series are set out in Table 2. External hernias continued to be the most common mechanism until the mid-20th century, when

Table 2. Causes of intestinal obstruction expressed as percentages of the total in each series (1888-1996).

First author	Years of data collection	Adhesions / bands	Hernia	Intussusception	Tumour	Volvulus	Others	No. of cases
Gibson [150]	1888-98	19	35	19	-	12	15	1000*
Burgess [104]	1913-22	-	65	13	14	-	8	1278
Souttar [61]	1920-24	18	46	21	12	2	1	3064
Miller [52]	1924-29	28	28	12	5	10	17	342
Vick [62]	1925-30	7	49	12	13	0.2	?19	6892
Becker [125]	1940-49	41	30	7	10	6	6	1007
Nemir [158]	1940-52	36	25	2	23	4	10	358
Smith [121]	1942-53	30	10	3	27	3	27	1252
Tendler [112]	1947-53	49	35	4	4	5	4	684
Barling [159]	1950-53	38	20	3	12	5	22	306
Waldron [160]	1944-56	41	12	4	14	6	23	493
Bevan [164]	1960-75	16	19	2	30	5	29	414
Laws [162]	1963-72	69	8	1	10	-	12	465+
Nelson [165]	1962-83	31	23	1	30	5	7	279#
Fevang [163]	1960-95	54	30	E	E	3	16	1007+
McEntee [127]	1985-86	32	25	-	26	4	14	228
Miller [166]	1986-96	68	3	-	5	25	-	1001+

* Gibson's was a collected series

Operative cases only

+ Small bowel obstruction only

E Excluded from series

their decline was overtaken by the rising incidence of adhesive obstruction. By then a policy of elective repair had reduced the incidence of strangulated hernia, although not yet in less developed countries [151]. The incidence of adhesive obstruction in the early years was greater than might have been expected because many cases of early postoperative obstruction (mostly post-appendicectomy) were operated upon and included in this category. Intussusception declined remarkably, explained partly by infants becoming concentrated in paediatric surgical units, and partly by there seeming to have been more cases in adults in the 19th century.

Adhesive obstruction

As the numbers of abdominal operations have increased, late postoperative obstruction due to adhesions has become the major cause of small bowel obstruction. Seror et al [152] in 1993 analysed 297 admissions for adhesive obstruction in 227 patients, of whom 73% responded to conservative treatment, with mortality for the whole series of 1.7%. The median period of conservative treatment in patients coming to operation was two days and none responded after five days.

There is concern at the economic burden of treatment for adhesions [153, 154]. Fortunately, the increasing use of laparoscopic surgery may gradually reduce the incidence of adhesive obstruction. In the operative management of adhesion obstruction, the application of a bio-resorbable membrane has potential to reduce subsequent adhesion formation [155].

Conclusions

When an operation was very high risk it could be considered only when the patient had deteriorated, at which stage the result was going to be poor, a situation persisting into the late 19th century. Opinion then switched to immediate operation but adherence to the 'toxaemia' theory delayed acceptance of fluid depletion and bowel distension as factors in the continuing mortality of 30-60%.

Enlightenment came in the 1930s, with intravenous fluids and suction decompression (the now ubiquitous 'drip and suck'), plain radiographs, improved anaesthesia, blood transfusion and, later, antibiotics. By the 1950s mortality rates were down to 10-20%, later reaching single figures for small bowel obstruction. A policy of selective conservative management was controversial because of the risk of missing strangulation.

Meanwhile, the case mix had shifted, with many fewer strangulated hernias and with adhesions predominating among small bowel causes. Now, laparoscopic surgery offers the potential for shorter stay and perhaps fewer recurrences of adhesive obstruction.

Biographical footnote on Owen Wangensteen

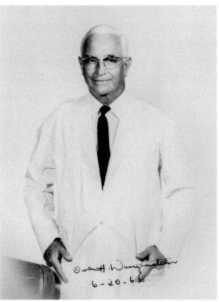

Figure 15. Owen H. Wangensteen (1898-1981). *Reproduced with permission from the National Library of Medicine, Bethesda, Maryland, USA.*

Owen Wangensteen was born in Lake Park, Minnesota in 1898 into a farming family of Norwegian stock. He was one of four siblings whose mother died when he was seven; he developed a close bond with his father. All three brothers helped on the farm, Owen perhaps more than the others: "They learned to hunt, and I learned to work. And I think I got the best of the deal." Indeed, he was set on becoming a farmer, but his father felt that all his children should have higher education. One event seems to have settled the matter. During his junior year at high school their herd of 50 sows were unable to farrow their young. The veterinary surgeon could offer no solution, but then Owen successfully performed a manual delivery for a litter of five piglets; during the following three weeks he delivered a total of over 300. This convinced him that he should become a veterinarian, but his father prevailed upon him to study medicine.

After obtaining a BA from the University of Minnesota he enrolled in the medical school and graduated first in his year in 1922. He had initially been attracted to internal medicine but the lectures given by Dr. Arthur Strachauer convinced him that "surgery was where the action was". At the end of his internship in Minnesota there was no surgical fellowship available, so he accepted one in medicine and this included an introduction to research. He spent 1924 with Dr. William Mayo at the Mayo Clinic, with the opportunity to visit the nearby animal farm and research laboratories. He then returned to the University of Minnesota to complete his dissertation on "The undescended testis: an experimental and clinical study". In 1925, he obtained a PhD in surgery; a classmate reported that: "The examiners finally gave up. They could not ask anything he could not answer." On completion of his training he was offered a place in a practice in South Dakota at four times his then salary but he declined saying that it was "impossible for me to leave the University", which indeed he never did, apart from a year in Europe.

A vacancy then arose, on the resignation of Dr. Strachauer, for the Headship of the Department of Surgery. Three candidates, including Owen Wangensteen, were interviewed but the other two withdrew on the basis that "there is nothing here and never will be". The Dean of the Medical School was keen for Wangensteen to be appointed, but he was only 31 and held the lowly rank of instructor. The problem was solved by promotion to Assistant Professor and his being sent on a study tour to Europe, working with De Quervain (Kocher's successor) and Ascher. On the recommendation of Dr. William Mayo, he visited famous clinics in Germany. He also met Lord Moynihan, who advised him to read Shakespeare. On returning to Minnesota he was promoted to Associate Professor, and in 1930 he became Chairman of Surgery, at the early age of 32.

He launched the Department into the intensive study of intestinal obstruction, which in 1932 had a mortality of over 30%. The programme involved the promotion of auscultation, plain abdominal films and intravenous fluids, and especially the introduction of nasogastric and later naso-intestinal suction. He demonstrated that the 'lethal factor' in simple obstruction was bowel distension (including the closed loop effect), not the previously accepted 'toxin'. As a result, mortality rates fell to 5-10% and these methods remain the norm 70 years later. For this crucially important work he received the Samuel D. Gross Prize in 1935. Nevertheless, gastric suction was not readily accepted by publishers; the first paper on suction drainage was rejected by two journals and had to be repackaged under the innocuous title of "The early diagnosis of acute intestinal obstruction with comments on treatment, with a report of successful decompression of three cases of mechanical bowel obstruction by nasal catheter suction siphonage". In the third edition of his book *Intestinal Obstruction*, he describes how the first edition had been rejected by the three publishers.

The Department's research flourished in many other directions, notably in the development of techniques for open heart surgery and in the management of cancer. Inevitably, not all of his enthusiasm prospered, for example, gastric freezing for duodenal ulcer proved ineffective and dangerous, but it was well worth trying. He was author of over 800 original articles.

When he started in 1930 there was one surgical fellow in the department, increasing to 100 by the time of his retirement in 1967. Each had a programme tailored to his needs, with encouragement of original thought and what we would now call evidence-based medicine. Practical training was started in the lab: "The young surgeon who, during his pursuit of a research problem, has learned to operate with safety upon a dog, is a surgeon to whom operations in man can be trusted." Logical, but no longer acceptable. Of his trainees, 110 became full professors and 38 were departmental chairmen.

In 1937 he co-founded the journal *Surgery*, continuing as co-editor until his retirement in 1970, a remarkably long innings. In 1940, to provide trainees with a surgical audience for their research presentations, he proposed the inclusion of a 'Surgical Forum' at meetings of the Society of University Surgeons. The Surgical Forum has grown to occupy about 25 sessions at each meeting of the American College of Surgeons.

After retirement from clinical surgery in 1967 he developed his interest in surgical history. With his wife, Sarah, in 1978 he published *The Rise of Surgery: from Empiric Craft to Scientific Discipline*.

Acknowledgement

Not having had the privilege of knowing Dr. Wangensteen, I have drawn heavily upon information from tributes published in *Surgery* and *Digestive Surgery*.

References

1. Power D'A. Epoch making books in British Surgery: I. A system of surgery by Master John Arderne. *Br J Surg* 1927; 15: 1-9.

2. Adams F. The genuine works of Hippocrates. London: Sydenham Society, 1849.

3. Ashhurst J. On laparotomy, or abdominal section, as a remedy for intussusception; with tables showing the results of the operation in cases of this affection, and in those of other forms of acute obstruction of the bowels. *Am J Med Sci* 1874; 68: 48-64.

4. Wangensteen OH, Wangensteen S. Intestinal obstructions. In: *The rise of surgery.* Folkestone: Dawson, 1978: 106-41.

5. Petit J-L. Traité des maladies chirurgicale et des opérations que leur convenient, ouvrage posthume. *Paris* 1790; 2: 273-358.

6. Maunoury LJ. Considérations sur l'étranglement interne du canal intestinal. Paris thesis quoted by Veillard L. *Union Méd* 1857; 11: 371-3.

7. de Ronsil A. *A dissertation on hernias, or ruptures.* London, 1748.

8. Cheselden W. *The anatomy of the human body,* 11th edn. London, 1778.

9. Pott P. *Treatise on ruptures.* London: Hawes Clarke & Collins, 1763: 73-120.

10. Lawrence W. A treatise on rupture. London, 1816.

11. Jones CW. *A series of lectures on the most approved principles and practice of surgery derived from the lectures delivered by Astley Cooper,* 2nd edn. Syder CM, Ed. London: Highley, 1821: 279-80.

12. Browne JW. Practical remarks relative to the subject of strangulated hernia. *Br Med J* 1883; 2: 912-3.

13. Frankau C. Strangulated hernia: a review of 1487 cases. *Br J Surg* 1924; 10: 779.

14. Sydenham T. *The works of Thomas Sydenham.* Trans Latham RG. London: Sydenham Society, 1848; 1(68): 194-202.

15. Brown BW. On intestinal obstructions. *Assoc Med J* 1853; 1: 117-23.

16. Hutchinson J. Notes on intestinal obstruction: its diagnosis and treatment. *Br Med J* 1878; 2: 305-7.

17. Brinton W. *Intestinal obstruction.* London: Churchill, 1867.

18. Bryant T. The mode of death from acute intestinal strangulation and chronic intestinal obstruction. *Br Med J* 1884: 2: 1001-5.

19. Gordon TE. A case of haemorrhagic infarction of the small intestine: successful resection. *Br Med J* 1898; 1: 1447-8.

20. McGlannan A. Intestinal obstruction. *JAMA* 1915; 65: 673-5.

21. Hausler RW, Foster WC. Studies of acute intestinal obstruction. *Arch Int Med* 1924: 34: 97-107.

22. Scott HG, Wangensteen OH. Blood losses in experimental intestinal strangulations and their relationship to degree of shock and death. *Proc Soc for Expt Biol and Med* 1932; 40: 748-51.

23. Van Zwalenburg C. Strangulation resulting from distension of hollow viscera. *Ann Surg* 1907; 46: 780-6.

24. Morrison R. Notes on a case of intestinal obstruction: with comments on bursts of the intestine. *Br J Surg* 1918; 6: 135-9.

25. Wangensteen OH. The early diagnosis of acute intestinal obstruction with comments on pathology and treatment. *Western J Surg Gyn Obstet* 1932; 40: 1-17.

26. Cohn I. The toxic factor in closed loop obstruction. *Am J Surg* 1962; 104: 482-9.

27. Treves F. *Intestinal obstruction; its varieties with their pathology diagnosis etc.* London: Cassell, 1884.

28. Treves F. *Intestinal obstruction.* London: Cassell, 1901.

29. Murphy JB. Ileus. *JAMA* 1896; 26: 15-22.

30. Richardson EP. Acute intestinal obstruction: a study of a second series of cases from the Massachusetts General Hospital. *Boston Med Surg J* 1920; 183: 288-98.

31. Southam AH. Treatment of ileus following operations. *Lancet* 1928; 214: 41-2.

32. Cope Z. A history of the acute abdomen. London: Oxford University Press, 1965.

33. Amussat JZ. Quelques réflexions pratiques sur les obstructions du rectum. *Gaz Méd Paris* 1839; 7: 1-8.

34. Hawkins CH. Case of stricture of the colon successfully treated by operation. *Med-chir Trans* 1852; 35: 85-126.

35. Hilton J. *Hilton's rest and pain,* 6th edn. London: Bell, 1953: 298-99.

36. Barbette P. *Opera chirurgico-anatomica.* Leyden 1672: 381-2.

37. Gay J. On intestinal obstruction by the solitary band. Read at a meeting of the Medical Society of London, 1861; *Roy Coll Surg Engl*; Tracts 578(1).

38. Nélaton A. (In discussion). *Union Méd* 1851; 5: 344.

39. Hutchinson J. A successful case of abdominal section for intussusception. *Med-chir Trans* 1874; 57: 31-75.

40. Teale TP. On exploration of the abdomen in obstruction of the bowels. *Br Med J* 1879; 1: 41-3.

41. Bryant T. On the surgical treatment of intestinal obstruction, with two cases of enterotomy. *Lancet* 1878: 1; 674-5.

42. Parker R. Intestinal obstruction. *Br Med J* 1883; 2: 669-72.

43. Fitz RH. The diagnosis and medical treatment of acute intestinal obstruction. *Trans Am Congress of Physicians and Surgeons* 1888; 1: 1-42.

44. Senn N. *Intestinal Surgery.* Chicago: Keener, 1899: 28.

45. Treves F. An address on some rudiments of intestinal surgery. *Br Med J* 1898; 2: 1385-90.

46. Kocher T. Intestinal obstruction. *Br Med J* 1898; 2: 1298-1300.

47. Elliott JW. Management of certain critical cases of intestinal obstruction with a report of cases. *Ann Surg* 1905; 42: 668-77.

48. Holmes T. Experience of St. George's Hospital in laparotomy. *Br Med J* 1895; 2: 125-8.

49. Burgess AH. An address on acute intestinal obstruction. *Lancet* 1929; 1: 857-9.

50. Tuttle HK. The mortality of intestinal obstruction: a study of 150 cases coming to operation or autopsy. *Boston Med Surg J* 1925; 192: 791-5.

51. Deaver JB, Ross GG. The mortality statistics of 276 cases of intestinal obstruction. *Ann Surg* 1915; 61: 198-203.

52. Miller CJ. A study of 343 surgical cases of intestinal obstruction. *Ann Surg* 1929; 89: 91-7.

53. Murphy FT, Brooks B. Intestinal obstruction: an experimental study of the causes of symptoms and death. *Arch Int Med* 1915; 15: 392-412.

54. Dragstedt LR, Dragstedt CA, McLintock JT, *et al*. Intestinal obstruction II: a study of the factors involved in the production and absorption of toxic materials from the intestine. *J Exp Med* 1919; 30: 109-21.

55. Williams BW. The importance of toxaemia due to anaerobic organisms in intestinal obstruction and peritonitis. *Br J Surg* 1926; 14: 295-322.

56. Whipple GH, Stone HB, Bernheim BM. Intestinal obstruction II: a study of a toxic substance produced by the mucosa of closed duodenal loops. *J Exp Med* 1913; 17: 307-23.

57. Bonney V. Faecal and intestinal vomiting and jejunostomy. *Br Med J* 1916; 1: 583-5.

58. Moynihan B. *Abdominal operatons*, 4th edn. Philadelphia: Saunders, 1926: 128-59

59. Primrose R. Discussion on intestinal obstruction. *Br Med J* 1925; 2: 999.

60. Taylor W. The treatment of primary acute intestinal obstruction. *Br Med J* 1925; 2: 993-5.

61. Souttar HS. Discussion on acute intestinal obstruction. *Br Med J* 1925; 2: 1000-2

62. Vick RM. Statistics of acute intestinal obstruction. *Br Med J* 1932; 2: 546-8.

63. Van Beuren FT, Smith BC. The status of enterostomy in the treatment of acute ileus. *Arch Surg* 1927; 15: 288-97.

64. Codman EA. Intestinal obstruction. *Boston Med Surg J* 1920; 182: 420-4, 451-8.

65. Holden WB. Intestinal obstruction: a survey of 135 personal cases. *Arch Surg* 1926; 16: 882-6.

66. Brill S. The mortality of intestinal obstruction. *Ann Surg* 1929; 89: 541-8.

67. O'Shaughnessy WB. *Report on the chemical pathology of the malignant cholera: containing analyses of the blood, dejections etc of patients labouring under that disease in Newcastle and London*. London: Highley, 1832.

68. Matas R. A clinical report on intravenous saline infusion in the wards of the New Orleans Charity Hospital from June 1888 to June 1891. *New Orleans Med and Surg J* 1891; 19: 1-93.

69. Hey Groves EW. *A synopsis of surgery*, 4th edn. Bristol: John Wright, 1914.

70. Hartwell JA, Hoguet JP, Beekman F. An experimental study of intestinal obstruction. *Arch Int Med* 1914; 13: 701-36.

71. Wilkie DPD. Experimental observations on the cause of death in acute intestinal obstruction. *Br Med J* 1913; 2: 1064-7.

72. Orr TG, Haden RL. Reducing the surgical risk in some gastrointestinal conditions. *JAMA* 1925; 85: 813-4.

73. Whipple AO. Safety factors in the treatment of acute intestinal obstruction. *Boston Med Surg J* 1927; 197: 218-22.

74. Armour JC, Brown TG, Dunlop DM, *et al*. Studies on high intestinal obstruction: the administration of saline and other substances by enterostomy below the site of obstruction. *Br J Surg* 1931; 18: 467-78.

75. Gamble JL, Ross SG. The factors in the dehydration following pyloric obstruction. *J Clin Invest* 1925; 1: 403-23.

76. Penfield WG, Teplitsky D. Prolonged intravenous infusion and the clinical determination of venous pressure. *Arch Surg* 1923; 7: 111-24.

77. Mattas R. The continued intravenous 'drip'. *Ann Surg* 1924; 79: 643-61.

78. Newland HS. Remarks on acute intestinal obstruction. *Br Med J* 1932; 2: 539-40.

79. Burgess AH. Acute intestinal obstruction. *Br Med J* 1932; 2: 542-4.

80. Gatch WD, Culbertson CG. Circulatory disturbances caused by intestinal obstruction. *Ann Surg* 1935; 102: 619-35.

81. Wangensteen OH, Paine JR. Treatment of acute intestinal obstruction by suction with the duodenal tube. *JAMA* 1933; 101: 1532-9.

82. Coller FA, Bartlett RM, Bingham DLC, *et al*. The replacement of sodium chloride in surgical patients. *Ann Surg* 1938; 108: 769-82.

83. Wangensteen OH, Rea CE, Smith BA, *et al*. Experiences with employment of suction in the treatment of acute intestinal obstruction; a reiteration of the indications, contra-indications and limitations of the method. *Surg Gynecol Obstet* 1939; 68: 851-68.

84. Borow M, Aquilizan L, Krausz A, *et al*. Use of CVP as an accurate guide for body fluid replacement. *Surg Gynecol Obstet* 1965; 120: 545-52.

85. Schilling JA, McCord AB, Clausen SW. Potassium loss in experimental intestinal obstruction. *Surg Gynecol Obstet* 1951; 92: 1-13.

86. Paine JR. The history of the invention and development of the stomach and duodenal tubes. *Ann Int Med* 1934. 8: 752-63.

87. Levin AL. A new gastro-duodenal catheter. *JAMA* 1921; 76: 1007.

88. Grey Turner G. Discussion on acute intestinal obstruction. *Br Med J* 1925; 2: 1001-2.

89. Westermann CWJ. Über die Anwendung des Dauermagenhebers bei der Nachbehandlung schwerer Peritonitisfälle. *Zentralbl Chir* 1910; 37: 356.

90. Wangensteen OH, Rea CE. The distention factor in simple intestinal obstruction; an experimental study with exclusion of swallowed air by cervical oesophagostomy. *Surgery* 1939; 5: 327-39.

91. Abbott WO, Johnston CG. Intubation studies of human small intestine: a non-surgical method of treating, localising and diagnosing obstructive lesions. *Surg Gynecol Obstet* 1938; 66: 691-7.

92. Smith BC. Experiences with the Miller-Abbott tube. *Ann Surg* 1945; 122: 253-9.

93. Bizer LS, Liebling RW, Delany HM, *et al*. Small bowel obstruction: the role of non-operative treatment in simple intestinal obstruction and predictive criteria for strangulation obstruction. *Surgery* 1981; 89: 407-13.

94. Fleshner PR, Siegman MG, Slater GI, *et al*. A prospective randomised trial of short versus long tubes in adhesive small bowel obstruction. *Am J Surg* 1996; 170: 366-70.

95. Rohovsky S, Bleday R. Small bowel obstruction. In: *Oxford Textbook of Surgery*, 2nd edn. Morris P, Wood WC, Eds. Oxford: Oxford University Press, 2000: 1345-9.

96. Monks GH. Studies in the surgical anatomy of the small intestine and its mesentery. *Ann Surg* 1905; 42: 543-69.

97. Wangensteen OH. New operative techniques in the management of bowel obstruction. *Surg Gynecol Obstet* 1942; 75: 675-92.

98. Savage PT. Discussion on small bowel obstruction. *Proc Roy Soc Med* 1958; 51: 507-8.

99. Baker JW. A long jejunostomy tube for decompressing intestinal obstruction. *Surg Gynecol Obstet* 1959; 109: 518-20.

100. Mayo W. Report of a case of volvulus of the sigmoid flexure of the colon successfully reduced after abdominal section. *Ann Surg* 1893; 18: 28-9.

101. Bailey H, Love McN. *A short practice of surgery*. London: HK Lewis, 1959: 559-60.

102. Schwarz G. Die Erkennung der tieferen Dünndarmstenosen mittels des Röntgenverfahrens. *Wien Klin Wchnschr* 1911; 24: 1386-94.

103. Case JT. Roentgen studies after gastric and intestinal operations. *JAMA* 1915; 65: 1628-34.

104. Burgess AH. Discussion on the treatment of obstruction of the colon. *Br Med J* 1923; 2: 547-56.

105. Paterson HJ. Acute intestinal obstruction. *Br Med J* 1932; 2: 546.

106. Ochsner A, Granger A. The röentgen diagnosis of ileus. *Ann Surg* 1930; 92: 947-54.

107. Rabwin MH, Carter RA. Acute intestinal obstruction - its diagnosis by the flat X-ray film. *Californian Western Med* 1930; 33: 483-6.

108. Wangensteen OH. The value of diagnostic criteria for the choice of therapeutic procedure in the management of acute intestinal obstruction: experimental and clinical observations. *Radiology* 1940; 35: 680-8.

109. McKittrick LS, Saris SP. Acute mechanical obstruction of the small bowel. *New Engl J Med* 1940; 222: 611-22.

110. Samuel E, Smith R. *Acute intestinal obstruction*. London: Arnold, 1948: 54-81.

111. McIver MA. Acute intestinal obstruction. *Arch Surg* 1932; 25: 1106-24.

112. Tendler MJ, Cartwright RS. Acute intestinal obstruction - a re-evaluation of therapy: review of thirty-one years at a university hospital (1923-1953). *J Louisiana State Med Soc* 1956; 108: 4-10.

113. Vick RM. Discussion on intestinal obstruction. *Br Med J* 1925; 2: 999-1000.

114. The report of the Confidential Enquiry into PeriOperative Deaths. Nuffield Provincial Hospitals Trust and The King Edward's Hospitals Fund for London. London, 1987.

115. Orr TG. The therapeutic management of intestinal obstruction. *Surgery* 1937; 1: 838-47.

116. Aird I. Morbid influences in intestinal obstruction and strangulation. *Ann Surg* 1941; 114: 385-414.

117. Smith R. *Acute intestinal obstruction*. London: Edward Arnold, 1948: 4.

118. Shires T, Adwan KO. A review of advances in management of mechanical obstruction of the small intestine. *Am Surg* 1958; 24: 432-8.

119. Leigh OC, Diefendorf RO. The Miller-Abbott tube in surgery. *JAMA* 1942; 118: 210-4.

120. Stewardson RH, Bombeck CT, Nyhus LM. Critical operative management of small bowel obstruction. *Ann Surg* 1978; 187: 189-93.

121. Smith GA, Perry JF, Yonahero EG. Mechanical intestinal obstructions: a study of 1252 cases. *Surg Gynecol Obstet* 1955; 100: 651-60.

122. Cooke RV. Discussion on small bowel obstruction. *Proc Roy Soc Med* 1958; 51: 503-7.

123. Silen W, Hein MF, Goldman L. Strangulation of the small intestine. *Arch Surg* 1962; 85: 137-45.

124. Ellis H. Mechanical intestinal obstruction. *Br Med J* 1981; 283: 1203-4.

125. Becker WF. Intestinal obstruction. *Southern Med J* 1955; 48: 41-6.

126. Wolfson PJ, Bauer JJ, Gelernt IM, *et al.* Use of the long tube in management of patients with small-intestinal obstruction due to adhesions. *Arch Surg* 1985; 120: 1001-6.

127. McEntee G, Pender D, Mulvin D, *et al.* Current spectrum of intestinal obstruction. *Br J Surg* 1987; 74: 976-80.

128. Riveron FA, Farouk N, Obeid FN, *et al.* The role of contrast radiography in presumed bowel obstruction. *Surgery* 1989; 106: 496-501.

129. Donkier V, Closset J, Van Gansbeke D. Contribution of computed tomography to decision making in the management of adhesive small bowel obstruction. *Br J Surg* 1998; 85: 1071-4.

130. Franklin ME, Gonzalez JJ, Miter DB, *et al.* Laparoscopic diagnosis and treatment of intestinal obstruction. *Surg Endosc* 2004; 18: 26-30.

131. Bailey IS, Rhodes M, O'Rourke N, *et al.* Laparoscopic management of acute small bowel obstruction. *Br J Surg* 1998; 85: 84-7.

132. Wullstein C, Gross E. Laparoscopic compared with conventional treatment of acute adhesive small bowel obstruction. *Br J Surg* 2003; 90: 1147-51.

133. Tsumura H, Ichikawa T, Murakami Y, *et al.* Laparoscopic adhesiolysis for recurrent post-operative small bowel obstruction. *Hepatogastroenterology* 2004; 51: 1058-61.

134. Parker MC, Baines MJ. Intestinal obstruction in patients with advanced malignant disease. *Br J Surg* 1996; 83: 1-2.

135. Hardy JR. Medical management of bowel obstruction. *Br J Surg* 2000; 87: 1281-3.

136. Paul FT. Colectomy. *Br Med J* 1895; 1: 1136-9.

137. Muir EG. Right hemicolectomy. *Proc Roy Soc Med* 1947; 40: 831-3.

138. Sames CP. Resection of carcinoma of the rectum in the presence of obstruction. *Lancet* 1960; 2: 948-9.

139. Hughes ESR. Mortality of acute large bowel obstruction. *Br J Surg* 1966; 53: 593-4.

140. Gregg RO. The place of emergency resection in the management of obstructing and perforating lesions of the colon. *Surgery* 1955; 37: 754-60.

141. Fielding LP, Stewart-Brown S, Blesovsky L. Large bowel obstruction caused by cancer: a prospective study. *Br Med J* 1979; 2: 515-7.

142. Dudley HAF, Radcliffe AG, McGeehan D. Intraoperative irrigation of the colon to permit primary anastomosis. *Br J Surg* 1980; 67: 80-1.

143. Sjodahl R, Franzén T, Nyström P-O. Primary versus staged resection for obstructing colorectal carcinoma. *Br J Surg* 1992; 79: 685-8.

144. Stewart J, Finan PJ, Courtney DF, *et al.* Does a water-soluble contrast enema assist in the management of acute large bowel obstruction; a prospective study of 117 cases. *Br J Surg* 1984; 71: 779-801.

145. Young CJ, Solomon MJ. Acute malignant colorectal obstruction and self-expandable metallic stents. *ANZ J Surg* 2002; 72: 851.

146. Nadrowski LF. Pathophysiology and current treatment of intestinal obstruction. *Rev Surg* 1974; 31: 381-407.

147. Handley WS. Discussion on acute intestinal obstruction. *Br Med J* 1925; 2: 995-6.

148. Morton JJ. Factors determining the selection of operation in obstruction of the small intestine. *Ann Surg* 1932; 95: 848-58.

149. Miller LD, Mackie JA, Rhoads JE. The pathophysiology and management of intestinal obstruction. *Surg Clin N Am* 1962; 42(5): 1285-309.

150. Gibson CL. A study of one thousand operations for acute intestinal obstruction and gangrenous hernia. *Ann Surg* 1900; 32: 486-514.

151. Naaeder SB, Archampong EQ. Changing pattern of acute intestinal obstruction in Accra. *Wo Afr Med J* 1993; 12: 82-8.

152. Seror D, Feigin E, Szold A, *et al.* How conservatively can postoperative small bowel obstruction be treated? *Am J Surg* 1993; 165: 121-6.

153. Ray NF, Denton WG, Thamer M, *et al.* Abdominal adhesiolysis: inpatient care and expenditures in the United States in 1994. *J Am Coll Surg* 1998; 186: 1-9.

154. Miller G, Boman J, Shrier I, *et al.* Natural history of patients with adhesive small bowel obstruction. *Br J Surg* 2000; 87: 1240-7.

155. Becker JM, Dayton MT, Fazio VW, *et al.* Prevention of postoperative abdominal adhesions by sodium hyaluronidate based bio-resorbable membrane: a prospective randomised double blind multicentre study. *J Am Coll Surg* 1996; 183: 297-306.

156. Hudson RV, Smith R, Selbie FR, *et al.* The prognosis of acute intestinal obstruction. *Lancet* 1941; 1: 438-42.

157. Eliason EL, Welty RF. A ten-year survey of intestinal obstruction. *Ann Surg* 1947; 125: 57-65.

158. Nemir P. Intestinal obstruction: ten-year statistical survey at the Hospital of the University of Pennsylvania. *Ann Surg* 1952; 135: 367-75.

159. Barling EV. Intestinal obstruction. *ANZ J Surg* 1956; 25: 285-91.

160. Waldron GW, Hampton JM. Intestinal obstruction: a half century comparative analysis. *Ann Surg* 1961; 153: 839-50.

161. Davis SE, Sperling L. Obstruction of the small intestine. *Arch Surg* 1969; 99: 424-6.

162. Laws HL, Aldrete JS. Small-bowel obstruction: a review of 465 cases. *South Med J* 1976; 69: 733-4.

163. Fevang BT, Fevang J, Stangelend L, *et al.* Complications and death after surgical treatment of small bowel obstruction: a 35-year institutional experience. *Ann Surg* 2000; 231: 529-37.

164. Bevan PG. Adhesive obstruction. *Ann Roy Coll Surg Engl* 1984; 66: 164-9.

165. Nelson IW, Ellis H. The spectrum of intestinal obstruction today. *Br J Clin Pract* 1984; 38: 249-51.

166. Miller G, Boman J, Shrier I, *et al.* Etiology of small bowel obstruction. *Am J Surg* 2000; 180: 33-6.

Chapter 10

Intestinal reconstruction

David FL Watkin MChir FRCS

Emeritus Consultant Surgeon, Leicester Royal Infirmary, Leicester, UK

Bowel anastomosis

Anastomosis is an integral part of many gastro-intestinal operations, but it had a difficult birth. The issues to be resolved included the suture material, or other devices for approximation of the bowel ends, the placement of the sutures and the configuration of the join (side-to-side or end-to-end). Various methods were employed to minimise spillage of intestinal contents, extending to the use of a 'closed' technique.

Early attempts at bowel repair

Senn (Figure 1) reviewed the early attempts at suturing bowel, usually for stab wounds [1]. At first surgeons employed a continuous over-and-over 'glover's stitch', the ends of which were brought out through the wound to promote fistula formation in the event of leakage.

In the 13th century, Saliceto, treating strangulated hernias in Italy, sutured the bowel ends over a splint of animal bowel. His pupil Lanfranc [2] used a stent of animal trachea, as did Duverger in 1747; the trachea was passed about three weeks later. Ramdohr (1727) and Pott [3] (1756) described invagination of the proximal into the distal end, secured with a few

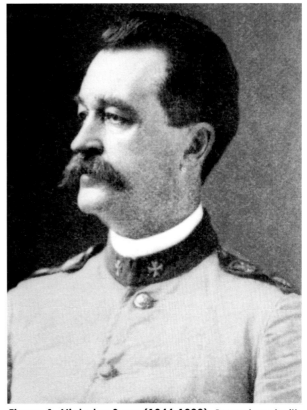

Figure 1. Nicholas Senn (1844-1909). *Reproduced with permission from the National Library of Medicine, Bethesda, Maryland, USA.*

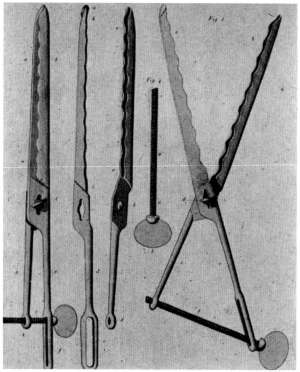

Figure 2. Dupuytren's enterotome for crushing the spur of an artifical anus. The instrument is shown closed, open, and dismembered into the two blades and screw. *Reproduced with permission from Oxford University Press. The Development of the Surgery of Acute Abdominal Disease. In: Pioneers in Acute Abdominal Surgery. Cope Z. London: Humphrey Milford, 1939: 19.*

dogs, everting the mucosa, and showed that sutures involving all layers are discharged into the lumen of the bowel.

Lembert, a pupil of Dupuytren, observed that serosa adhered to serosa and used interrupted inverting sutures in dogs in 1826, to take advantage of this [7]. His sutures either penetrated the mucosa or, if the bowel was thick, glided between the muscularis and the mucosa (the present meaning of Lembert sutures) (Figure 5). All the sutures were inserted before any was tied and, contrary to the then

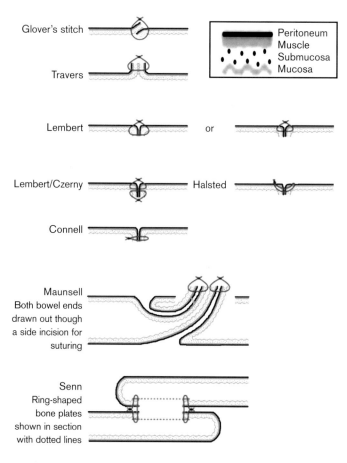

Figure 3. Anastomotic techniques. *Courtesy of the Medical Illustration Department, Leicester Royal Infirmary, Leicester, UK.*

sutures which were brought out through the wound; such apposition of mucosa and serosa is not favourable for union.

However, most surgeons in the 18th century, including those of the French Royal Academy, took the safer option of creating a double stoma. They hoped for spontaneous closure of the fistula, encouraged by traction on a suture through the adjacent anti-mesenteric borders to break down the spur. Later, Dupuytren (Figure 5, Chapter 12), who had a referral practice in closure of these fistulae, devised an enterotome for this purpose [4] (Figure 2).

Anastomotic techniques (Figure 3)

Cooper [5] (Figure 3, Chapter 9) and Travers [6] (Figure 4) experimented with bowel anastomosis in

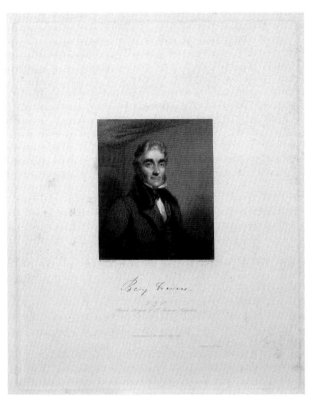

Figure 4. Benjamin Travers (1783-1858). *Reproduced with permission from the Wellcome Library, London.*

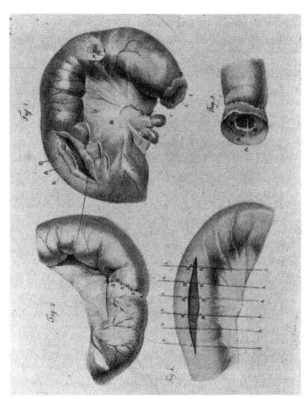

Figure 5. Lembert's drawing of his anastomosis. *Reproduced with permission from Oxford University Press. The Development of the Surgery of Acute Abdominal Disease. In: Pioneers in Acute Abdominal Surgery. Cope Z. London: Humphrey Milford, 1939: 21.*

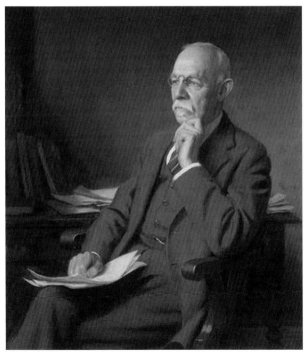

Figure 6. William Stewart Halsted (1852-1922). *Reproduced with permission from The Alan Mason Chesney Medical Archives of The Johns Hopkins Medical Institutions.*

accepted practice, the sutures were cut close to the knots. Lembert did not have a surviving patient from this procedure, but Dieffenbach did in 1836 [4]. Serosal contact remained a principle of intestinal anastomosis until linear stapling was introduced.

In the early 1880s, German surgeons, building on Lembert's method and with the aid of antisepsis, published new techniques of anastomosis. Kocher [8] (Figure 14, Chapter 12), dealing with strangulated hernias, emphasised that the line of section must be through healthy bowel. Czerny [9] (Figure 16, Chapter 4) added an inner row of sutures, uniting mucosa and muscularis to reduce the risk of leakage, the knots being buried under the Lembert sutures. Rydygier [10] used a continous suture for each of the two layers.

Halsted (Figure 6), in 1887, on the basis of animal experiments, identified the submucosa as the important layer: "The submucosa is found to be an exceedingly tough, fibrous membrane. It is air-tight and watertight, and is the skin in which sausage meat is stuffed." [11] He believed that leakage from penetration of the bowel was responsible for troublesome adhesions and developed a technique of circular anastomosis using interrupted horizontal mattress ('quilting') sutures, placed extra-mucosally to include the submucosa. Pouting of the mucosa was prevented by the insertion of 'presection' sutures to fix the submucosa before dividing the bowel. He considered that a second layer would cause ischaemia.

Bowel anastomosis in the latter part of the 19th century was marred by frequent leakage. This and the time required for suturing led to the development of various ingenious alternatives. Senn, in Chicago, clamped the bowel together with open centred plates of decalcified bone, placed within the lumen and approximated with four sutures [1]; the bone was later passed rectally. Within a year the method was being used in London, but it was only suitable for lateral anastomosis.

Abbe replaced Senn's bone plates with bundles of catgut but later, in 1892, reverted to simply suturing the anastomosis, as he found that this provided a larger opening and could be achieved as expeditiously [12]. He usually employed a side-to-side anastomosis, using two layers of continuous silk: an inner over-and-over suture uniting all layers and an outer continuous Lembert suture.

Discussion centred on two risks: that a second layer of sutures produced a partial 'diaphragm' which might cause obstruction; and that these sutures penetrating the bowel might result in leakage, particularly if the knots were on the outside.

Maunsell, a surgeon from New Zealand who moved to London, devised a complicated solution in 1892. This was inspired by the spontaneous cure of intussusception by sloughing of the intussuscipiens. He brought out both bowel ends through a side incision a few centimetres from one end, enabling the anastomotic sutures to be tied on the luminal surface. The anastomosis was then returned to the lumen and the side incision was closed [13]; the penalty was the need to close this additional incision. Nevertheless, it

enjoyed some currency on both sides of the Atlantic over the following few years.

M.E. Connell [13] employed a continuous inverting all-layers loop-on-mucosa stitch in dogs and ten years later F.G. Connell [14] used a single layer of interrupted horizontal mattress sutures, with the knots on the mucosa, in 64 patients. The continuous version has generally been used as the inner of two layers, overcoming the objection of penetration of the bowel. Many surgeons have used it only to turn in the mucosa at the corners of the inner layer of an anastomosis.

In 1892, Murphy (Figure 7) listed the reported problems: "The suture was imperfectly applied; the bowel sloughed through the line of suture; the invagination increased ... until complete obstruction was produced; openings in the bone discs and plates were not in apposition; the ends of the bone plates caused pressure ... and perforation; the catgut sutures were too rapidly absorbed; prolonged operation produced fatal shock." [15]

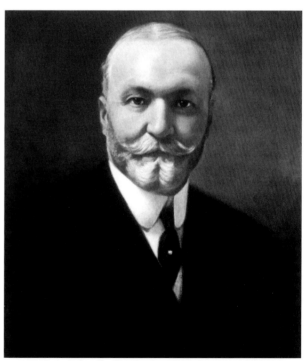

Figure 7. John B. Murphy (1857-1916). *Reproduced with permission from the National Library of Medicine, Bethesda, Maryland, USA.*

He then introduced his anastomotic button (Figure 8). A purse-string was inserted around each lateral incision or bowel end and mushroom-shaped devices were inserted into these, the purse-strings were tied and the two components were clipped together. After the serosal surfaces had united the button sloughed away, with the in-turned bowel edges, and was passed rectally.

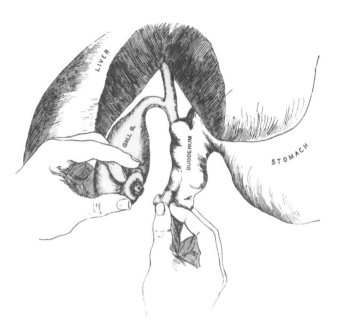

Figure 8. Murphy's button in use for cholecysto-enterostomy. *Reproduced with permission from the National Library of Medicine, Bethesda, Maryland, USA.*

Murphy described extensive animal trials and successful use of the button in three patients for cholecystojejunostomy and three for gastro-enterostomy, emphasising speed: "It takes about as long to describe the operation as to perform it." Similar devices were developed by Jaboulay [16], Boerema [17] and in 1985, Hardy described a biodegradable version [18].

There remained many uncertainties; Halsted, in his last publication, enquired whether two layers were better than one and whether continuous suturing was as good as interrupted [19]. In 1926, Moynihan summarised developments: "There are probably no pages in the history of surgery that are so grossly encumbered with the description of useless methods of work as are those dealing with the subject of suture of intestinal wounds." [20] His preference, which was perhaps the consensus, was for a two-layered anastomosis, using an inner continuous Connell suture and an outer Lembert suture. He commented that "mechanical appliances are no longer necessary". What would Moynihan have thought of stapling?

Gambee, in 1951, advocated anastomosis using a single layer of interrupted sutures, the posterior wall knots being on the mucosa, but the anterior wall closed with all-layer inverting sutures knotted on the serosal surface [21]. Latterly, this has been widely adopted, but with a preference for extra-mucosal sutures, giving serosal apposition.

Suture materials

Goldenberg [22] documented the early history of suture materials. Initially, silk, linen, cotton or occasionally wire was used. Catgut was unreliable until 1881 when Lister developed a process of chromicisation [23]. Thereafter, opinion was divided between silk and catgut until synthetic fibres became available. Finally, synthetic materials, hydrolysing over a suitable period of about 30 days, provided the ideal suture for intestinal anastomosis.

In the early reports straight needles were used, "not too small or they would be difficult to thread" [11]. Curved needles proved more convenient for bowel work, but they still had to be threaded at the table. Some surgeons knotted the suture at the needle to prevent it slipping, thereby increasing the trauma; alternatively, the Reverdin needle gripped the thread. Atraumatic needles came into use gradually in the 1950s, starting with the '441' (00 chromic catgut on a curved needle) and the dangerous glass vials were replaced by foil packs.

Control of faecal contamination

Prevention of contamination by bowel contents was particularly important in the 19th century, when peritonitis was such a serious threat. In 1883, Bishop summarised the means hitherto employed [24]: finger pressure by reliable assistants (Billroth, Péan); ligation of the bowel (Jaffe, Czerny); and forceps of various kinds, none of them designed for this purpose (Kocher and others). Rydygier used two iron rods, covered with rubber, tied with rubber at their extremities [10]. Halsted utilised two glass microscope slides "of the English pattern" tied together at their ends as a clamp; "through its glass blades the state of the circulation in the intestinal wall may be watched" [11]. Treves [25] (Figure 9) and Bishop produced occlusive clamps to control the contents of the bowel.

seven were applicable to end-to-end reconstruction. They had good results in animals, closing each end with a 'basting' stitch, applied over a crushing clamp, tightened, but not tied, after sliding the clamp out. The closed ends were then united by a circular continuous suture, after which the two basting sutures were withdrawn, restoring continuity to the lumen. Halsted [20], and Fraser [27] described similar techniques, cutting the purse-string closure of each end with, respectively, a guillotine ligature and a knife passed rectally. However, with increasing confidence in antibiotics these ingenious measures fell out of use.

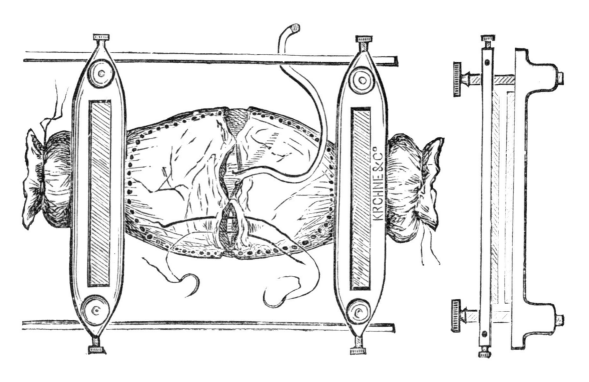

Figure 9. Treves' clamp for enterectomy or colectomy. *Reproduced from: Treves F. Intestinal obstruction; its varieties with their pathology diagnosis. Cassell PLC, a division of Orion Publishing Group, London, 1884: 481.*

In 1892, Murphy was using his own intestinal compression forceps [16] and many other designs followed, including Lane's twin clamp to align two hollow viscera for side-to-side anastomosis, but as late as 1951 Gambee was still using temporary catgut ligatures to control bowel contents [22].

Techniques were devised to avoid contamination by using an aseptic, or closed, anastomosis. Parker and Kerr [26] in 1908 reviewed 25 methods, of which only

Conclusions

Methods of anastomosis progressed as a result of the ingenuity of surgeons and in response to changing circumstances, as speed became less important and antibiotics protected against minor contamination. They are changing again with the availability of stapling, which is particularly advantageous in laparoscopic surgery.

References

1. Senn N. Enterorrhaphy; its history technique and present status. *JAMA* 1893; 21: 215-35.

2. Lanfranc. *Science of chirurgerie.* Translated by R Fleischacker. London: Early English Text Society, Kegan Paul Trench Trubner, 1894.

3. Pott P. *A treatise on ruptures*, 2nd edn. London: Hawes Clarke & Collins, 1763: 118-20.

4. Cope Z. *Pioneers in acute abdominal surgery.* London: Oxford University Press, 1939: 17-24.

5. Cooper A. *The anatomy and surgical treatment of inguinal and congenital hernia.* London: Longman, 1804: 35-6.

6. Travers B. *An enquiry into the process of nature in repairing injuries to the intestine.* London: Longmans-Green, 1812: 109-45.

7. Lembert A. Mémoire sur l'entéroraphie, avec la description d'un procédé nouveau pour pratiquer cette opération chirurgicale. *Répert Gén d'Anat et Physiol Path* 1826; 2: 100-7.

8. Kocher T. Zur methode der darm-resektion bei eingeklemmter gangränäser hernie. *Zentralbl Chirurgie* 1880; 29: 465-9.

9. Czerny V. Aus der Heidelberger chirurgischen klinic: zur darmresection. *Berliner Wochenschrift* 1880; 45: 637-42.

10. Rydygier. Ueber circuläre darmresection mit nachfolgender darmnaht. *Berliner Klinische Wochenschrift* 1881; 41: 593-5.

11. Halsted WS. Circular suture of the intestine - experimental study. *Am J Med Sci* 1887; 94: 436-61.

12. Abbe R. Intestinal anastomosis and suturing. *Med Record* 1892; 41: 365-70.

13. Connell ME. An experimental contribution looking to an improved technique in enterorrhaphy whereby the number of knots is reduced to two or even one. *Med Record* 1892; Sept 17: 335-7.

14. Connell FG. Through-and-through intestinal suture with report of additional cases. *American Medicine* 1903; 5: 135-42.

15. Murphy JB. Cholecysto-intestinal, gastro-intestinal, entero-intestinal anastomosis and approximation without sutures. *Med Record* 1892; 42: 665-76.

16. Beer E. Jaboulay's anastomotic button: an experimental study. *Ann Surg* 1905; 42: 744-754.

17. Linschoten H. *The Boerema Button in total gastrectomy for carcinoma.* Antwerp: Bussum, 1970.

18. Hardy TG, Pace WG, Maney JW, *et al.* A biofragmentable ring for sutureless bowel anatomosis. *Dis Colon Rectum* 1985; 28: 484-90.

19. Halsted WS. Blind-end circular suture of the intestine. *Ann Surg* 1922; 75: 356-64.

20. Moynihan BH. *Abdominal operations*, 3rd edn, Vol 1. Philadelphia: Saunders, 1916: 384-405.

21. Gambee LP. A single layer open intestinal anastomosis applicable to the small as well as the large intestine. *Western J Surg Obstet Gyn* 1951; 59: 1-5.

22. Goldenberg IS. Catgut, silk and silver - the story of surgical sutures. *Surgery* 1959; 46: 908-12.

23. Lister J. President's address. *Trans Clin Soc London* 1881; 14: 43-63.

24. Bishop ES. On methods of occlusion in enterectomy. *Br Med J* 1883; 2: 867-9.

25. Treves F. *Intestinal obstruction; its varieties with their pathology diagnosis* etc. London: Cassell 1884: 481.

26. Parker EM, Kerr HH. Intestinal anastomosis without open incision by means of basting stitches. *Johns Hopkins Hospital Bulletin* 1908; 19: 132-7.

27. Fraser J, Dott N. Aseptic intestinal anastomosis with special reference to colectomy. *Br J Surg* 1924; 11: 439-54.

Chapter 11

The history of mechanical sutures in surgery

Felicien M Steichen MD FACS
Professor of Surgery, New York Medical College, New York, USA

The original pioneers

If one were to accept the definition of a pioneer as the person who explores new ways and then creates ingenious means to satisfy the demands resulting from his or her exploration, the task of this writer would be simple. Originally, there are only two people who would satisfy this definition in the development of mechanical sutures or metal staples used to join tissues in surgical procedures: one the surgical explorer and conceptual innovator, the other the ingenious and talented manufacturer advancing from concept to realisation of a new instrument.

The first mechanical suture instrument using staples was the result of a close collaboration between the surgeon and innovator Hûmer Hültl of Budapest (Figure 1) and the manufacturer Victor Fischer [1].

Lajos Adam, Hültl's assistant, presented the instrument at the Second Congress of the Hungarian Surgical Society in late May 1908 [2], after it had been used successfully for distal gastrectomy, in one patient on May 9th, 1908. This patient was part of a series of 83 patients, operated on over a period of three years preceding this presentation, in which the distal gastrectomy had been performed by conventional means.

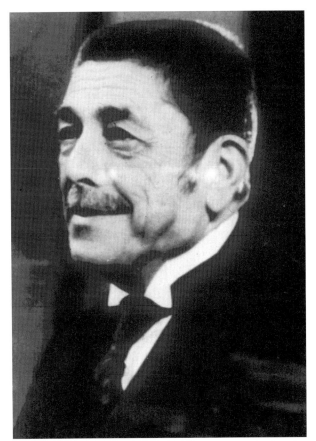

Figure 1. Hûmer Hültl (1868-1940). *Courtesy of J. Sandor MD, Budapest, Hungary.*

By 1909, Hültl had successfully operated on 21 patients using his stapling instrument [3]. Ten operations were for gastric carcinoma. The technique of stapled closure of stomach and duodenum was favourably compared to manual sutures, while the duration of open viscera and hence the exposure of the peritoneal cavity to contamination was greatly reduced. Hültl's concern for asepsis, together with his aim to improve efficiency of operative techniques and hence accept the bioengineering challenge to achieve these goals, were the motivating forces in his quest to conceive and then create this new instrument. He did so with the help of Victor Fischer, who was a frequent visitor in the operating suite of the hospital.

While the instrument was heavy (3.5kg) and its assembly and loading with staples tedious and time consuming, Hültl and Fischer had from the start defined the principles that have been essential for the successful use of mechanical sutures ever since: compression and immobilisation of the tissues to be stapled in a first step, followed by the placement and B formation of the fine wire staples, similar to those we use today, in a second step.

The only exception to the fine metal wire staples was introduced by von Petz and maintained by Friedrich and Nakayama, who preferred the broad, flat 'German Silver' staples, while they carefully respected all the other, essential features described earlier.

Hültl's instrument placed two double rows of fine wire staples, so that the stomach or duodenum could be transected, leaving a staggered, double row of staples on each side of the section. Hültl was Surgeon-in-Chief at the St. Stephen's Hospital and at the St. Rokus Hospital in Budapest, the institution in which Semmelweis once worked and taught. While Semmelweis was not very successful in having the principles of asepsis accepted during his lifetime, a historian's imagination could easily speculate that Hültl's concern for asepsis represented recognition and continuation of the great obstetrician's legacy. The wards and operating rooms in which he worked were impeccably clean. He used tincture of iodine for skin preparation and was the first in Hungary, and probably amongst the first in Europe, to use face masks and sterile gloves, first of cotton and later of

rubber. Manual sutures consisted of individually placed silk stitches. After each placement he discarded needle and holder out of the operating field, to be washed and sterilised for reuse.

Hültl was considered to be an elegant and skillful surgeon, a stimulating teacher, a colourful innovator and an encyclopaedic master of the surgical literature. He spoke English, German and French fluently, besides his native Hungarian. He attracted many visitors to his clinic, including Leon Ginzburg, the longtime Surgeon-in-Chief at Beth Israel Hospital and Roland Grausman, Attending Surgeon at Mount Sinai Hospital, in New York, who worked in succession as assistants in Professor Hültl's Department between 1922 and 1924.

However, no human endeavour remains the monopoly of one person, certainly not when it pertains to science in the service of mankind, and Hültl's generous teaching and support of other innovators bears witness to this. Even though the principles of successful mechanical suturing had been recognised and definitively established by Hültl and Fischer, there remained many pioneering opportunities in such areas. Ever improving materials, adaptation of instrument profiles to changing and expanding surgical techniques, and advances in biomedical technology all needed to be addressed. The first one to take advantage of such an opportunity was Aladar von Petz (Figure 2), also of Budapest, whose name and instrument were long identified with stapling of the gastrointestinal tract by most surgeons [3, 4].

Von Petz had had considerable experience with the Hültl-Fischer instrument and also with the 'sewing machine' of Florian Hahn, an ingenious mechanical sewing instrument, using needle and thread, that never appeared, however, to have gained wide acceptance beyond its author and a few surgeons familiar with its use [5, 6].

Von Petz presented his instrument at the Eighth Annual Meeting of the Hungarian Surgical Society on September 21st 1921. This instrument, significantly lighter and mechanically simpler than Hültl's, was produced by Jetter and Scheerer of Tüttlingen, and as in the Hültl instrument, a bar was driven forward by manually activating a wheel (an improvement over Hültl's crank), to push the staples in sequentially against the grooves in the anvil arm of the instrument, achieving the, by now, familiar B-shape of the staples.

At the time of the official introduction of this instrument, von Petz was a young assistant in the Second (and rival) Surgical Clinic in Budapest, directed by Professor Kuzmik. Because of the competition between the two clinics, it had been expected that there would be a heated discussion between the old master and his younger colleague. As told by Robicsek [1], Hültl arrived early, asked the nervous von Petz to hand him his instrument and then tried it out on his own leather spectacle case. He inspected the suture line carefully and with the statement "it is better", he congratulated von Petz and left the room. The gracious yielding of the old chief to the young assistant was generous, but perhaps not entirely appropriate, since the use of double staggered rows of fine wire staples, initiated by Hültl, has prevailed over the use of flat, single file, German silver staples. Von Petz later moved to Berlin as Professor of Surgery at the Charité Hospital.

In the wake of these two instruments, Sandor [7], Tomoda [8, 9], Nakayama (Figure 4) [10, 11], Uchiyama [12] and Jascalevich [13, 14] developed instruments that offered special features and/or improvements, that would, however, not qualify to remove any one of them from the repertoire of variations on a common theme by either Hültl or von Petz.

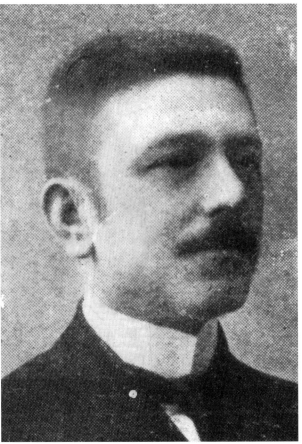

Figure 2. Aladar von Petz (1888-1956). *Courtesy of J. Sandor MD, Budapest, Hungary.*

Württemberg and consisted essentially of a giant Payr clamp (Figure 3).

The two rows of single file, flat, German silver staples were loaded into one arm of the instrument

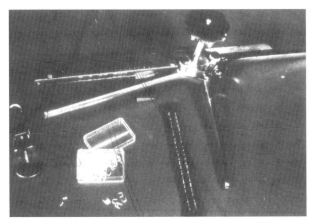

Figure 3. The von Petz clamp. *Reproduced from the author's private collection.*

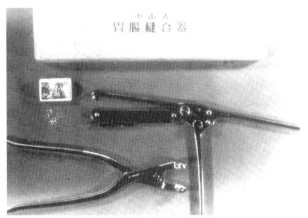

Figure 4. Stapling machine designed by Komei Nakayama. *Reproduced from the author's private collection.*

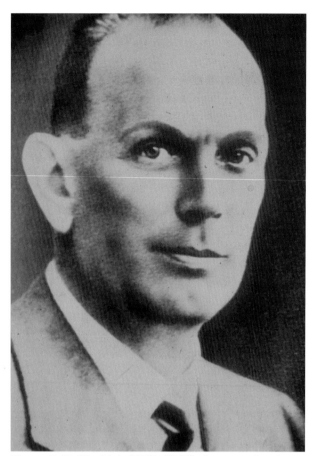

Figure 5. H. Friedrich (1893-1944). *Courtesy of Professor Hans Beger, Ulm, Germany.*

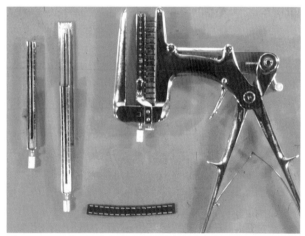

Figure 6. Friedrich and Neuffer's stapling instrument. *Reproduced from the author's private collection.*

The last members of the group of original pioneers in surgical stapling are clearly Friedrich (1893-1944) (Figure 5) and his associate, Neuffer (1892-1968), of

Ulm, who presented in 1934 an instrument [15] that represented a clear departure from and a significant advance over their two predecessors (Figure 6).

While they continued to use the coarse, flat German silver staples, they had drastically changed the configuration of the instrument, in collaboration with Heinrich C. Ulrich (1895-1967), an instrument manufacturer in Ulm. The instrument company, founded by Ulrich, offered the Friedrich-Neuffer instrument in its catalogue and at the German Surgical Congress until quite recently.

With compression of the operator friendly handles, the jaw of the instrument carrying the staple cartridge, slides along the vertical arm against the fixed horizontal jaw of the L-shaped instrument, harbouring the grooves of the anvil. The tissues held between both jaws are compressed and immobilised in this fashion, as the usual first step. After releasing a switch located in the articulation of the handles, a second compression of the handles initiates and completes the second step of driving the staples in two parallel Indian file rows and closing them in the now familiar B-shape. The sophisticated mechanism of the double compression, to achieve both steps of a staple procedure, has only recently been reproduced by contemporary instrument manufacturers. Another major advance was the provision of removable and exchangeable cartridges that could be preloaded, allowing the repeated use of the instrument in a single operation. The staple lines, as for the Hültl and von Petz instruments, were considered as haemostatic, but temporary seals that were always inverted below conventional, manual sutures.

The Soviet Russian group of pioneers

A major step in the advance of mechanical sutures was the systematic research and development of stapling instruments at the Scientific Institute for Experimental Surgical Apparatus and Instruments in Moscow, probably initiated during the mid- and late 1940s and continued during the 1950s and 1960s. This effort was not only highly significant because of the scope of technological innovations and use of new materials to satisfy every conceivable surgical application, but also because of the introduction of the new and equally pioneering concept of quality assurance in operations, requiring the sealing and anastomosing of human tissues, especially in emergency situations.

Quality health care, even if all other factors such as funding, personnel, facilities and transportation were equally accessible and available, was complicated by the sheer landmass of the previous USSR, spanning over two continents and 12 of the 24 time zones and extending from the arctic ice to the Gobi desert. Furthermore, the tremendous sacrifices in human beings and material goods, and wellbeing during the great 'patriotic' war of 1941-1945 made a tenuous situation much worse. Even today, after the amputation of Ukraine, Byelorussia, Georgia and the '-istan' Republics, the Russian Federation covers 6.5 million square miles (17 million square kilometers), 1.8 times the size of the US and is composed of 21 autonomous republics and 68 autonomous territories and regions, presenting a continued challenge to the equal distribution of goods and services.

To return from these geopolitical considerations to the realities of surgical services in the 1950s and 1960s, it appears that the planners of that time held the view that if the technical act of sealing and joining tissues could be rendered independent of the level of surgical skills available in a given situation, especially in emergency and bad weather conditions prohibiting transportation to a distant centre of experts, the outcome of operations on thoracic and abdominal viscera could be greatly improved across the USSR. This reasoning led to the expansion of the Moscow Institute and its intense research and development of mechanical suture instruments; a project that involved, during its peak activity, some 204 surgical investigators and clinicians, basic scientists, engineers, metallurgists, designers, draftsmen, machinists and laboratory technicians. The *a priori* reasoning holding that the result of a stapled anastomosis in healthy tissues could be of high quality and represent a standard unequalled by a manual anastomosis, performed by the same surgeon skilled in both techniques, was brilliantly vindicated by a co-operative study, comparing both techniques in operations on the stomach and rectum. Details of randomisation were not recorded, but there was no disadvantage caused by stapling in a series of several

thousand gastrectomies, nor in a series of several hundred of compared colorectal resections [16, 17].

Surprisingly, the first instrument to gain notoriety in the West and demonstrate the impetus given by the Moscow Institute to the study, construction and use of stapling instruments, was the vascular, anastomotic stapler by Gudov [18] and in its wake, a whole series of vascular stapling instruments, championed by Androsov [19-22]. However, while these instruments produced anatomically perfect, widely patent, everting end-to-end and end-to-side anastomoses, their beautiful but complicated engineering consisting of many parts, as well as their tedious and time-consuming assembly and loading, created admiration for the machine rather than for its purpose and performance.

Since the edges of the vessels to be joined had to be everted, which did not seem to be suitable for rigid arteriosclerotic arteries, it was most suited to joining fairly normal vessels, such as in organ transplantation. Its use was limited, considering that hand-sewn anastomoses of normal vessels are easy for the expert and much faster to perform than the assembly of the vascular instrument.

However, the vascular stapler became an attention leader, attracting interest to a whole variety of Russian instruments, designed for every possible use, the extreme of which could be found in an experimental stapler for the human cornea. We will only consider here the broad categories of instruments that proved their worth as practical, regularly useful, representing a model for continued refinements and leading to improvements or even new avenues in surgical technique.

Instruments for terminal and tangential linear closure of bronchi, pulmonary vessels and parenchyma, and elements of the gastrointestinal tract, vastly improved by their American counterparts, are shown in Figure 7. The purpose of drawing attention to the bronchial stapling instruments causing eversion, is in marked contrast to the historic principles by Lembert and Dieffenbach, described in Chapter 10, namely the principle of inversion. The safety of eversion has been confirmed over the years in gastrointestinal stapling, ever since widespread use.

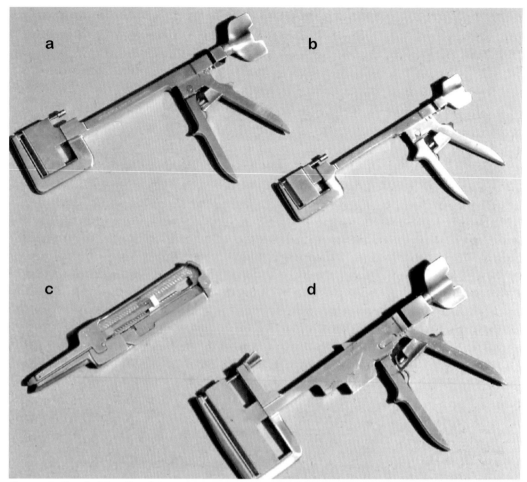

Figure 7. The first family of American produced instruments: a) Linear closing instrument (TA 55). b) TA30. c) Linear anastomosing instrument (GIA). d) TA 90. *Reproduced from the author's private collection.*

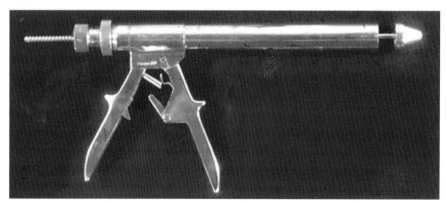

Figure 8. Early end-to-end oesophagogastric stapler ('Russian gun'). *Reproduced from the author's private collection.*

Figure 7 also shows the instrument for the creation of a side-to-side anastomosis, and Figure 8 shows an instrument for inverting, end-to-end, circular anastomoses in the gastrointestinal tract.

Over the years, the names of Gudov [18], Androsov [19-25], Amosov [26], Berezovsky [26], Ananiev [27], Bobrov [28], Geselevitch [29], Gritsman [27, 28, 30], Babkin [33], Kalinina [31-35], Petrova [36] and Svinkin [37] have been associated with this very extensive effort and reform of surgical techniques and should be considered as pioneers, both as creators of new instruments and as developers of new surgical techniques.

The modern day pioneers

In 1958, rumour had it that Russian scientists and physicians had successfully preserved blood up to three years and then transfused it into patients with therapeutic benefit. If true, this purported advance was not only of great scientific importance, but also had some strategic significance. In May of 1944, a German spy in England had apparently predicted within a three-day span the date of the allied invasion of Normandy, by observing the unusually busy rounds of Red Cross ambulances collecting blood all over England, Wales and Scotland, in mid and late May. By simply consulting a regular textbook, he learned about the average survival of red blood cells. From the observation of massive blood collections, he concluded that the assault on Europe was about to take place and from the knowledge of red cell survival, he calculated correctly the short span of time during which this invasion would occur. Apparently, the German high command gave little credence to this information, which obviously did not pinpoint the area of invasion in any event. It can only be speculated that western spies in the USSR were well aware of this story and watching, amongst other suspicious activities, for an abnormally active blood collection drive, before spy satellites of the then super-powers and of many lesser powers rendered this kind of intelligence collection obsolete.

In any event the National Research Council of the US, under the leadership of Margaret Sloan, its Executive Secretary, decided to send a delegation of

scientists to the USSR in the autumn of 1958, in order to confirm the veracity of the rumour and, if real, explore as much as possible its scientific merits. Any interest by other agencies in Washington was at best marginal to the main mission. The delegation was guided by Dr. Ivan Brown, surgeon-scientist at Duke University, with well established research credentials in freezing and preserving blood and tissues, in hypothermia and in diving medicine. Also in the delegation were: Dr. Mark Ravitch (Figures 9 and 10; Figure 6, Chapter 13) who had started the blood bank at the Johns Hopkins Hospital in 1940 and who spoke fluent Russian; Dr. Clement Finch, Professor of

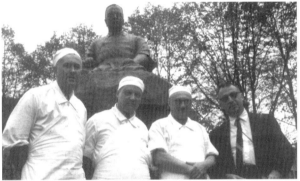

Figure 9. Mark Ravitch with Professor Petrovsky and staff under the statue of Petrovsky's father (1958). *Reproduced from the author's private collection.*

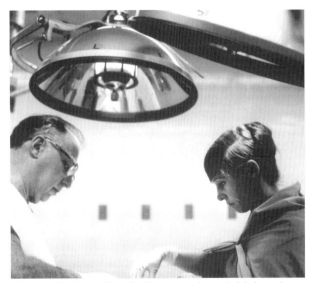

Figure 10. Operating in the experimental laboratory. Mark Ravitch assisted by Turi Josefsen, Vice President of the United States Surgical Corporation. *Reproduced from the author's private collection.*

Medicine at the University of Washington in Seattle and expert on the preservation of red cells and their changes during storage; and finally Robert Pennell PhD, Chemist at the Harvard Blood Characterization and Preservation Laboratory.

The details and circumstances of their trip to Russia were described by Mark Ravitch in the deliberate and delightful style that was so much his own and were reproduced in the 'Festschrift' in his honour in *Surgical Rounds* of May 1990 [38].

After a short stay in Moscow, the four American scientists arrived in Kiev, to visit the Transfusion Institute in that city, one of the main goals of their trip. However, it soon became obvious that there was either no such Institute or that the authorities would not allow the American visitors to see it, because - as it appeared to the visitors - they preferred not to expose any possible deficiencies. To cut the long story of the rumour short, the Americans were told sometime later in secretive confidence that on one occasion a female research assistant had given a transfusion of six-month-old blood to a patient without any ill effect. The 'informer' gave some importance to the fact that this mishap was perpetrated by a woman and that it was never repeated.

As a consolation for the missed Transfusion Institute, the two surgeons were offered a visit to the Institute of Thoracic Surgery, an area of special interest to both Brown and Ravitch. Here they were received very openly by Dr. Amosov, the Surgeon-in-Chief, who gave them a very honest report of his mortality, bronchial fistula rates, and sputum conversion in patients with pulmonary tuberculosis; the latter represented at the time the main activity of any general thoracic surgery department. He invited the two American surgeons to his operating suite the following day, where they were able to witness his masterful use of surgical stapling in a pneumonectomy and in a tissue-saving parenchymal resection for a localised tuberculous lesion, after the pulmonary parenchyma had been compressed and sealed by a double, staggered line of staples.

Both American surgeons were impressed and attempted through official channels to obtain one or several stapling instruments, to no avail. They returned to Moscow and then went to Leningrad, now St. Petersburg, where during a café house conversation,

a young university student told Ravitch that stapling instruments were made in the Red Guard factory, just outside Leningrad. At that point, Ravitch remembered that he had seen earlier that day a store that sold surgical instruments in the Nevskii Prospect, one of the main avenues; this was a highly unusual circumstance in a country where at the time, all health care was controlled by the State and procurements were at least theoretically processed through bureaucratic requisitions. However, the following morning, both Brown and Ravitch were able to acquire a UKB bronchial stapler each, the only stapler in stock at the store, for hard cash.

On his return to home base in late September 1958 at the Baltimore City Hospital, an affiliate of the Johns Hopkins University, Ravitch and his associates first acquired a feel for loading and using the instrument in the experimental laboratory, before starting their clinical application in bronchial closures on patients operated mostly for sequellae of pulmonary tuberculosis [39]. In their 1964 report on 139 pulmonary lobectomies and segmentectomies mostly for tuberculosis, they were able to report a bronchial fistula rate of some 4.6%, a significant reduction of a rate of some 14% in manual bronchial closures in operations for tuberculosis [40]. While the UKB stapler continued to be in use, Ravitch explored the opportunity of acquiring various other Russian instruments, and did in fact buy the linear and circular stapling instruments, for extensive research activities in the laboratory.

In 1963, Leon Hirsch (Figure 11), representing a group of what might best be characterised as venture capitalists, noticed a strange metal object used as a paper weight in a patent broker's office. When he inquired as to the nature of this object, he was told that this was a Russian surgical stapler and that the patent lawyer had been retained by the Russian government to market the instrument in the US. Leon Hirsch was also told that three American surgeons were familiar with Russian staplers. Of the three, the only one to respond to Hirsch's call was Mark Ravitch whom Hirsch visited at the Baltimore City Hospitals. A 15-minute meeting, accorded by Ravitch, stretched into lunch and well into the afternoon, while Ravitch discussed Russia and the use of staplers in surgical procedures.

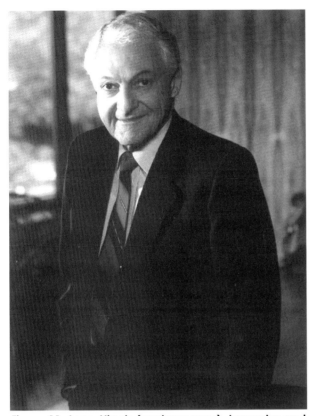

Figure 11. Leon Hirsch (contemporary). Innovator and leader of new industrial designs in operative surgery. *Reproduced from the author's private collection.*

Hirsch was fascinated by Ravitch's tales of Russia and demonstrations in the dry laboratory of stapling instruments. The use of exchangeable staple cartridges had been demonstrated ever since Friedrich, but since the Russian instruments were finished by hand, their various parts, including the cartridges were not interchangeable. In addition, those instruments that accepted a cartridge had to be partially disassembled in order to replace the spent cartridge with a newly loaded one, specifically tuned for that stapler. However, the chief problems with the Russian stapler were the incorporation of the many moving parts and to advance and form the staples within the basic instruments, which created problems with cleaning, maintenance and breakage. The recognition that cartridges could be created that would be usable in any given series of instruments, that would be preloaded, pre-sterilised, colour-coded for size and disposable, in addition to containing all the moving parts, reduced the stapler to a shell that could house, position and activate the staples contained in the cartridge [41]. Examples of their use at extreme ends of the gastrointestinal tract are shown in Figures 12 and 13 below.

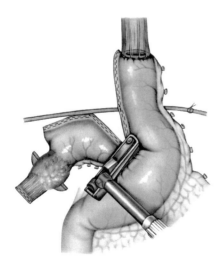

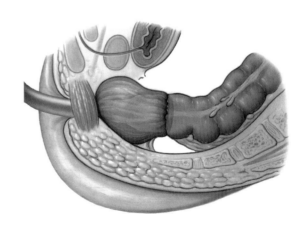

Figure 12. Oesophagogastrostomy for cancer. *Reproduced from the author's private collection. Mechanical sutures in operations on the esophagus & gastroesophageal junction. Steichen FM, Wolsch R. Ciné-Med, Inc., 2005; Figure 111-15C: 117.*

Figure 13. Low anterior resection using an end-to-end stapling device. *Reproduced from the author's private collection. Mechanical sutures in operation on the small and large intestine & rectum. Steichen FM, Wolsch R. Ciné-Med, Inc., 2004; Figure V-20 F: 111.*

This led to the birth of the United States Surgical Corporation, for which Dr. Ravitch and his associates declined any commercial interest, in order to be free, to investigate the products "and report the findings exactly, good or bad" [42]. Turi Josefsen, originally from Norway and pictured earlier in Figure 10 with Dr. Ravitch, was an instrumental player in the Corporation, having started with the company at the bottom, soon rising to Executive Vice President in a very short time. As an extremely hard-working, highly intelligent person and despite no formal surgical training, it was apparent to all visitors to the animal laboratory that she had superbly skilful hands in the operating theatre. Visitors assumed that she was a fully trained surgeon, when she ran the national training and educational programmes.

The rest is history, with many contemporary variations on a common theme. To summarise, the author's modern day pioneers in surgical stapling are:

♦ Mark M. Ravitch, for having recognised the tremendous potential of mechanical sutures and their impact on the art of our specialty;
♦ Leon C. Hirsch, a layman who was curious about a new way of doing things in operative surgery and then demonstrated fortitude and tenacity to bring industrial concepts to the operating room; and
♦ Turi Josefsen, who joined this adventure early and then headed an educational effort to instruct and train a corps of company representatives, who would always put teaching and training ahead of commercial considerations.

Biographical footnote on Mark Ravitch

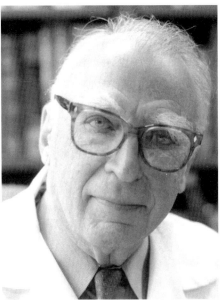

Figure 14. Mark Ravitch (1910-1989).
Reproduced with permission from Elsevier ©
2004. Naef AP. The mid-century revolution in
thoracic and cardiovascular surgery: Part 3.
Interact Cardiovasc Thorac Surg 2004; 3: 3-
10.

Mark M. Ravitch was born in New York City on September 12th 1910, of Russian immigrant parents. His college education was obtained at the University of Oklahoma in Norman, Oklahoma, where he graduated in 1930 with a Bachelor's degree in Zoology. He then attended the Johns Hopkins School of Medicine in Baltimore where he achieved his MD degree in 1934. After a surgical internship at the Johns Hopkins Hospital 1934-1935, he spent one year as an intern in the Pediatric Department at the Harriett Lane Hospital of Johns Hopkins University. He next returned to the Department of Surgery as an assistant resident 1936-1942, and resident surgeon from 1942 to 1943, under the guidance of Alfred Blalock (1899-1964), Surgeon-in-Chief at the Johns Hopkins Hospital, who had become a reputed scientist, teacher and major leader in cardiac surgery.

During World War II (1939-1945), Dr. Ravitch was a Major in the Medical Corps of the US Expeditionary Forces in Europe (1943-1946) and after his tour of military duty, returned to Johns Hopkins as the trusted right hand of Alfred Blalock. He became Director of the newly created Division of Pediatric Surgery and also Director of the Blood Bank which he had brought into being from scratch. Dr. Ravitch was soon recognised as a 'teacher extraordinaire', a scholarly commentator on medical and political historical affairs.

In 1952, Dr. Ravitch was next appointed Director of the Department of Surgery at the Mount Sinai Hospital and a Clinical Professor of Surgery at Columbia University, in New York City. He returned to Baltimore in 1956 as Surgeon-in-Chief of the Baltimore City Hospitals, now the Bayview Medical Center of the Johns Hopkins Medical Institutions. Some ten years later, he followed the call to become Professor of Surgery and Director of the Department of Pediatric Surgery at the University of Chicago, but in 1969, he moved to Pittsburgh, Pennsylvania, as Surgeon-in-Chief at the Montefiore Hospital and also Professor of Surgery at the University of Pittsburgh. Here the Department of Surgery was directed by Henry T. Bahnson, a friend and fellow graduate of the Hopkins Surgical Residency from post-war years, who had become a major innovator in cardiac surgery.

Dr. Ravitch retired in 1986 but continued to be very active as a teacher, author, editor, historian and raconteur. He died on March 1st 1989 at the age of 78 years. He had become a member of all the prestigious scientific societies related to his vast medical, surgical and human interests in the US and abroad. He was the author of the two-volume book *A Century of Surgery*, which was a brilliant account of the first 100 years of the American Surgical Association, of which he was the President in 1981.

Ravitch's many contributions to the art and science of modern surgery, in such a variety of specialties, clearly demonstrated his status as a truly great 'general surgeon'. In paediatric surgery, he was an authority on congenital diaphragmatic hernia, the techniques for correction of chest wall deformities and also the reduction of intussusception in infants and children which avoided open operation.

In colorectal surgery, he was an innovator in sphincter-saving operations in the management of inflammatory bowel disease and familial polyposis, by proposing and developing the concept of mucosal stripping to reduce or eliminate the incidence of recurrent disease, yet preserving sphincter function. This concept was later adopted by Sir Alan Parks (Figure 8, Chapter 13), the English colorectal surgeon who was noted for his technique of ileal pouch-anal anastomosis described in that chapter, and by Franco Soave (Figure 11, Chapter 16) of Genoa for his pull-through procedure in Hirschsprung's disease.

Last but not least, he was the original pioneer in modern surgical stapling as described in this chapter. The techniques developed by the widespread use of these instruments have changed operative procedures in all aspects of surgery, one outstanding example again being sphincter preservation with the use of the circular anastomosing instrument (Figure 8).

Mark Ravitch was above all a passionate teacher, mentor and role model, especially for young academic surgeons. He was a scholar with an encyclopaedic knowledge, as well as being a distinguished historian and critical, political commentator. One of his biographers, Enrico Nicolo MD from Pittsburgh, wrote: "As Mark Ravitch turned back to find his surgical companions in the great past, we too may turn back to find in Mark Ravitch a companion and a friend."

References

1. Robicsek F. The birth of the surgical stapler. *Surg Gynecol Obstet* 1980; 150: 579.
2. Hültl H. Kongress der ungarischen gesellschaft fur chirugie, Budapest 1908. *Pester Med Chir Presse* 1909; 45: 108-10.
3. von Petz A. Zur technik der magenresektion, ein neuer magen-Darmnahapparat. *Zentralbl Chir* 1924; 51: 179.
4. von Petz A. Aseptic technique of stomach resections. *Ann Surg* 1927; 86: 388.
5. Hahn F. Nahapparat fur magen-und dickdarmresektionen, 39-ter Kongress, Vierter Sitzungstag. *Deutsche Gesellsch Chir* 1910; 1: 293.
6. Hahn F. Nahapparat fur magen-und darmresektionen. *Muench Med Wochenschr* 1911; 58(36): 1919-20.
7. Sandor S. Magen-darmnaht mit metallklammern nach Hültl und ein neues nahinstrumen. *Zentralbl Chir* 1936; 63: 1334.
8. Tomoda M. Ein neuer magen-darmnahapparat. *Zentralbl Chir* 1937; 64: 1455.
9. Tomoda M. Eine neue modifikation der magenresektions-technik mit eigenem magen-darmnahapparat. *Zentralbl Chir* 1937; 64: 1584.
10. Nakayama K. Simplification of the Billroth I gastric resection. *Surgery* 1954; 35: 837.
11. Nakayama K, Tamiya T, Yamamoto K, Akimoto S. A simple new apparatus for small vessel anastomosis (free autograft of the sigmoid included). *Surgery* 1962; 52: 1918.
12. Uchiyama H, Tokunaga T, Kajisa T. Gastro-pseudo-esophagoplasty following total or subtotal mediastinal esophagectomy: evaluation of antethoracic or presternal gastroesophageal reconstruction. *Ann Surg* 1962; 156: 727.
13. Jascalevich ME. A new stapler for gastric operations. *Surgery* 1967; 62: 1100.
14. Jsscalevich ME. The gastrectomy operation revisited with automated suturing devices. *Arch Surg* 1972; 105: 524.
15. Friedrich H. Ein neuer magen-darm-nahapparat. *Zentralbl Chir* 1934; 61: 504.

16. Androsov PI. Apparat zum vernahen des magenstumpfes und die erfahrung bei seiner klinischen anwendung. *Zentralbl Chir* 1965; 92: 436.

17. Androsov PI. Experience in the application of the instrumental mechanical suture in surgery of the stomach and rectum. *Acta Chir Scan* 1970; 136: 57.

18. Gudov WF. A method for the application of vascular sutures by mechanical means. *Khirurgiia* 1950; 12: 58.

19. Androsov PI. New method of surgical treatment of blood vessel lesions. *Arch Surg* 1956; 73: 902.

20. Androsov PI. Operations in cases of aneurysms. Restoration of continuity of arteries by means of grafts, without isolating the aneurysmatic sac. *Arch Surg* 1956; 73: 911.

21. Androsov PI. Blood supply of mobilized intestine used for an artificial esophagus. *Arch Surg* 1956; 73: 917.

22. Androsov PI, Babkin SI, Beliakov PD, Klemina EP, Kriuchkova GS. Apparat dlia mekhanicheskoi pereviazki sosudov (Apparatus for mechanical ligation of blood vessels). *Nov Khir Appar* 1957; 1: 86.

23. Androsov PI. *Atlas of Surgical Operations by Means of Suturing Instruments*, 2nd Edition. Moscow: V/O Medexport, Vneshtorgizdat: 19.

24. Androsov PI. *New Surgical Instruments and their Clinical Use.* Moscow: V/O Medexport, 1962.

25. Androsov PI, Potekhina LA, Savchenko ED, Strechopytov AA, Thliakova SA, Sheinber SA. A new method of suture of bronchial stump. *Khirurgia* 1955; 8: 66.

26. Amosov NM, Berezovsky KK. Pulmonary resection with mechanical suture. *J Thorac Cardiovasc Surg* 1961; 41: 325.

27. Ananiev MG, Antochina NV, Gritsman Yu Ya. Apparatus for tissue suture with tantalum staples. *Eksp Khirurg (Moskova)* 1957; 2: 28.

28. Bobrov BS, Gritsman Yu Ya. Particulars of use of the apparatus for side-to-side gastrointestinal anastomoses. Results of experimental studies, in New Surgical Apparatus and Instruments and Experience with their Use. Moscow, 1960.

29. Geselevitch AM, Gorkin NS. *New Instruments and Equipment for Chest Surgery.* Moscow: V/O Medexport, 1961.

30. Gritsman Yu Ya. *Tantalum Mechanical Sutures for Gastric Resection.* Moscow: Medgiz, 1961.

31. Kalinina TV. Mechanical sutures for intestinal and esophagointestinal anastomoses, Proceedings II Congress of Kazakstan Surgeons, Alma Ata, 1960.

32. Kalinina TV. The use of mechanical sutures for the creation of anastomoses between the rectum and the small or large intestine. *Klin Khir (Kiev)* 1966; 10: 56.

33. Kalinina TV, Babkin SI, Kasulin VS, Astafiev GV. Mechanical sutures for esophago-intestinal (gastric) anastomoses. *Clin Surg Moscow* 1962; 8: 81.

34. Kalinina TV, Kasulin VS. A modified PKS-25M apparatus. *Khirurg Moscow* 1966; 42: 141.

35. Kalinina TV, Kasulin VS. Peculiarities of the PKS-25M instrument for suturing the esophagus to the intestine or to the stomach. *Klin Khir (Kiev)* 1967; 5: 86.

36. Petrova NP, Rabinovich JJ, Kapitanov NN, Bogomolova OR. Employment of two new stapling devices (Models SB-2 and US-18) in experimental combined resections of the bronchus and the pulmonary artery. *Ann Thorac Surg* 1975; 19: 67.

37. Svinkin EK. Extension of the indications for the use of the suture instruments of the NZhKA, in Experiences in the Clinical Use of New Surgical Apparatus and Instruments. Moscow: Meditsina, 1964.

38. Ravitch MM. The great Australian staple caper. *Surgical Rounds* 1990, May: 45-78.

39. Ravitch MM, Brown IW, Daviglus GF. Experimental and clinical use of the Soviet bronchus stapling instrument. *Surgery* 1959; 46: 97.

40. Ravitch MM, Steichen FM, Fishbein RH, Knowles PW, Weil P. Clinical experience with the Soviet mechanical bronchus stapler, (UKB-25). *J Thorac Cardiovasc Surg* 1964; 47: 446.

41. Hirsch LC. Personal recollections. *Surgical Rounds* 1990; May: 79.

42. Steichen FM, Ravitch MM. *Stapling in Surgery.* Chicago-London: Year Book Medical Publishers, Inc., 1984.

Chapter 12

The story of appendicitis

Michael KH Crumplin FRCS

Honorary Curator and Archivist at the Royal College of Surgeons of England

Honorary Consultant Surgeon, Wrexham Maelor Hospital, Wrexham, UK

Introduction

Acute appendicitis remains a most frequent acute abdominal emergency. There are in excess of 50,000 hospital admissions with this disease in England and Wales each year. The evolution of management of the disease has been fraught with ignorance, delay and prejudice. This was a result of:

◆ inattention to the organ's existence and function;

◆ attributing inflammatory disease of the appendix to the caecum;

◆ inappropriate late surgical referral;

◆ reticence to undertake simple early surgery, in the hope of natural resolution;

◆ lack of antibiotics, parenteral fluid and nutritional support in early times.

Early history

The earliest reference to acute appendicitis may have been found in the peritoneal cavities of Egyptian mummies from the Byzantine era by finding adhesions in the right iliac fossa [1].

Since Hippocrates, some physicians had named pains in the right lower quadrant 'Iliac passion' or 'colic'.

According to Adams, acute appendicitis may have been recorded by Aretaeus the Cappadocean in 30 AD [2]. Leonardo da Vinci was the first to illustrate the vermiform appendix in 1507 (Figures 1 and 2).

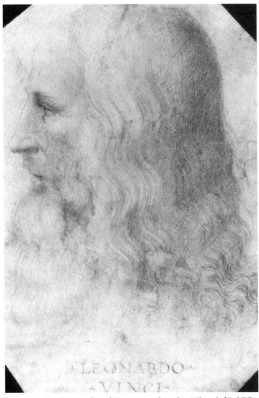

Figure 1. Portrait of Leonardo da Vinci (1452-1519). *Reproduced with permission from The Royal Collection Picture Library, Windsor Castle. © HM Queen Elizabeth II.*

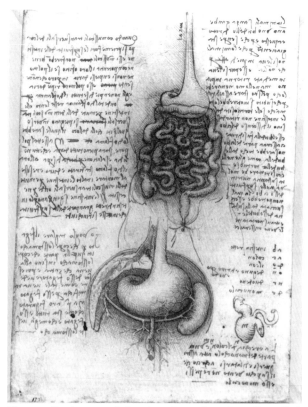

A description of the appendix was provided by the anatomist, Berengario de Carpi in 1521 [3]. Erasmus, the Dutch scholar and teacher, a great companion of Sir Thomas More, gave a fascinating personal account of what may well have been an appendicular abscess, from which he thankfully recovered!

Soon after Leonardo's drawing, Vesalius, in 1543, drew for his major anatomical work *De Humani Corporis Fabrica*, the second recorded illustration of the appendix. Figure 3 shows the appendix labelled as 'O'.

Later, in 1719, Giovanni Morgagni illustrated the appendix in his book *Adversaria Anatomica* (Figure 4).

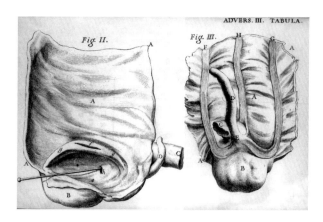

Figure 2. Leonardo's drawing showing the first illustration of the human appendix. *Reproduced with permission from The Royal Collection © 2005, Her Majesty Queen Elizabeth II.*

Figure 4. Morgagni's illustration of the appendix base with a probe lying in the orifice of the vermiform appendix. *Courtesy of the President and the Heritage Department of The Royal College of Surgeons of England.*

A probe is shown, inserted into the lumen of the organ, and the confluence of the taeniae at the base of the caecum is clearly demonstrated.

In 1711, Lorenz Heister, a pupil of Boerhaave and later Professor of Surgery in Altdorf, wrote up the first pathological account of acute appendicitis, though not published until 1755.

Amyand's appendicectomy

There should be little controversy over who performed the first appendicectomy. Although the surgery was not conventional, credit must go to

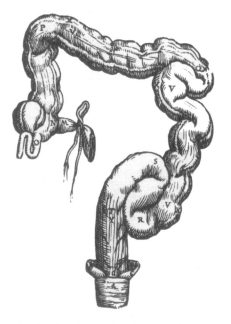

Figure 3. Anatomical drawing by Vesalius of the large intestine including the appendix. *Reproduced with permission from the Classics of Surgery Library (Gryphon Editions), New York, USA.*

Claudius Amyand (1681-1740) of Huguenot descent, who was Serjeant Surgeon to the King and was one of the founders of St. George's Hospital (Hyde Park Corner). Creese's biography, surprisingly [4], rather denigrates his capabilities.

Amyand performed the operation on the 6th of December 1735, at St. George's Hospital. The patient was 11-year-old, Hanvil Anderson. The child had presented with an irreducible swelling in the right groin, with a chronic faecal fistula discharging between the scrotum and thigh. At exploration, without anaesthesia, the hernia sac was opened and the appendix found perforated by a pin. The appendix was partially removed, and the wound healed without mishap. Not surprisingly, the hernia recurred! The young patient suffered the operation bravely which lasted half an hour. The surgeon commented, "this operation proved the most complicated and perplexing I ever met with", he continued "t'is easy to conceive that this operation was as painful to the patient, as laborious to me." [5]

Hutchinson, in his account of what he calls 'Amyand's hernia' [5], commented that if Littré's hernia was worthy of an eponym, then it was an historical oversight, not only to have credited Amyand with the first appendicectomy, but to have omitted naming an inguinal hernia containing the appendix, 'Amyand's Hernia'.

In 1759, in Paris, Mestivier [6] performed a post mortem on a 45-year-old patient following drainage of an appendicular abscess (containing a pint of 'mauvaise qualité' pus) by another surgeon. He found the caecum normal and an encrusted pin penetrating the appendix.

John Hunter (1767), John Parkinson (1812) and Francois Melier in Paris (1827), all described fatal case reports or autopsy findings. The recognition of the appendix as a source of inflammatory disease was not followed-up, as there were inappropriate theories in Europe that effectively blocked logical thought for about 50 years.

Dupuytren's dogma

Goldbeck, a German student at the University of Heidelberg, in 1830, wrote an MD thesis, describing 80 cases of inflammatory conditions occurring in the right iliac fossa. He ascribed these changes as being secondary to inflammatory changes in the mucosa of the caecum and named them 'typhlitis', or 'perityphlitis' [7]. Albers, a surgeon from Bonn, seemed to agree with Goldbeck's ideas [8]. Unfortunately, the flawed concept of pericaecal inflammation was championed by a powerful and iconoclastic figure - Guillaume Dupuytren (Figure 5).

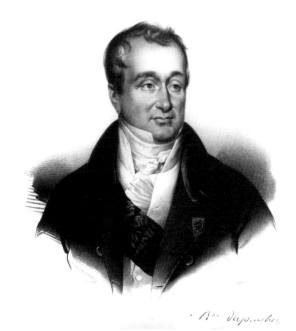

Figure 5. Guillaume Dupuytren (1777-1835). *Reproduced with permission from the National Library of Medicine, Bethesda, Maryland, USA.*

He forbade the term 'appendicitis' to be used by his staff on pain of dismissal. Dupuytren advised waiting for the late stages of fluctuation or local emphysema before draining an abscess in the right iliac fossa. This influential giant of a man, known by his peers as the "dictator of surgery in Paris", formed the basis of comment by John B. Deaver in 1905, who stated: "A knowledge of the pathology of the vermiform appendix slumbered nay even hibernated from the time of Melier (1827) until the time of Fitz (1886), and is one of the most remarkable things in the whole of the history of medicine."

Glimmers of light

Despite a stasis of thinking by surgeons and pathologists, Bright and Addison, from Guy's Hospital in 1839, recognised that appendicitis was the cause of most of the inflammatory conditions in the right iliac fossa [9].

Two important developments were to offer opportunities to ease the therapeutic difficulties. Firstly, the introduction of general anaesthesia in 1846, demonstrated by Morton in the Massachusetts General Hospital and later, the use of antiseptic principles, including the use of phenol, reported by Lister in 1865, described in Chapter 3.

In 1848, Henry Hancock (1809-1890) of the Charing Cross Hospital and President of the Medical Society of London presented the case of a 30-year-old pregnant lady who had peritonitis and was delivered of her stillborn child. On the twelfth day of the illness, under anaesthesia, pus, gas and faecoliths were drained from an appendicular abscess. The patient recovered [10].

Across the Atlantic, Willard Parker [11] (1800-1884), Professor of Surgery in New York, had drained an appendix abscess in 1843 and three more in 1867. He carried out these procedures earlier, thus challenging the customary advice to wait for crepitus and fluctuation. Kelly and Hurdon, in 1905, after reviewing 141 cases of appendicitis reported up to 1860, considered the condition not uncommon [12].

A German surgeon, Kronlein, working in Zurich pursued Johann von Mikulicz's recommendation of early appendicectomy. He was not successful in his surgical efforts, however, after two attempts in 1884. In 1885, a British surgeon, Sir Charters Symonds, employing the retroperitoneal approach, removed a calculus from the lumen of the appendix, in a patient who had had recurring attacks of appendicitis [13].

Developments across the Atlantic were shortly to make their mark. Before this, however, and unknown to all, a British surgeon had beaten all to the post and had become the first to excise the organ during an attack of acute appendicitis.

Tait's modest triumph

This accolade goes to Lawson Tait (Figure 6), a leading abdominal surgeon from Birmingham. Unfortunately, the case was not published until ten years later, in 1890. In 1880, Tait had operated on a 17-year-old girl with appendicitis. He used a vertical abdominal incision, removed the inflamed organ after burying its stump [14], and the patient recovered. Tait regarded appendicectomy a considerable risk, and seldom repeated the operation [15].

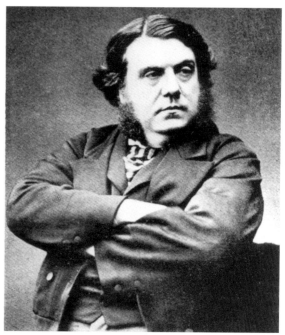

Figure 6. Lawson Tait (1845-1899). *Reproduced with permission from the Wellcome Library, London.*

Shepherd had found it difficult to give Tait the credit for the first successful removal [16]. In 1889, Tait reported a case of 'recurrent' appendicitis, which he treated by splitting, not removing, the organ [17]. He remarked in this report that he had previously removed the organ in two cases. Four years after Tait's operation, in 1884, a physician to the London Hospital, Dr. Samuel Fenwick, although fully aware of the poor results of late surgery wrote: "theoretically it would seem much better if we could cut down on the appendix as soon as the diagnosis was tolerably certain, tie it above the seat of perforation and remove from its neighbourhood any concretion or decomposing material that might be the cause of irritation." [18] Not long after this, a similar thought process was to launch progress and fundamentally change ideas in the US.

American adventures

If Tait's exploits received less adulation than they deserved, in a like manner American progress was not appreciated in Europe.

Timely efforts were made to spread the gospel of early diagnosis and management in the US. Willard Parker, mentioned above, recognised the complications and pathological progression of appendicitis, describing gangrene, ulceration and abscess formation. Having recommended drainage of abscesses, between day five and 12, he had managed to reduce his mortality from 50% to 15%, over a 15-year period [19]. According to Chen and Chen [20], Parker felt there was neither medical nor surgical treatment at that time for peritonitis following perforation. He believed the chance of cure could only come from abscess formation, and successful drainage. Parker and his management of the disease were to have influence over a young attending medical student, Charles McBurney.

J.B. Murphy, from Chicago, having successfully drained a 'peri-typhlytic' abscess on his own laboratory assistant at Cook County Hospital 1885, was to perform his first appendicectomy in 1889. In the spring of 1886, Hall of New York removed an inflamed appendix from a strangulated inguinal hernia, thus repeating Amyand's operation and thus performed the first American (serendipitous) appendicectomy [21].

A momentous turning point was a public lecture by a much travelled pathologist-physician Reginald Fitz. Fitz (Figure 7) was Shattuck Professor of Pathology at Harvard University, and Physician at the Massachusetts General Hospital. At the inaugural meeting of the American Association of Physicians in Washington on the 18th June 1886, he effectively started to bury the myth of typhlitis. He said, "It seems preferable to me to use the term 'appendicitis' to express the primary condition." Thus was born the term appendicitis [22]. He studied 257 cases of perforation of the appendix at post mortem, and compared these cases with 209 patients with typhlitis or perityphlitis.

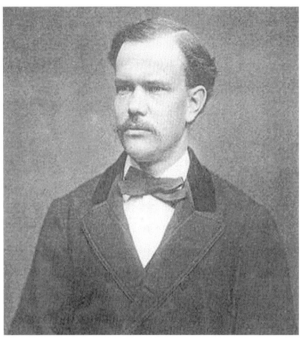

Figure 7. Reginald Heber Fitz (1843-1913). *Reproduced with permission from the National Library of Medicine, Bethesda, Maryland, USA.*

He proceeded to review 176 patients with the disease, of whom 60 (34%) had perished before the sixth day. He then queried Willard Parker's dictum that the operation should be performed between the fifth and twelfth day. He consequently recommended surgery at the latest by day three [23]. Now there was an accurate pathological concept and also an exhortation for earlier surgery. Henry Sands who held the Surgical Chair in New York, however, advocated a conservative approach. In 1888, he diagnosed a case of appendicitis, took out two faecoliths and repaired the organ with sutures! The patient recovered.

McBurney (Figure 8) was to take matters further, and studied the anatomical variations of the appendix, on cadavers. The area of maximal tenderness with appendicitis was immortalised by McBurney [24] who, in 1889, read his paper to the New York Surgical Society. He defined it as being "in every case the seat of greatest pain, determined by the pressure of one finger has been very exactly between an inch and a half and two inches from the anterior spinous process of the ilium on a straight line drawn from that process to the umbilicus".

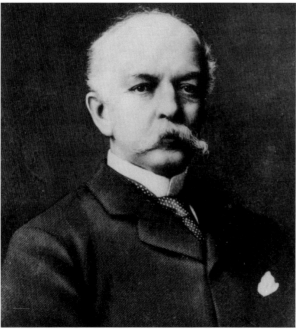

Figure 8. Charles McBurney (1845-1913). *Reproduced with permission from the National Library of Medicine, Bethesda, Maryland, USA.*

This was later simplified to become the junction of the lateral one third and medial two thirds along the same line; Figure 9 shows McBurney's point and possible positions of the appendix encountered at operation.

Following the death of Sands, McBurney was given the Chair of Surgery in New York. He was a vigorous believer of Fitz's doctrines and was in turn supported by Murphy. Murphy taught that "removal of the appendix at the first sign of inflammation was the way to permanent cure". Remarkably, Murphy's own results in 2000 cases gave an astoundingly low mortality of 2%! Other reports filtered in from Fowler, Cutler and Deaver. As some reports had such low mortality rates, it would have been interesting to know the normal appendicectomy rate! Most series around this time registered surgical mortality at 20-30%, and for perforations around 80%.

A Canadian surgeon was to be the first in the North American continent to perform a successful appendicectomy, preceding Hall by three years, in 1883. Abraham Groves practised in Fergus, Ontario, and on May 10th successfully removed the inflamed

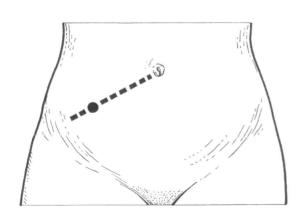

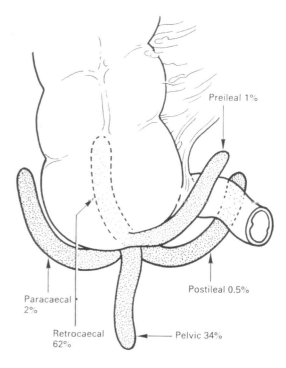

Figure 9. McBurney's point and appendix positions. *Illustration to show McBurney's point and the sites of the appendix. Reproduced with permission from Elsevier. Burnand and Young. The New Aird's Companion in Surgical Studies. Edinburgh, London, Madrid, Melbourne, New York, and Tokyo: Churchill Livingstone, 1992.*

appendix from a 12-year-old boy. Groves did not report the case, until it was mentioned in his autobiography in 1934 [25].

In 1900, George R. Fowler (Figure 10) advised nursing patients with appendicitis head up (by 75cm) to allow pus to track to the pelvis and localise there, where it could be drained through the vagina or rectum [26]. It was tragic that this fine surgeon himself died from a perforated appendicitis.

A regimen of conservative management was propounded by Dr. A.J. Ochsner of Chicago in 1902 [27], and also by Sherren (Figure 11) from London in 1905 [28]. Sherren, incidentally, was an excellent technical surgeon and described his triangle of hyperaesthesia, when the inflamed organ lay in contact with the peritoneum. This expectant treatment, if survived, would allow appendicectomy to be safely undertaken later.

This conservative approach became known as the 'Ochsner-Sherren' regimen. The regimen consisted of nil by mouth, gastric lavage, and nutrient enemas. No doubt, this was an unsafe plan for many. However, in remote rural areas where there was limited surgical expertise, this may have afforded the best chance of survival.

European progress

Predictably, there was to be unseemly delay in the progress of these advances in the old countries. Although Frederick Treves, Lawson Tait and Mayo Robson all had experience of abdominal surgery, the first British review of diseases of the appendix was written by a physician, Dr. Herbert Hawkins in 1895 [29]. In 1886, Barlow and Godlee operated on a case of acute appendicitis, merely draining the peritoneal

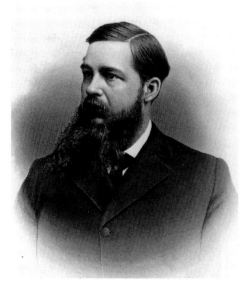

Figure 10. George Ryerson Fowler (1848-1906). *Reproduced with permission from the National Library of Medicine, Bethesda, Maryland, USA.*

a

b

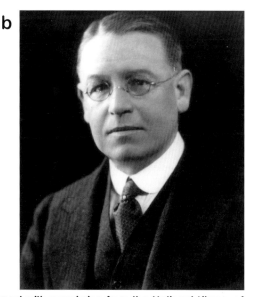

Figure 11. a) Albert Ochsner (1858-1925). *Reproduced with permission from the National Library of Medicine, Bethesda, Maryland, USA.* b) James Sherren (1872-1945). *Reproduced with permission from the Royal London Hospital Medical College Library.*

cavity, via a lower midline incision [30]. Frederick Treves, who championed interval surgery for appendicitis, first operated on a patient for the disease in 1887. He didn't remove the organ, but divided an adhesion, which had kinked the organ. He supported Fitz's ideas and declared the term 'typhlitis' obsolete. In 1888, Sir Dyce Duckworth proffered the recommendation that the organ should be removed in early life, but stubbornly denied the term 'appendicitis'.

It may be that the first interval appendicectomy was carried out by Lane of Guy's Hospital in 1888 [31]. Treves and Swallow successfully dissected out a mucocoele in 1889 [32]. In 1899, Duckworth and Langton successfully removed a gangrenous appendix by ligating the organ at its healthy base [33]. They were criticised for advocating early operation!

Sir Berkeley Moynihan believed that patients with perforated appendicitis were almost certainly going to die. In 1896 he successfully treated a 13-year-old boy, just by draining a large abscess via two incisions [34].

Therapeutic conundrums were not easily settled in many European minds. Some patients survived conservative surgery and there were still significant risks following surgical intervention. Resuscitation, antibiotics, the provision of good fluid balance, imaging and improved surgical techniques had yet to arrive.

In 1900, J.S. Riddell [35], writing in the *Scottish Medical Journal* observed that "no case of perforative appendicitis if left to nature recovers, but with operation the patient has a chance".

The Royal Seal of approval

Probably the most famous case of appendicitis was that of the longstanding Prince of Wales (Figure 12), (later King Edward the VII) at the time of Queen Victoria's death in 1901; Edward was 59 years old. His coronation was scheduled for June 26th 1902.

Sequence of events:

June 12th. Prince Edward developed abdominal pains and Sir Francis Laking, the Royal Physician was consulted. Overnight the Prince's pains grew worse.

June 13th. Another physician, Sir Thomas Barlow, was consulted, but the Prince improved and moved to Windsor.

June 18th. Despite the Prince's fear of surgeons, Frederick Treves (Figure 13), who had a special interest in the disease, was summoned. Treves found signs of localised appendicitis, but the patient was improving.

June 23rd. Edward travelled to London to host a dinner with coronation guests. Having indulged in a seven-course dinner with six different wines, his pains returned with a vengeance.

June 24th. The following morning, Frederick Treves, Lord Lister, Sir Thomas Barlow, Sir Francis

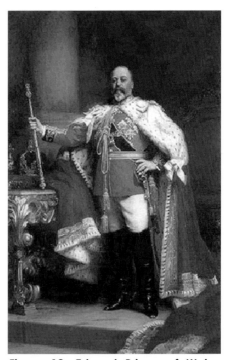

Figure 12. Edward Prince of Wales (1841-1910). *Reproduced with permission from Brigadier Ritchie and the New Club in Edinburgh.*

Laking, and Sir Thomas Smith agreed that surgery was indicated. The future King avowed that he must attend the coronation and had to "keep faith with my people and go to the Abbey". Treves replied "then, Sir you will go as a corpse". Edward relented and consented to surgery. The operation was carried out in Buckingham Palace at 12.30pm. The general anaesthetic was given by Sir Frederick Hewitt. An incision was made in the plump right iliac fossa and an abscess was drained. The appendix was not found so two rubber drains were inserted. The patient's recovery was uncomplicated. The coronation was postponed, no doubt at considerable financial loss to the exchequer [36].

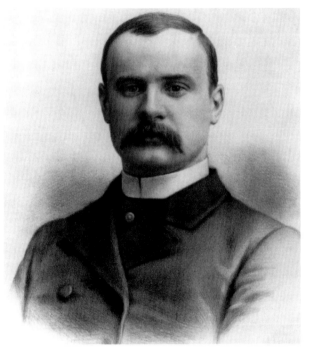

Figure 13. Frederick Treves (1853-1923). *Reproduced with permission from the Wellcome Library, London.*

Treves had seven sleepless nights after the operation, but was made a baronet for his services. He wasn't an enthusiast for early surgery and, ironically, lost his own daughter from acute appendicitis.

A new century dawns (1900-1950)

Between 1900 and 1950, there evolved a better understanding of fluid balance, resuscitation, surgical technique and the introduction of the first antibiotics.

Those patients who succumbed to appendicitis during this period were still dying from sepsis, dehydration and delay in diagnosis.

In 1905, Sir Hugh Lett at the London Hospital, reported the overall mortality from appendicitis to be 26%, but in a cohort of 166 patients with general peritonitis the mortality was 76% [37]. In 1929, Ogilvie astutely questioned some other work from the London Hospital that seemed to promulgate expectant treatment (i.e. Ochsner-Sherren's regimen, or using the Fowler position). He observed that contemporary mortality in patients with general peritonitis at St. Thomas's Hospital was 70% with conservative treatment, whereas with surgery, it was 29%. He noted the escalating mortality in cases of appendicitis, where there was delay in surgery. For the first six days the death rates were 5.9%, 9.2%, 20.9%, 23.5%, 29.4%, and 33.3% respectively [38].

Kocher's influence in Europe was appreciable. Recognised as a surgical giant, he had achieved 4% mortality for thyroidectomy (with no modern aids!). He, as many other eminent surgeons of the time, advised surgery in the early stages of the disease, but noted the Swiss surgeon, César Roux, who found no abnormal pathology in 39% of appendicectomy specimens [39]! Kocher, somewhat teutonically stated that the interval operation "is entirely devoid of danger", and that "the patient can leave his bed and follow his occupation after eight days" [40]. He quoted a paper by Ochsner, in 1904, giving an impressive mortality rate for early disease of 1.9%, abscess 3.4%, and peritonitis 30% [41].

Surgical modifications

There was to be some debate and jostling for the optimum abdominal incision for appendicectomy.

A small incision over the appendix seemed ideal and the 'gridiron' (named after a frame of cross beams used to support a ship during repair) approach was and still is the most popular. According to Strohl [42], this incision was proposed simultaneously at a meeting of the Chicago Medical Society in 1894, by Dr. Lewis McArthur of Chicago and McBurney from New York. McArthur's paper was deferred, McBurney's paper appearing in the *Annals of Surgery*. McBurney received the credit, but he graciously acknowledged the idea also came from McArthur [43].

In 1897, William Henry Battle of St. Thomas's Hospital introduced a vertical pararectus incision, which, in the days before muscle relaxants, placed the surgeon nearer to the appendix than the midline approach [44]. Kocher (Figure 14) like Senn, made a gridiron incision for early appendicitis [45], and like Fowler, employed a vertical incision along the linea semilunaris for severe cases [46, 47]. Another advantage of a vertical incision was the ability of the surgeon to perform a more thorough treatment of the disease. Kocher irrigated the peritoneal cavity after laparotomy for peritonitis [47], a practice later championed by Crile. Others believed that such lavage was dangerous as it might spread the infection.

Next came the transverse incision. Harrington claimed that J.W. Elliot from Boston first described this [48]. In 1905, A.E. Rockey, of Portland, Oregon, described a transverse incision with vertical muscle cutting [49]. The following year, G.G. Davis of Philadelphia, advocated division of the lateral portion of the rectus sheath as well as cutting the external oblique splitting the fibres of the two deeper muscles. The eponym for this transverse approach - the 'Rocky Davis' incision is still used in the US [49]. The 'Fowler-Weir' approach was described by Harrington. This was a medial extension of the Fowler incision, dividing the lateral part of the rectus sheath. Figure 15 demonstrates some of the older incisions before relaxant anaesthesia.

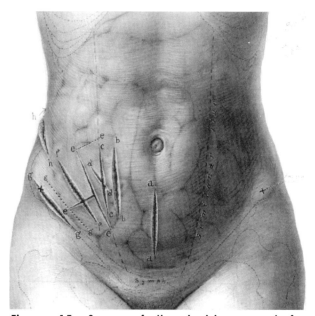

Figure 15. Some of the incisions used for appendicectomy. a) Median incision. b) Battle's incision. c) Lennander and Schüller (vertical incision). d) Morris. e) Fowler's oblique incision with extensions. f) McBurney. g) Sonnenburg, solid line - skin incision, dotted line - deep incision along Poupart's ligament. h) Edebohls' incision for both kidney and appendix. *Reproduced from Kelly HA, Hurdon E. The vermiform appendix and its diseases. Philadelphia: WB Saunders & Co, 1905.*

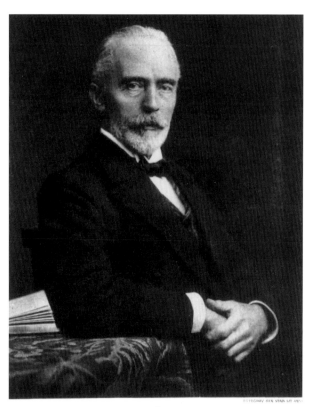

Figure 14. Theodor Kocher (1841-1917). *Reproduced with permission from the National Library of Medicine, Bethesda, Maryland, USA.*

After consideration of the various incisions, another therapeutic dilemma was that of the management of the contaminated appendicular stump. Options either lay between ligation or adding inversion. Kocher crushed the stump before ligation [47], Fowler preserved a thick cuff [50], and Treves often closed the stump in two layers or later transfixed the stump more than once [51]. Dawbarn had suggested a purse-string suture (so named after the tightened string at the neck of a tobacco pouch 'tabaksbeutel') to obviate the chance of a faecal fistula [52]. In 1926, concerns were raised at the Southern Surgical Association that there had been postoperative bleeding from the caecum after insertion of the purse-string suture. In 1985, Engström and Fenyö found that neither stump ligation nor inversion was superior [53].

As the first 50 years of the 20th century progressed, it was relevant to review results before the influence of antibiotic therapy. Heneagie Ogilvie, in 1929, demonstrated that apart from patients with severe infection (peritonitis), results were reasonable. His review may not, however, have reflected those of the entire surgical community (Table 1). Surgical outcomes from 1934 to 1950 pass through the introduction of antibiotics and improved fluid balance.

Table 1. Heneagie Ogilvie's results in 1929.

Infection localised to appendix	0.9%
Local peritonitis	6.2%
Abscess	4.6%
General peritonitis	20.5%

Table 2. Mortality and stay in hospital (1934-1950).

	Mortality	Stay/days
1934-1937	5.4%	18 days
1940-1943	4.3%	18 days
1940s	Antibiotics	
1943-1950	2.3%	15 days

These show an improvement in mortality (5.4%-2.3%) with peritonitis, but a considerable length of stay in hospital (Table 2). One consequence of this was that, of seven deaths after mild appendicitis, six were from pulmonary embolism. Table 3 demonstrates the fall in mortality between 1934 and 1950.

Table 3. Mortality relative to severity of disease (1934-1950).

Disease severity (various series)	Patient Nos.	Overall Mortality	Reduction in mortality Between 1934 and 1950
Group 1 Inflammation, confined to appendix	1958	0.35%	No change
Group 2 Appendicitis + localised peritonitis	1933	2.2%	Improved mortality (3.5%→ 0.78%)
Group 3 Appendicitis + abscess	935	8.7%	Improved mortality (10.8%→7.9%)
Group 4 Appendicitis + general peritonitis	330	23%	Improved mortality (36%→12%)

Barnes *et al* [54] reviewed 5,800 cases of appendicitis managed at the Massachusetts General Hospital from 1937-1959. They chose to look at mortality rates before and after 1946, as they considered that by this year, there should have been an impact on survival brought about by antibiotics and blood transfusion (Table 4). It should be added, however, that these results also must have been influenced by other factors such as improved fluid balance and anaesthetic technique.

Table 4. Mortality of perforated appendicitis (before and after the routine use of antibiotics and blood transfusion).		
Author and publication year	**Before 1946**	**After 1946**
Babcock (1959)	17%	1.7%
Stafford and Cantrell (1955)	14.2%	4.9%
Gilmour (1952)	13.7%	5.4%
Barnes *et al* (1962)	11.3%	3.8%

The next 50 years (1951-2001)

The number of patients to die from this disease in the UK would more than halve between 1974 and 1999 (Table 5). Just before the turn of the 21st century in the UK, only 11 patients were dying of the disease each month.

Table 5. Mortality of appendicitis (number of deaths each year [1974 1999]).				
Date	**1974**	**1980**	**1990**	**1999**
Deaths	282	179	148	133

We next should consider the improvements and philosophies of more recent times. The policy of precautionary appendicectomy (i.e. "if in doubt - take it out") was becoming *de rigueur*, for it was in the minds of many surgeons that it was safer to remove a normal organ, than risk delaying surgery, which would lead to more perforations and greater risk of severe sepsis.

Whilst septic complications decreased over this period, Jones reported they still occurred following removal of a non-inflamed appendix, which soon promulgated an attitude towards minimising removal of a normal organ, which was occurring in 20-30% of cases [55]. Not only might septic complications arise after a negative exploration, but also there could be the occasional patient who might present with other penalties of unnecessary surgery.

To minimise the serious sequelae of sepsis would require a detailed understanding of the local organisms and a design for efficient antibiotic prophylaxis. Veillon and Zuber, in 1898, described the frequent occurrence of non-sporing anaerobes in appendicitis [56]. It was also realised that pure *E. coli* infections were odourless [57]. In the mid-1970s there were publications demonstrating a 90% incidence of *Bacteroides* species in post-appendicectomy wound infections [58], and a dramatic reduction in wound sepsis (0% against 19%) when placebo was compared with prophylactic intrarectal metronidazole [59].

About one third of acute general surgical admissions have non-specific abdominal pain, many being children. Of these, one third suspected of appendicitis, improve spontaneously. Acute non-specific abdominal pain, reported in 1969, by Jones from Aberdeen [60], and confirmed by a study from Rang in Oxford in 1970 [61], found this condition to be the sixth and tenth most frequent causes of admission to hospitals in Oxford in both female and male patients. The assessment of patients with appendicitis may often call for a high degree of surgical diagnostic acumen. Repetitive careful observation, preferably by the same clinician, is crucial to best outcome. This is what Kocher advised many years previously [41].

Today, serial white blood counts (or CRP levels) can be useful adjuncts to frequent clinical appraisal. Walker found that a delay in diagnosis of 24 hours before surgery usually did not affect the perforation rate or length of stay [62]. Perforation rates were about 50% both in infancy and in patients above 75 years of age, and 10% between the ages of 10 and 40 years. In the UK, two thirds of all deaths from this disease are in patients less than four or greater than 64 years of age (Table 6).

Table 6. Mortality at extremes of age.

Year	Age 0-4 yrs (no of deaths)	Age 65+ yrs (no of deaths)	Total deaths (all ages)	% of total deaths made up by the young and elderly groups
1974	9	172	282	64
1980	3	129	179	74
1990	2	101	148	70
1999	1	95	133	72

Diagnosis is less certain in female patients, in patients at extremes of age, or those who have an appendix sited in the retrocaecal, or retro-ileal positions, lying over the pelvic brim and in cases of malrotation. How might diagnostic accuracy improve? There was some hope with increasingly sophisticated imaging techniques. Ultrasound and computer assisted tomography, however, are both observer-dependent, expensive and are not routinely used [63, 64]. The major value of pelvic ultrasound is for problems with female internal genitalia. Neither computer-assisted diagnosis nor scoring systems so far have had much success. As far as the latter are concerned, the Alvarado score [65] is simple, encompassing six clinical and two laboratory parameters.

Laparoscopy, long since a routine procedure of the gynaecologists, began to make an impact on the management of the disease. In 1975, Sugarbaker et al [66] studied the use of the procedure in the diagnosis of acute abdominal pain. Its main benefit would be in female patients. There is a much higher positive 'hit' rate when laparoscopy is used to diagnose appendicitis amongst men and children, as other studies have shown.

A general surgeon form the Netherlands, Kok [67], bridged the gap between open and laparoscopic appendicectomy in 1977 using laparoscopically-assisted appendicectomy. Through two 10mm ports he examined the abdomen in general and the caecum in particular. Most of the work was done laparoscopically; management of the stump was dealt with externally. At first he removed obviously inflamed appendices, but became more aggressive in those who had recurrent right-sided pains of less certain origin.

His peers were not so enthusiastic about removing so many apparently normal appendices, but 15 years

and 1214 appendicectomies later [68], he believed he had cured about 80% of their original symptoms.

Kurt Semm (Figure 16), a gynaecologist, introduced total laparoscopic appendicectomy in 1988 (Figure 17) [69]. Take-up of the technique has been patchy, partly because of the speed and simplicity of open operation appendicectomy and, initially, laparoscopic skills were not widespread.

New dilemmas emerged with the use of the laparoscope. Who should have a laparoscopy? If the appendix appears to be normal, should it be

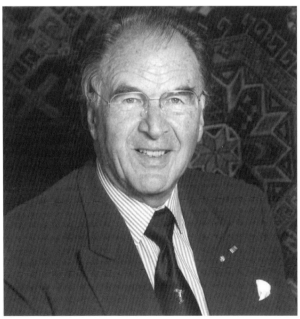

Figure 16. Kurt Semm (1927-2003). *Reproduced with permission from the Society of Laparoendoscopic Surgeons. Mettler L. Historical Profile of Kurt Karl Stephan Semm, Born March 23, 1927 in Munich, Germany, Resident of Tucson, Arizona, USA since 1996. JSLS 2003; 7(3): 185-8.*

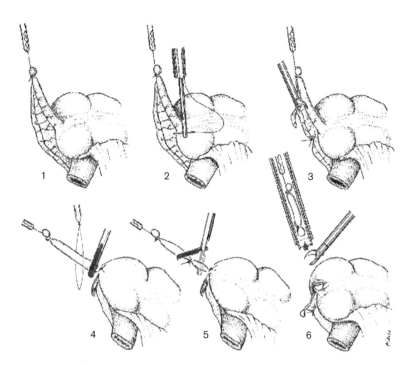

Figure 17. Laparoscopic appendicectomy. *Reproduced with permission from George Thieme Publishers. Semm K. Endoscopic Appendicectomy. Endoscopy 1983; 15: 62.*

removed? Which way should the organ be removed? It now seems reasonable to laparoscope all young female patients who might have appendicitis.

To help answer the question regarding removal of a normal organ, a series of patients from Holland was studied [70]. One hundred out of 109 patients with apparently normal appendices were followed for a median period of 4.4 years. Two developed appendicitis and nine had recurrent abdominal pain. Confusingly, another problem emerged that not all 'normal-looking' organs are so. Grunewald and Keating reported on 43 normal-looking appendices in 1993. Eleven, (almost 25%!) had changes of inflammation [71]. Bearing this in mind, also the possibility of occult neoplastic appendicular disease such as carcinoid and lymphoma, the removal of the normal organ, with due care and appropriate antibiotic prophylaxis could be justified in low-risk patients.

There seemed to be little to choose between open and laparoscopic removal of the appendix. Cochrane reviews, comparing open against minimal access operations, have shown that given improved laparoscopic skills there was less wound sepsis, postoperative pain and stay in hospital with laparoscopic removal. There have been some concerns, however, regarding deep abdominal sepsis in the laparoscopic group. This finding has not been confirmed by Attwood, who emphasised the crucial and simple surgical manoeuvre of thorough abdominal lavage to prevent intra-abdominal sepsis [72]. In Britain, pressure on theatre time, costs and patchy consultant experience with laparoscopic skills, appear to be limiting this procedure [73].

So, the assessment of appendicitis has left us with some inescapable precepts. Repeated clinical appraisal, minimal expensive tests, where the positive yield is low, employing laparoscopy in appropriate cases, giving suitable prophylactic antibiotics, and performing careful, well-consented surgery, will bring optimal results.

Conclusions

Appendicitis is still a dangerous disease. It has taken just over 100 years to bring about improvements. Attention to detail in this relatively minor clinical problem is important. This mission is well illustrated in the words of Helen Keller: "I long to accomplish a great and noble task, but it is my chief duty to accomplish small tasks as if they were great and noble."

References

1. Bett WR. Appendicitis. In: *A short history of some common diseases*. Bett WR, Ed. London: Oxford University Press, 1934: 162-7.
2. Adams F. The extant works of Aretaeus the Cappadocean. The Sydenham Society, 1856.
3. Benedictus H de. Berengario De Carpi Commentaria cum amplissimus additionibus super anatomica. *Mundini cum textu ejusdem in pristinum et verum nitorem vedacto*. Bonnniae Impression, 1521.
4. Creese PG. The first appendicectomy. *Surg Gynecol Obstet* 1953; 97: 643-52.
5. Hutchinson R. Amyand's hernia. *J Roy Soc Med* 1993; 86: 104-5.
6. Seal A. Appendicitis; a historical review. *Can J Surg* 1981; 24: 427-33.
7. Goldbeck G. Ueber eigen thümliche entzundliche Geschwültze in der rechten Hüftbeingegend. Thesis by JA Kranzbüller Worms, 1830.
8. Albers JFH. Geschichte de Blindamen zünchung Beob Geb. *Path Anat* 1837; 2: 1.
9. Bright R, Addison T. *Elements of the practice of medicine.* London: Longmans Green & Co Inc., 1839.
10. Hancock H. Disease of the appendix caeci cured by operation. *Lancet* 1848; 2: 380-1.
11. Parker W. An operation for abscess of the appendix vermiform caeci. *Med Rec NY* 1867; 2: 25-7.
12. Kelly HA, Hurdon E. *The vermiform appendix and its diseases.* Philadelphia: WB Saunders & Co, 1905.
13. Symonds CJ. Mr Symonds' case of removal of calculus. *Trans Clin Soc London* 1885; 18: 285.
14. Tait L. Surgical treatment of typhlitis. *Birmingham Med Rev* 1890; 27: 26-34.
15. Tait L. An account of two hundred and eight consecutive cases of abdominal section performed between Nov 1st 1881 and December 31st 1882. *Br Med J* 1883; i: 300-8.
16. Shepherd JA. Lawson Tait and acute appendicitis. *Lancet* 1956; 2: 1301-2.
17. Tait L. A case of recurrent perityphlitis successfully treated by abdominal section. *Br Med J* 1889; ii: 763.
18. Fenwick S. Clinical lectures on cases of difficult diagnosis. Perforation of the appendix vermiformis. *Lancet* 1884; ii: 987.
19. Parker W. An operation for abscess of the appendix vermiform caeci. *Med Rec NY* 1867; 2: 25-7.
20. Chen TS, Chen PS. *The history of gastroenterology. Essays on its development and accomplishments.* Carnforth, UK: Parthenon publishing group, 1995: 186.
21. Hall RJ. Suppurative peritonitis due to ulceration and suppuration of the vermiform appendix: laparotomy and resection of the vermiform appendix: toilet of the peritoneum: drainage: recovery. *NY Med J* 1886; 43: 662-3.
22. Fitz RH. Perforating inflammation of the vermiform appendix with special reference to its early diagnosis and treatment. *Trans Assoc Am Physicians* 1886; i: 107-44.
23. Fitz RH. Perforating inflammation of the vermiform appendix; with special reference to its early diagnosis and treatment. *Am J Med Sci* 1886; 92: 321-46.
24. McBurney C. Experience with early operative interference in cases of disease of the vermiform appendix. *NY Med J* 1889; 50: 676-84.
25. Grove's Autobiography. Harris CW Abraham Groves of Fergus; the first elective appendicectomy? *Can J Surg* 1961; 4: 405-10.
26. Fowler R. *A treatise on appendicitis.* Philadelphia: JB Lippincott Company, 1900.
27. Ochsner AJ. *A handbook of appendicitis,* 2nd Ed. Chicago: GP Englehard & Co., 1906.
28. Sherren J. The causation and treatment of appendicitis. *Practitioner* 1905; June: 833.
29. Hawkins HP. *On diseases of the vermiform appendix.* London, 1895.
30. Barlow T, Godlee RJ. *Med Times London* 1886; 2: 85.
31. Lane A. Acute appendicitis, a historical survey by John Shepherd. *Lancet* 1954; 2: 302.
32. Treves F, Swallow JD. A case of relapsing typhlitis treated by the removal of the vermiform appendix. *Lancet* 1889; i: 267.
33. Duckworth D, Langton J. Removal by operation of a gangrenous appendix vermiformis containing a faecal concretion. *Med Chir Trans* 1889; 72: 430.
34. Moynihan BGA. Case of acute perforative appendicitis, followed by septic peritonitis; abdominal section; recovery. *Lancet* 1896; ii: 1806.
35. Riddell JS. Appendicitis. *Scot Med J* 1900; 6: 214-22.
36. Courtney JF. The celebrated appendicitis of Edward VII. *Med Times* 1976; 104: 176-81.
37. Lett H. The present position of acute appendicitis and its complications. *Lancet* 1914; i: 295-302.
38. Ogilvie WH. In peritoneum and large intestine. *Recent Advances in Surgery* 1929; 1: 260-5.
39. Makin S. Operations on the vermiform appendix - appendicectomy - indications for the operation. In System of Operative Surgery, 1909.
40. Kocher T. Operations for disease of the appendix. *Chirurgische Operationslehre Jena* (1892), 4th Ed. 1903; 156.
41. Kocher TH. *Textbook of Operative Surgery,* 3rd Ed. Styles HJ, Paul CB. London: Adam and Charles Black, 1911: 645.
42. Strohl EL, Diffenbaugh WG. The historical background of the gridiron or muscle splitting incision for appendicectomy. *Ill Med J* 1969; 135: 287-8.
43. McBurney C. The incision made in the abdominal wall in cases of appendicitis, with a description of a new method of operating. *Ann Surg* 1894; 20: 38-43.
44. Battle WH. A contribution to the surgical treatment of diseases of the vermiform appendix. *Br Med J* 1897; 1: 965-7.
45. Kocher TH. *Textbook of Operative Surgery,* 3rd Ed. Styles HJ, Paul CB. London: Adam and Charles Black, 1911: 639.
46. Fowler GR. Observations on appendicitis. An analysis of 169 personally observed cases of appendicitis. *Ann Surg* 1984; 19: 546-65.
47. Kocher TH. *Textbook of Operative Surgery,* 3rd Ed. Styles HJ, Paul CB. London: Adam and Charles Black, 1911: 642.
48. Harrington FB. Hernia following appendicitis. *Boston Med Surg J* 1899; 141: 105-8.

49. Rockey AE. Transverse incisions in abdominal operations. *Med Rec* 1905; 68: 779-80.

50. Fowler GR. *Ann Surg* 1894; 19: 634-8.

51. Treves F. Relapsing typhlitis treated by operation. *Proceedings of the Royal Medical and Chirurgical Society* 1888; 71: 165-72.

52. Dawbarn RHH. A study in technique of operation upon the appendix. *Int J Surg* 1895; 8: 139-43.

53. Engström L, Fenyö G. Appendicectomy: assessment of stump invagination v. simple ligation. A prospective randomised trial. *Br J Surg* 1985; 72: 071-2.

54. Barnes AB, Behringer GE, Wheelock FC, Wilkins EW. Treatment of appendicitis at the Massachusetts General Hospital (1937-1959). *JAMA* 1962; 245: 122-7.

55. Jones PF. Acute abdominal pain in childhood with special reference to cases not due to appendicitis. *Br Med J* 1969; 1: 284-6.

56. Veillon and Zuber. Recherches sur quelque microbes strictement anaérobies et leur role en pathologie. *Archive de Médécine Expérimentale et d'Anatomie Pathologique* 1898; 10: 517-45.

57. Altemeier WA. The cause of the putrid odor of perforated appendicitis with peritonitis. *Ann Surg* 1938; 107: 634.

58. Leigh DA, Simmons K, Norman E. Bacterial flora of the appendix fossa in appendicitis and postoperative wound infection. *J Clin Path* 1974; 27: 997-1000.

59. Willis AT, Ferguson IR, Jones PH, *et al.* Metronidazole in prevention and treatment of *Bacteroides* infections after appendicectomy. *Br Med J* 1976; I(3): 18-20.

60. Jones PF. Suspected acute appendicitis - trends in management over 30 years. *Br J Surg* 2001; 88: 1570-7.

61. Rang EH, Fairbairn AS, Adeson ED. An enquiry into the incidence and prognosis of undiagnosed abdominal pain treated in hospital. *Br J Prev Soc Med* 1970; 51: 24-47.

62. Walker SJ, West CR, Colmer MR. Acute appendicitis; does removal of a normal appendix matter? What is the value of diagnostic accuracy and is surgical delay important? *Ann Roy Coll Surg Eng* 1995; 77: 358-63.

63. Douglas CD, MacPherson NE, Davidson PM, Gani JS. Randomised control trial of ultrasonography in diagnosis of acute appendicitis incorporating the Alvarado scale. *Br Med J* 2000; 32: 919-22.

64. Patel AG. Editorial - managaing acute appendicitis. *Br Med J* 2002; 325: 505-6.

65. Chan MYP, Tan C, Chiu MT, Ng YY. Alvarado Score: an admission criterion in patients with right iliac fossa pain. *J Roy Coll Surg Ed Ire* 2003; 1(1): 39-41.

66. Sugarbaker PH, Sanders JH, Bloom BS, Wilson RE. Preoperative laparoscopy in the diagnosis of abdominal pain. *Lancet* 1975; i: 442-5.

67. Kok HJM de. A new technique for resecting the non-inflamed not-adhesive appendix through a mini-laparotomy with the aid of the laparoscope. *Archivum Chirurgicum Nederlandicum* 1977; 29: 195-8.

68. Kok HJM de. Laparoscopic appendectomy: a new opportunity for curing appendicopathy. *Surgical Laparoscopy & Endoscopy* 1992; 2(4): 297-302.

69. Semm K. Endoscopic appendicectomy. *Endoscopy* 1983; 15: 59-64.

70. Van den Broek WT, Bijnen AB de, Ruiter P, Gouma DJ. A normal appendix found during diagnostic laparoscopy should not be removed. *Br J Surg* 2001; 88: 251-4.

71. Grunewald B, Keating J. Should the 'normal' appendix be removed at operation for appendicitis? *J Roy Coll Surg Ed* 1993; 38: 158-60.

72. Attwood SEA, Hill ADK, Murphy PG, Thornton J, Stephens RB. A prospective randomised trial of laparoscopic versus open appendectomy. *Surgery* 1992; 112: 497-501.

73. Noble H, Gallagher P, Campbell WB. Who is doing laparoscopic appendicectomy and who taught them? *Ann Roy Coll Surg Eng* 2003; 85(5): 331-3.

Chapter 13

The surgery of inflammatory bowel disease

John Nicholls MD FRCS EBSQ (Coloproctology)
St. Mark's Hospital, Harrow, UK

Surgery of ulcerative colitis

There are ancient references to the bloody flux which dealt a mortal blow to King Herod as related in the Acts of the Apostles. Aritaeus born in the 1st century AD refers to dysentery caused by ulcerations of the bowel. Sydenham [1] mentions it in his *Observationes Medicae* but offers no useful comment. Diarrhoea in pre-modern times was often lethal as the well documented cholera epidemics of the 19th century in Western Europe showed. Through pioneers such as Snow and Rudolph Virchow, public health measures to identify transmission and subsequently, control of cholera, confirmed its infectious nature. This progress would not have been possible without the work of earlier pioneers such as Budd, but particularly of Pasteur who effectively founded the sciences of microbiology and immunology. With the identification of the bacterium responsible for tuberculosis by Robert Koch in 1871, an explosion in microbiology occurred during the next 30 years; numerous bacterial species were identified somewhat analogously to the identification of genes and their mutations, that we have witnessed in the last 15 years. The late 19th century was a time of logarithmic progression in science and technology.

During this period it began to be appreciated that there was a group of patients with inflammation of the large bowel which did not seem to be due to infection. Cruveilhier [2] (Figure 4, Chapter 6), in his pre-photographic treatise on anatomical pathology in 1832, probably described a case, but it was Wilks who, with Moxon in their Lectures on Pathological Anatomy 1875 [3], began to identify ulcerative colitis. In their words "cases of true idiopathic colitis are rare and stand, as we have said, in the same relation to true dysentery as croup does to diphtheria". Subsequently, Hale White of Guy's Hospital in 1888 described 11 cases at post mortem of ulcerative disease of the colon [4]. He recognised the previous description by Nothnagel in 1884 [5] and noted that neither "he nor Nothnagel had observed any case in which ulceration was preceded by submucous pus as would occur in infective colitis". By 1900, it was accepted that there was a discrete disease entity separate from infection [6] and by the early 1900s clinical outcomes of ulcerative colitis were being described.

Diagnosis had been made easier by the introduction of lighted proctoscopy developed by Strauss in Germany. By allowing inspection of an internal epithelial surface, it is understandable that the medical approach adopted was analogous to that of the dermatologist. Herschell and Abrahams [7] in 1914 advised dental treatment, pancreatic extracts, diets and irrigants administered during sigmoidoscopy, in which the rectum was distended to allow a tube to be advanced into the sigmoid. There was no mention of surgery. Perhaps this was for good reason, as the early figures from the London Teaching Hospitals showed an uncommonly high mortality (Table 1) [8].

Table 1. Mortality from ulcerative colitis in the London Hospitals (1884-1908) [8].			
Hospital	n	Mortality	Recovered
Guy's	55	40	15
Westminster	42	19	-
St. George's	19	9	-
St. Mary's	19	8	-
St. Thomas'	80	40	-
UCH	51	13	38

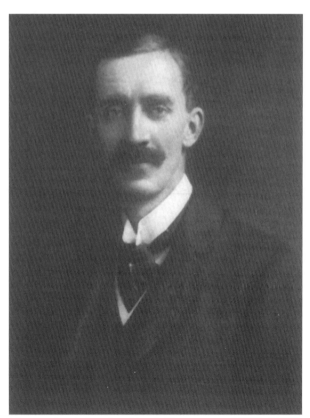

Figure 1. John Lockhart-Mummery (1875-1957). *Reproduced with permission from St. Mark's Hospital, Harrow.*

Surgery at the time took the form of appendicostomy, originally described by Keetly in 1895 and carried out by Weir in 1902 [9]. Appendicostomy was not really surgery as we understand it today. It was a device to allow access to the large bowel for local treatment, to gain greater exposure to the inflamed mucosa. It was, however, the first example of invasive treatment and it retained its adherents up to the 1940s. In 1914, Lockhart-Mummery [10] (Figure 1) described ulcerative colitis in his book. "Until recently," he wrote "ulcerative colitis was a disease of the post mortem table." He described confusion with a diagnosis of tropical dysentery and included in the differential diagnosis Bright's disease, gout, specific infection including amoeba and Shiga's dysentery, enteric fever, ischaemia and interference with the innervation of the colon. Histopathologically, it was characterised by inflammation and pseudo-polyps were recognised. Erroneously, full-thickness inflammation was also included. He also described the clinical manifestations of acute, relapsing and chronic disease. The results of treatment in 60 patients of average age of 37 years with an equal sex distribution, showed a lower mortality among those having appendicostomy. Of 27 such patients there were six (22%) deaths compared with 25 (78%) deaths among 33 patients not operated on.

In 1911 there was an international conference in Brussels. This was 'La Belle Époque' when for example Stanislaw Kadensky, subsequently to become Sir Stanford Cade, came to London as a refugee owing to the outbreak of the First World War. Having completed his medical studies in Belgium but not qualified, he was examined in French for his final degree in London by English members of the Conjoined Board of the Royal Colleges. At the Brussels Congrès de Chirurgio in 1911, ulcerative colitis was discussed. Pizoud recounts the management of bowel rest and irrigations. It was felt that ileosigmoidostomy, coming into the picture at this early stage, was a serious operation. The same themes are pertinent to us today regarding the indications for surgery, including failed medical treatment and severe bleeding. Medical treatment included calcium chloride irrigations, auto vaccines and serums. In a statement which might be familiar to us now, Pizoud declared: "Nous ne hesitons pas a ecrire aujourd'hui que l'on n'intervient ni assez souvent ni assez tot." We are still faced with the same dilemma between medical and surgical care and the difficult dividing line between them.

The First World War years resulted in many doctors in Western Europe and later in the US enlisting in the armed forces. It is probable that practice and progress in ulcerative colitis became retarded as priorities were dictated by the "War to end all wars". The war stimulated medical advance including blood transfusion, greater understanding of trauma, and greater confidence of surgical intervention. Sadly it resulted in the cultural diminution of Germany but it also led to the rise of medicine in the US. The language of science gravitated to English and the subsequent medical literature in ulcerative colitis reflected this.

Surgical measures

From local irrigation via appendicostomy, treatment developed with the idea of defunctioning taking root. Colostomy went back well into the 19th century, but ileostomy was relatively new. Brown in 1913 [11] described its use in various conditions and ulcerative colitis was only one of many indications. The first patient survived the operation but died three months later. Despite this, a strategy of management was launched which was followed over the next three decades into the 1940s. Clinical responses were often observed but mortality was high. Rupert Corbett [12], surgeon to St. Bartholomew's Hospital, in his Presidential Address on ulcerative colitis to the Section of Proctology of the Royal Society of Medicine in 1945, identified fulminating colitis with a high mortality stating that most patients will die without surgery. He emphasised the high mortality of ileostomy and discussed the difficulty in the timing of surgery in cases of chronic colitis. Anal sepsis, subsequently to be identified with Crohn's disease, was recognised, and arthritis, cutaneous lesions and carcinoma were accepted as complications of the disease. Carcinoma had been reported in detail, particularly by Bargen [13] of the Mayo Clinic, from the 1920s onwards. Cattell [14] gave an incidence of 33% and Counsell and Dukes (1952) [15] of 11%. This factor became a major element in the future, often

intense discussion of colectomy with ileorectal anastomosis as opposed to proctocolectomy.

Diversion was not just carried out through external ileostomy. Internal ileosigmoid anastomosis had been described from the late 19th century by Wiesinger and Giordano and it was shortly to be applied to ulcerative colitis. Estor and Etienne [16] in 1914, reported a series of 46 patients having ileocolostomy or ileosigmoidostomy either using a suture technique or the Murphy button. Resolution of symptoms was reported in 34 patients. The same authors described the use of colectomy and maintained that it should have a larger place in practice. They reported three patients with ulcerative colitis treated by colectomy and urged that it should be used earlier rather than later. Reinhof [17] reported cases treated by ileosigmoidostomy, one of whom was a 40-year-old female who did badly after an initial terminal ileostomy, despite irrigations with potassium nitrate solution. A side-to-side ileosigmoidostomy at the rectosigmoid junction was then performed and this resulted in considerable improvement leaving the patient with a bowel frequency of only twice per day.

By the early 1940s, appendicostomy was regarded as producing no more than temporary improvement. This was effectively signalled in the UK by a debate held at the Royal Society of Medicine in 1940 [18]. At this, Norbury and Gabriel of St. Mark's Hospital spoke in favour of appendicostomy giving the results of 52 patients with five deaths and gradual improvement in health in about 50% of the survivors. On the other side, Ogilvie and Hurst spoke against. They maintained that there was no evidence that appendicostomy resulted in any improvement compared with medical treatment alone. For Ogilvie, surgery was not indicated for fulminating colitis, but he recommended a staged approach for chronic disease including ileostomy, colectomy with subsequent anastomosis. In his view, resection of disease was an important feature of treatment. Arthur Hurst, founder of the British Society of Gastroenterology, then got up and stated that medical treatment gave good results in most cases; appendicostomy was of little value. When surgery was indicated he felt that ileostomy was the operation of choice. Subsequent colectomy with or without restoration of intestinal continuity should be judged on these merits. He said: "I regard surgery on the individualised lines I have described, as the most important advance in the treatment of ulcerative colitis in the last ten years."

Hurst's balanced approach probably was ahead of its time. Thus Bargen of the Mayo Clinic in his book entitled *The Modern Management of Colitis* [13] felt that surgery should be used very sparingly, although he recognised that ileostomy often gave marked temporary improvement while having no influence on healing. Of 696 patients treated medically, there were 69 deaths. The treatment included rest and restful recreation, diet, vitamins, nursing care, drugs, transfusions, irrigations and instillations, supportive measures, removal of infection, the parenteral administration of fluids and serum, and vaccine treatment. This last resulted from his research into the disease, whereby he had isolated a Gram-positive diplococcus [19] in the "vast majority of cases" and was able to reproduce similar lesions in rabbits by intravenous injection of pure cultures of the organism. Equine anti-diplococcus serum was part of his treatment.

During the 1930s, the strategy of defunctioning began to move towards resection. Rankin [20] of the Mayo Clinic in 1939 advocated ileostomy as a prelude to colectomy but regarded it to be futile in acute disease. He reported 82 patients. Those with acute colitis had a mortality of 31.7%. Among the series, however, there were 12 patients who had a colectomy with only one death. Cave and Thompson [21] in 1941 reported the mortality resulting from surgery from the same institution. During the period of review, 696 patients had been treated medically with 81 (12%) deaths and 175 had undergone surgery with 67 (40%) deaths, including 22 from peritonitis and 16 from carcinoma. The mortality of emergency surgery was 50% compared with 9% for elective. Thirty-eight (39%) of 98 patients undergoing ileostomy died, while the mortality among ten patients having a colectomy was slightly less at 30%.

Cattell [22] (Figure 2) of the Lahey Clinic on the other hand reported 12 patients having total or subtotal colectomy with only one death, suggesting that excision might be safer than diversion. This possibility was further illustrated by Lahey [23]. In 70 patients

having an ileostomy, mortality was 22% compared with two deaths in 34 having a total colectomy of whom 30 were well at the time of reporting. Strauss and Strauss [24] who between 1915 and 1944 had treated 104 patients by surgery, felt that ileosigmoidostomy had no place, owing to the failure of patients to thrive, and continued haemorrhage due to the persisting colon. They had two deaths among 11 complete colectomies with only four among 40 patients treated by ileostomy alone. The idea of primary colectomy with ileostomy, subsequently followed by ileosigmoid anastomosis or rectal excision began to take root.

Cattell [25] reported his huge experience for the time to the Section of Proctology of the Royal Society of Medicine in 1953. He maintained that surgery was required in 60% of patients with ulcerative colitis and set out the indications as acute fulminating colitis, haemorrhage, fistula, perforation, infectious arthritis, obstruction, malignancy and intractability to medical treatment. Between 1928 and 1952, 871 patients with

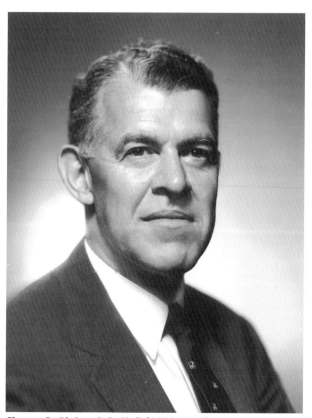

Figure 2. Richard Cattell (1900-1964). *Reproduced with permission from the Lahey Clinic Archives.*

ulcerative colitis had attended the Lahey Clinic. Of these, 413 underwent surgery with an increase from 25% to 47% over the period. The mortality had fallen from 23% in 194 patients operated on from 1928 to 1946 to 5% in 219 treated from 1947 to 1952. Of the 413, 355 had had an ileostomy and 58 a partial colectomy without ileostomy. Up to 1946, 78 total colectomies had been performed as a second stage after an initial ileostomy and from 1947 onwards this had risen dramatically to 267. Analysis of outcome during the previous six years suggested that mortality of a two-stage approach including colectomy with ileostomy followed by rectal excision was double that of a three-stage strategy, including initial ileostomy, followed by colectomy, followed by rectal excision.

Thus, by the end of World War II, the surgery of ulcerative colitis, had evolved from local treatment via appendicostomy, to diversion, on to staged resection after initial diversion.

The importance of colectomy

The modern era of colitis surgery began with the publication of the classic work of Miller (Figure 3) and colleagues from Montreal. We do not know how many patients treated by ileostomy alone had a satisfactory outcome in terms of quality of life, including the capacity for work and social activity. With mortality as the most important endpoint, these aspects must have seemed only secondary. Colectomy as the primary procedure must have changed this. Miller, Gardner and Ripstein [26, 27] measured the protein content in the stool of colitic patients and found that losses per 24 hours could be as high as 200g or more. This led to the conclusion that leaving the colon as in a simple defunctioning ileostomy procedure did not affect the nutritional deficit of the patient. They therefore carried out a primary colectomy without any preceding defunctioning and reported a mortality of 4.4% in 69 patients treated by colectomy with ileostomy as the first operation, including only one death in 17 patients with acute fulminating colitis.

In a series of 24 patients with severe acute colitis, there was no mortality [27] and Ripstein *et al* [28] reported a mortality of 4% in a larger series of 72 patients from the same institution. The technique involved removal

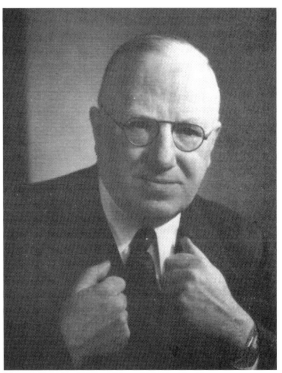

Figure 3. Gavin Miller (1893-1964). *Reproduced with permission from The Royal College of Surgeons of England.*

of the entire colon to the lower sigmoid leaving the distal sigmoid exteriorised through a stab wound in the left lower quadrant. No attempt at anastomosis was made since where this had been tried in the past, there was a high mortality due to peritonitis. Following this, the postoperative course was said to be smoother than after ileostomy alone, due to absence of the blood and protein loss from the diseased, now resected, large bowel. Subsequently, the rectum could be removed or used for anastomosis where it was felt indicated.

As an example of practice of the time, Counsell and Goligher [29] in 1952 described the surgical treatment of ulcerative colitis at St. Mark's Hospital. Of 90 patients, 60 had had an ileostomy with 13 (22%) deaths. There were 14 primary colectomies followed by a subsequent rectal excision and four patients who had a one-stage proctocolectomy.

While primary colectomy became the treatment of choice for acute disease for many surgeons at the time [28], Crile and Thomas [30] described an alternative approach to fulminating colitis, which involved the creation of an ileostomy in line with previous practice, but in addition this was combined with one or more colostomies. It was maintained that this approach was less traumatic and furthermore, a successful outcome left the patient with the colon intact. Although popular among a few surgeons, this operation did not stand the test of time.

The ileostomy enigma

Construction of an ileostomy had posed problems since the exteriorised terminal ileum was liable to dessication leading to stenosis and retraction causing mechanical dysfunction and skin damage. Attempts had been made to mitigate these complications by epithelialisation using split skin grafting. A satisfactory solution was achieved, however, by the introduction of the everted spout technique described by Brooke (Figure 4) [31].

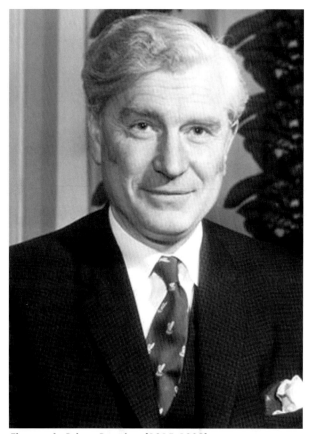

Figure 4. Brian Brooke (1915-1998). *Reproduced with permission from The Royal College of Surgeons of England.*

This avoided stenosis in most cases and considerably ameliorated the life of the patient. Developments of stoma appliances resulted from the research and development programmes of commercial organisations which led to the marketing of adhesive appliances in their various forms. Turnbull saw the need for professional support for 'ostomates' and was instrumental in founding enterostomal therapy as a specialist branch of nursing. There are now departments of stoma therapy in most hospitals throughout the world.

Following the foundation of the American Proctologic Society in 1899, there had been a joint meeting with the Section of Proctology of the Royal Society of Medicine founded in 1912 in London in 1924. Delegates went by ocean liner and it was not until 1959 that the third joint or bi-partite meeting was held. In this year the American Proctological Society had changed its name to the American Society of Colon and Rectal Surgeons with accreditation boards changing from the American Board of Proctology to the American Board of Colon and Rectal Surgery. How timely then to discuss the surgery of ulcerative colitis. Even in 1959 some delegates travelled by sea. The reception in London appeared to be greatly appreciated by the Americans, whose President Dr. Karl Zimmerman led the visiting party. Henry Thompson of St. Mark's Hospital, as President of the Section of Proctology of the Royal Society of Medicine, led the hosts. The dinner at the Guildhall attended by the Lord Mayor was particularly memorable.

The speakers included G.W. Ault, I.P.M. MacDougall, B.N. Brooke, R.S. Corbett, S.T. Ross, G. Gordon-Taylor and H.R. Reichmann [32]. Brooke [33] reported a 5% mortality for proctocolectomy and at the Lahey Clinic; this was 2% according to Ault [34]. The question of cancer was dealt with. Of 500 cases reported worldwide, sufficient detail for analysis was available in 286. Of these, 221 had died within five years, 13 (4.2%) had survived for more than five years and 70 (23%) were still alive within five years. This was a seminal meeting which resulted in a statement recommending optimal surgery for ulcerative colitis. The conclusion was that proctocolectomy with ileostomy was the procedure of choice for chronic disease. Its mortality was low, the patient regained normal health, the cancer risk was abolished and life with an ileostomy was more than manageable.

While these outcomes still apply today, it was already apparent that complications of the ileostomy were significant. Brooke's own figures for revisional operations were 10% in the first five years increasing to 14.5% from 6-15 years. In comparison, the UK Midlands Surgeon's figures were 12.5% and 35% respectively [33]. Counsell and Goligher [29] experienced retraction or prolapse in 20% of patients with an ileostomy. The cumulative complication rate of ileostomy is still relatively high today.

Escape from ileostomy?

Was Lahey's dictum "once an ileostomy, always an ileostomy" true and accepted? Ileostomy avoidance as a desirable endpoint began its history in the 1930s. The mainstream development of the surgery of ulcerative colitis was, as described, chiefly concerned with the reduction of mortality and restoration of health. In this context, the pioneers of ileostomy avoidance were searching for something, which at the time was only of secondary importance. Nevertheless, they sowed the seed of a development that became the main focus of the patient only when surgery was safe enough to enable it to be applicable in clinical practice.

Ileorectal anastomosis

The first development was colectomy with ileorectal or ileosigmoid anastomosis. Early reports did not result in its adoption in clinical practice. It was obviously a feared operation, no doubt owing to the high mortality of major surgery in an ill patient and to the danger of anastomotic breakdown. One of the pioneers of this operation was Hugh Devine from Melbourne, later Sir Hugh Devine. In 1943, he described a four-stage operation to create an ileorectal anastomosis after colectomy (Figure 5) [35] (the emphasis was on avoidance of peritoneal contamination):

1. The first stage involved division of the terminal ileum and sigmoid colon bringing four stomas out on to the anterior abdominal wall.
2. The next was a side-to-side anastomosis using an enterotome.
3. Next, the resulting stoma was closed.
4. At the fourth stage, the defunctioned colon was removed.

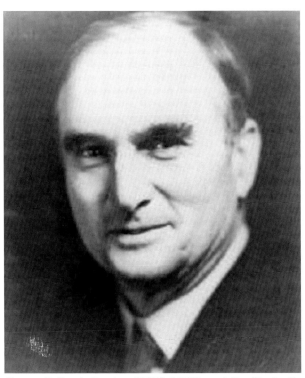
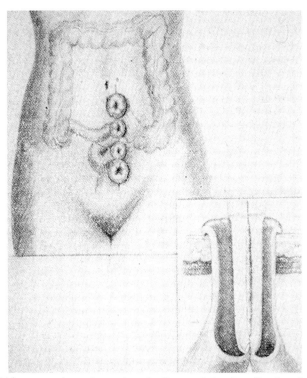

Figure 5. Hugh Devine (1878-1959) and the illustration of his procedure. *Reproduced with permission from the Royal Australasian College of Surgeons.*

Subsequently, the four-stage procedure became reduced to three and then to two stages, with the colon being removed during the first stage. This operation was taken up by other surgeons with caution. Even in 1959, Corbett [36] maintained that ileostomy alone was extremely useful in the acutely ill patient, although by that time he had treated 17 patients with colectomy and ileorectal anastomosis of whom 12 were well for up to ten years. In the UK, Stanley Aylett was the greatest advocate of colectomy with ileorectal anastomosis. He reported the results of 300 patients operated on between 1952 and 1965 [37]. They were divided into 53 fulminating, 134 acute and 113 chronic cases with respective mortalities of 17%, 5% and 3%. Of the operation survivors, 14 (5%) were converted to an ileostomy. There were ten non-operative deaths including three due to carcinoma. Of the total of 300, there were 259 survivors of whom 250 were said to be in good health. His last paper dealt with the cancer risk in the rectum [38] which was 5% over the long period of follow-up.

The subsequent reports of colectomy with ileorectal anastomosis [39-43] indicate a remarkable surgeon-related variable in case selection for the operation ranging from 10% to over 90%. Failure as defined by the need for proctectomy ranged from 10% to over 50%. As an example of the outcome of the procedure, Griffen et al [40] reported the results in 63 patients between 1948 and 1961. There were two postoperative deaths and 13 subsequent deaths including two from rectal cancer. The outcome in 43 survivors was good in 25, fair in eight and poor in ten patients.

Although colectomy with ileorectal anastomosis became an established surgical option, the introduction of restorative proctocolectomy greatly reduced its use. For example, the proportion of patients having colectomy with ileorectal anastomosis at St. Mark's Hospital fell from 25% during the pre-ileal pouch era to less than 10% afterwards [44]. Nevertheless, the operation had the advantage of being a one-stage procedure with fewer complications than restorative proctocolectomy.

In parallel with the development of colectomy with ileorectal anastomosis, removal of the large bowel with ileo-anal anastomosis began to evolve. Techniques for low anastomosis of the colon and ileum to the anus by Kraske [45], Hochenegg [46],

Maunsell [47], and Weir [48] had been described in the late 19th and early 20th century. Nissen [49] (Figure 20, Chapter 4) in 1933, during a meeting of the Berlin Surgical Society, reported a case involving an ileo-anal anastomosis in a 10-year-old boy with familial adenomatous polyposis. In a three-stage procedure, the large bowel was removed with an anastomosis made between the terminal ileum and the anal sphincter. The patient was continent. This case was referred to by Ravitch and Sabiston [50] in their classic paper on total proctocolectomy with anal ileostomy in dogs. Of 22 animals operated on without antibiotics, 11 died but the mortality was reduced to no deaths out of six further dogs given antibiotics.

A year later, Ravitch [51] (Figure 6) reported two patients with ulcerative colitis with a successful outcome. A few reports of the operation occurred over the next few years, of which that of Devine and Webb [52] was of particular interest, since it described the creation of a rectal muscular cuff through

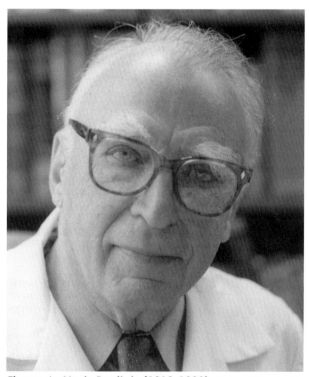

Figure 6. Mark Ravitch (1910-1989). *Reproduced with permission from Elsevier © 2004. Naef AP. The mid-century revolution in thoracic and cardiovascular surgery: Part 3. Interact Cardiovasc Thorac Surg 2004; 3: 3-10.*

mucosectomy by scissor excision, after submucous injection of saline solution. Two patients so treated had a satisfactory bowel frequency of two and six defaecations per 24 hours. The anastomosis could be made either endo-anally or via a posterior approach, as described by Best [53] in nine patients, only one of whom subsequently required conversion to an ileostomy.

Over the next 20 years, further reports of the so called 'straight' ileo-anal operation entered the literature. Martin et al [54] reported 17 patients who underwent straight ileo-anal anastomosis after total proctocolectomy. The rectum was denuded of its mucosa by a dissection carried out through the abdomen similar to the technique described by Soave [55] for the treatment of Hirschprung's disease. There were no operative deaths and two patients failed requiring an ileostomy. Complications included cuff abscess, pelvic sepsis and stricture of the anastomosis. Of the 13 patients who had had the temporary ileostomy closed, frequency of defaecation ranged from two to six times per 24 hours. Interestingly, only patients who had minimal involvement of the rectum were selected for this procedure. Telander and Perrault [56] reported 25 patients aged 11 to 25 years followed for a mean of 15 months. Stool frequency varied from five to 12 times per 24 hours. Three patients required further surgery and the functional results were judged as poor or fair in six patients, being good or excellent in the remainder.

The concept of mucosal proctectomy, which originated with the description by Devine and Webb [52], was taken further by Peck [57] who used it to treat the defunctioned rectal stump after colectomy. This removed the residual disease, avoiding an abdominal operation. Subsequently, he applied the method to sphincter preservation by relining the denuded rectum with a mucosal graft of terminal ileal mucosa [58]. He reported 29 patients, 12 with polyposis and 17 with ulcerative colitis, followed for three months to nearly eight years. There were two failures but no operative mortality. Of 23 evaluable patients, defaecation frequency per 24 hours was five for the polyposis patients and seven for the colitics. Nocturnal leakage occurred in 12 patients. This operation did not become part of routine surgical practice owing to its technical difficulty and to the simultaneous introduction of restorative proctocolectomy by Parks

and Nicholls [59]. It has, however, been resurrected recently with similar results, while avoiding the complication of pelvic sepsis [60].

While systemic return of health was achieved in most patients after straight ileo-anal anastomosis, function was not satisfactory in many. Frequency and particularly urgency of defaecation were common, the latter being a major disadvantage of the operation. Looking back now, the report of Valiente and Bacon [61] was a major step on the path to restorative proctocolectomy. They reviewed the literature of reports of the Ravitch and Sabiston operation. Of 34 cases, function was satisfactory in 20 and poor in 14, owing to frequency of defaecation, excoriation of the anal skin, fistula and abscess formation, and electrolyte imbalance. They speculated that if the frequency was reduced to a minimum, the above problems would not occur. They reported the reconstruction of an ileal reservoir in seven dogs. Only two survived but each had a low frequency of defaecation. The mortality of the animals was such, however, that in the discussion following the presentation of the paper, Turnbull commented that "somewhere in the future someone may perhaps solve this problem. I think that it is in the daydream stage at the present time".

'Continent ileostomy'

The concept of the reservoir as developed by Valiente and Bacon [61] was applied to clinical practice by Kock [62] who created a system whereby the ostomate would have a continent stoma. His research initially aimed to create a continent urostomy but he then applied the operation to ileostomy. In 1969 he reported the initial results of a reconstruction that consisted of an ileal reservoir with an inverted nipple valve of distal terminal ileum to create continence. Emptying the reservoir was effected by intubation of the stoma.

This worked variably depending on the experience of the surgeon. The most frequent complications included slippage of the valve and fistulation at the base of the valve to the exterior. Both required a major revision. Over his professional lifetime, Kock reduced these complications to below 10% [63]. Others did not achieve these results and a re-operation rate of 30%-40% for valve slippage was reported by Beahrs et al [64] and Gelernt *et al* [65]. While the application of this operation has declined owing to the introduction of restorative proctocolectomy, Philipson *et al* [66] found the assessment of patient health, biochemical and histological changes and microbiology demonstrated that an ileal reservoir in humans was compatible with satisfactory health. This was to become a major factor in the subsequent development of restorative proctocolectomy.

Ileo-anal pouch surgery

The demonstration of the technical possibility of ileo-anal anastomosis and the clinical outcome of the Kock continent ileostomy, led to the creation of the modern form of the ileo-anal procedure by Parks. Parks had himself developed the technique of endo-anal anastomosis. Combining this with total procto-colectomy and reservoir construction, he described proctocolectomy without ileostomy subsequently to be called restorative proctocolectomy (RPC) or ileal pouch-anal anastomosis (IPAA). The initial report of Parks' and Nicholls' first five cases [59] was amplified to 17 patients followed from two to 24 months [67]. There were no deaths and one patient (6%) had had the pouch removed. Bowel frequency ranged from 3-6 per 24 hours and continence was normal in 87%. Only 53% of the patients were able to evacuate spontaneously, however, the rest needing to do so by catheterisation. This problem was resolved by technical developments of reservoir design with the description of the J-reservoir by Utsunomiya *et al* [68]. Early evidence by Martin [69] favouring the reservoir reconstruction came from an uncontrolled comparison of 16 patients having a straight ileo-anal anastomosis with 14 having an ileal reservoir in addition. Respective frequencies of evacuation at 12 months were eight and four times per 24 hours.

The last 30 years have been the story of restorative proctocolectomy and its development. Other reports followed by Rothenberger *et al* in 1983 [70], Nicholls *et al* in 1984 [138] and by Metcalf *et al* [71] in 1985. The present state of the clinical results of the operation were reported in a symposium by Dozois *et al* [72]. Restorative proctocolectomy is now the most commonly used operation for ulcerative colitis accounting for over 70% of cases. Its history over the last 27 years has included technical questions of reservoir design [73], the method of forming the ileo-anal anastomosis and the use or not of a defunctioning ileostomy. Mucosal morphological changes within the reservoir have been recognised and found to be similar to those following the Kock reservoir reconstruction [74]. Techniques for salvage surgery have been developed and the long-term clinical outcomes have been clarified by Meagher *et al* [75], Fazio *et al* [76], Heuschen *et al* [77] and, Tulchinsky *et al* [78] along with quality of life assessments. It is now clear that failure defined as the need for a permanent ileostomy or indefinite defunctioning continues with the passage of time. Present data indicate that failure rates are about 5% at five, 10% at ten and 15% at 15 years [77, 78].

The indications for the operation have been modified over the last decades. Acute ulcerative colitis should be treated by an initial colectomy to be followed by restorative proctectomy later if the patient so wishes. Crohn's disease is not suitable for the operation, despite the results reported by Panis *et al* [79]. In the hands of all other authors, the failure rate in patients with Crohn's disease is up to 50% or more. Female fertility is reduced by at least 50% [80] and this factor must be taken into account when advising women of child-bearing age. Sclerosing cholangitis is a risk factor for pouchitis [81]. Prediction models for failure have been developed to assist patients in the decision-taking process [82].

The surgery of Crohn's disease

The history of the surgery of Crohn's disease has shown a different pattern to that of ulcerative colitis, since it tends to present with a localised anatomical pathology causing mechanical problems, such as obstruction or local perforation. There was no difficulty therefore in distinguishing the disease from dysenteric conditions as was the case with ulcerative colitis. With Crohn's disease, the distinction from tuberculosis was the essential aspect which identified it as a distinct pathological entity. Furthermore, by the time the classic description was published in 1932, abdominal surgery was considerably more advanced than it had been in the early years of the 20th century when ulcerative colitis was generally accepted as a discrete pathology. Thus the history of Crohn's disease is not associated with the evolution of surgical technique but more with the progressive understanding of its pathology. Initially described as affecting the terminal ileum, it gradually became apparent over the subsequent decades that Crohn's disease could involve any part of the gastrointestinal tract from the mouth to the anus. Treatment had therefore to be tailored to the localisation of the disease.

Perhaps the earliest description of Crohn's disease was made by Morgagni [83] (Figure 4, Chapter 12) in 1769, the year of the birth of Napoleon and Wellington. There were other reports of chronic obstructing intestinal disease in the 19th century. Coombe and Saunders [84] in 1813 described a "singular case of stricture and thickening of the ileum" in a young man who had suffered for many years with obstructive symptoms. A few years later in a treatise on "Pathological and practical researches on disease of the stomach, the intestinal canal, the liver and other viscera of the abdomen", Abercrombie [85] recognised a similar condition in 1828. In *Lectures on Pathological Anatomy*, Wilks and Moxon [3] described a case in 1875 with severe localised stenosis in the ileum.

An accurate description of Crohn's disease with results on the outcome of surgery was published by Dalziel in 1913 [86]. In the paper he began by recounting two cases with obstruction. The first was a doctor seen 12 years previously with intermittent obstructive symptoms for several weeks. At surgery, "the whole of the intestines, large and small alike" were contracted and rigid. There was no doubt that the wall of the whole intestine was chronically inflamed. Nothing could be done surgically and the patient died a few days later. Dalziel subsequently encountered further cases in which the disease was sufficiently localised to enable resection. He reported on nine patients, with "perfect recovery" postoperatively in seven and stated that he had no hesitation in resecting large portions of the intestine. The histopathology of three of the patients whose specimens were obtained from the ileum, jejunum and colon were examined in the Western Infirmary, Glasgow. They were reported in detail and demonstrated essentially the presence of transmural inflammation with coexisting chronic inflammation and

repair. Polymorphs, monocytes and giant cells were seen. In two patients no micro-organisms were found other than the ordinary bacterial flora of the gut.

Dalziel discussed the aetiology. Although the cases gave the impression of tuberculosis, the enlarged glands were not evidently caseous. The morbid pathology was "as similar as may be" to Johne's disease of cattle. Both are caused by an acid-fast bacillus but of different species. These could not be found in his cases in humans. Dalziel felt that he had described a new disease and suggested that previous cases were likely to have been erroneously described as tuberculosis: "My friends, the pathologists, prefer to call it hyperplastic enteritis." Others at about the same time had reported cases of colonic non-tuberculous granulomatous disease [87, 88].

Just before the classic paper of Crohn and colleagues (Figure 7), there were reports in the literature of almost certainly the same disease. Nuboer [89] described two cases of chronic phlegmonous ileitis in 1932, and Golob [90] in the same year reported a case of chronic infected granuloma of the terminal ileum and caecum. Non-specific granulomatous disease of the small intestine in four patients had been reported at Mount Sinai Hospital, New York in 1923 by the pathologists, Moschowitz and Wilensky [91], and Klemperer in the same department had recognised the existence of non-tuberculous non-caseating granulomatous disease in the 1920s.

Crohn's disease was, however, firmly established as a disease entity in 1932 by the publication by Crohn, Ginzburg and Oppenheimer (Figure 7) in the paper "Regional ileitis: a pathologic and clinical entity" [92].

The paper had been read before the Section of Gastroenterology and Proctology at the 83rd Annual Session of the American Medical Association in New Orleans on May 13th 1932. The publication appeared in the issue of the *Journal of the American Medical Association* dated October 15th 1932.

Ginzburg and Oppenheimer [93] had delivered a paper to the American Gastroenterological Association on the same subject, but the publication did not appear until 1933. Crohn, Ginzburg and Oppenheimer [92] described a disease of the terminal

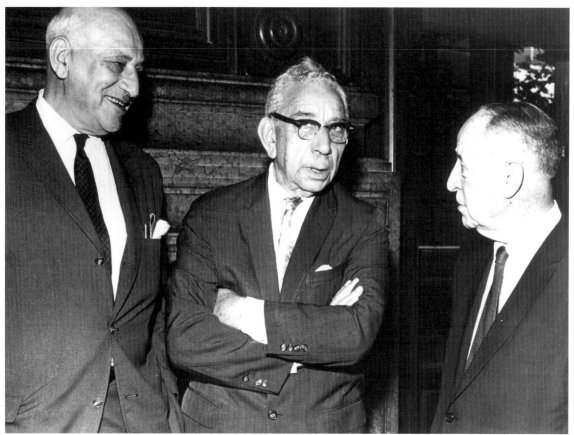

Figure 7. From left to right: Gordon D. Oppenheimer (1900-1974), Burrill Crohn (1884-1983) and Leon Ginzburg (1898-1988). *Reproduced with permission from the Mount Sinai Archives, Levy Library, New York, USA.*

ileum which belonged to none of the categories of recognised granulomatous inflammatory groups. They reported 14 patients, 13 of whom had been operated on by Dr. A.A. Berg, the previous Chief of Surgery at Mount Sinai. The pathological anatomy included full-thickness chronic inflammation, involvement of the terminal ileum most intensely at the ileocaecal valve, skip lesions in some cases, stenosis, chronic perforation and fistulation. The presence of giant cells in some cases was striking. The authors believed that these were the result of a foreign body reaction around particles of vegetable matter and were not an essential characteristic of the disease. Inoculation into rabbits, guinea pigs and chickens of material from lymph glands and intestinal wall was negative for tuberculosis and Lowenstein culture was negative. No patient had clinical tuberculosis. An abdominal mass was usually present and patients were often emaciated and anaemic. Barium enema in the 14 patients was negative but the barium meal showed

proximal ileal distension above a distal stricture. Transit was slowed and fistulae could be identified. Medical treatment was said to be 'purely palliative and supportive' and surgical resection would lead to 'complete cure'.

Early surgical results

Thirteen of the patients were restored to complete health either by resection and anastomosis or internal side-to-side ileo-transverse-colonic bypass after division of the intestine three feet above the ileocaecal junction and closing both ends of the ileum. There appeared to be two cases that developed progressive disease.

At the end of the original presentation to the learned society, Crohn, Ginzburg and Oppenheimer had called the disease "terminal ileitis", but J.A. Bargen of the Mayo Clinic felt that the word 'terminal' might convey to some the meaning of agonal. He suggested that 'regional' might be a better term and this was indeed adopted in the publication.

The paper by Ginzburg and Oppenheimer in 1933 [93] reported a larger group of 52 cases which included the 14 already published. Among the 38 (new) cases there were examples of chronic perforation and skip lesions and also of what they called 'localised hypertrophic colitis'. The possibility of colonic involvement had been raised by the earlier reports of Moynihan and Robson, and Nuboer, as well as by Klemperer and other pathologists at Mount Sinai Hospital. It was not long before colonic involvement was accepted as part of the same disease. Colp [94] reported a case with colonic involvement and shortly before, Bargen and Weber [95] had published evidence for a right-sided colitis. Crohn and Rosenak [96] and Crohn and Berg [97] reported further cases. At the same time it was shown that granulomatous chronic inflammation could involve the small intestine more proximally even to include the duodenum [98], and the stomach [99]. Involvement of the anus was subsequently described by Morson and Lockhart-Mummery [100, 101] and oral Crohn's disease became recognised in the 1960s and 1970s [102-104].

The original term 'regional ileitis' was thus no longer accurate and various other names were used including 'regional enteritis', 'granulomatous colitis' and 'transmural colitis', but none supplied an adequate anatomical pathological description of the disease. Alphabetical order determined the sequence of names in the classic paper and the term 'Crohn's disease' became accepted (more slowly in the US) as a convenient appellation which would be uniformly understood. It is interesting that Crohn himself persisted with the term 'regional ileitis' as evidenced by the second edition of his book dated 1958 and entitled *Regional Ileitis*.

Colonic Crohn's disease

Despite the descriptions of involvement of the colon by Crohn's disease, authorities such as Bargen of the Mayo Clinic considered colonic inflammation to be due to ulcerative colitis. In his book *The Modern Management of Colitis* dated 1943, he considered stricturing disease of the colon

to be an example of 'segmental ulcerative colitis' [13]. The barium enema contrast radiographs used to illustrate this condition are, however, typical of Crohn's disease. Even Crohn as late as 1965 [105] was reluctant to concede that involvement of the colon could occur in the absence of small intestinal disease. Others took a similar view [106, 107]. Even by the 1960s there was confusion between ulcerative colitis and Crohn's colitis. The clinical and pathological distinction between them was greatly clarified by Morson and Lockhart-Mummery [101]. Their work firmly established the clinical pathology of large bowel Crohn's disease and the often associated anal pathology. Subsequent work demonstrated an increasing prevalence of anal disease the more distal the intestinal involvement [108].

By the early 1970s there was some evidence that colonic Crohn's disease had become more frequent over the last 40 years. Thus Krause and colleagues in 1971 [109] showed an increase in the incidence of such cases without any diminution in the prevalence of ulcerative colitis.

The evolution of surgery

The evolution of surgery for Crohn's disease has differed according to the site of disease. In the early years surgery was regarded as the first-line treatment. All the original 14 patients had an operation [92]. The mechanical effect of the pathology resulting in obstruction or perforation lent itself to a surgical solution. Initially it was felt that the disease was a 'surgical' condition which was cured by operation. Within 20 years, however, the high incidence of recurrence following surgical resection began to be recognised. Van Patter and colleagues [110] reported recurrence after surgery in 80% of patients at 15 years and Crohn and Yarnis [111] found that over 80% of patients needed a subsequent operation. There is now a large literature on the incidence of recurrence after surgery [112-116]. As a result, physicians began to move more towards medical treatment, sometimes to the detriment of the patient with obstructing or perforating disease. Prolonged medication ran the risk of allowing the patient's condition to deteriorate presenting the surgeon with a more hazardous subsequent undertaking. Maintenance of an aggressive surgical strategy was, however, advocated mainly by Scandinavian surgeons [109, 117, 118] based on the argument that by early intervention serious complications, such as local perforation with abscess and fistula formation, could be avoided, thereby reducing the chance of surgical complications. In the last five years the introduction of biological anti-cytokine treatments has provoked a similar debate.

In practice, surgery was likely to be needed in the majority of patients at some time. Certainly in the era before anti-cytokine treatment, operation rates of 80% or more were reported in large series of patients treated initially by medical means [111, 112, 119, 120]. While the initial descriptions of surgical treatment dealt mainly with resection, some patients had undergone a bypass procedure. Of the original 14 patients reported by Crohn et al, three underwent a bypass owing to fistulation at the site of the disease in two and to a large inflammatory mass in one.

Bypass operations

Bypass with unilateral exclusion became commonly practised during the 1940s and 1950s. The procedure was popularised by the surgeons at Mount Sinai Hospital [121, 126]. Bypass surgery for Crohn's disease was popularised in the US when the then President Dwight Eisenhower underwent the procedure and did very well for the rest of his life. The risk of bypass was felt to be lower, while the results were thought to be similar. It became apparent, however, that the disease in the bypassed segment could progress resulting in a worsening of the patient's general condition. When bypass was compared with resection by others, however, it was clear that the latter was superior [122-125].

A further disadvantage of bypass was the incidence of carcinoma in the defunctioned segment with the passage of time, as reported by Greenstein et al from Mount Sinai Hospital in 1978 [127]. Carcinoma had already been reported in the terminal ileum of non-bypassed intestine [128].

Extent of resection

Thus by the 1970s resection had become the preferred surgical strategy. In the early years, resection aimed to remove the localised lesion to relieve obstruction or fistulation. When the high recurrence rates became known the strategy developed towards extensive excision of the diseased segment with ample margins of normal bowel above and below and wide excision of the mesentery. This was analogous to the concept of radical removal as applied to cancer and was advocated by Garlock and Crohn [121] and others [129, 130]. Histological involvement of the intestinal margin of the resected specimen was not associated with a higher recurrence rate than in cases where it was clear [131-133]. Repeated resections of small intestine led in some cases to short bowel syndrome and with the appreciation of this serious irreversible complication, the strategy of limited resection gradually prevailed. Evidence also emerged to indicate that limited resection with preservation of regional mesenteric lymph nodes, might be associated with a reduced incidence of recurrence.

Strictureplasty

The most extreme example of 'limited resection' was strictureplasty. This procedure had been used for the relief of tuberculous strictures of the intestine [134] and was applied to Crohn's disease by Lee in 1982 [135]. Seven patients were described. All showed improvement judged by gain of weight and relief of symptoms. Subsequent experience with strictureplasty [136, 137] showed its value in relieving obstructing symptoms in the long term for patients selected on the criteria of multiple short segment strictures and those with an already short small intestine. Strictureplasty has also been combined with resection according to the distribution and the extent of disease [138].

Biographical footnote on Sir Alan Parks

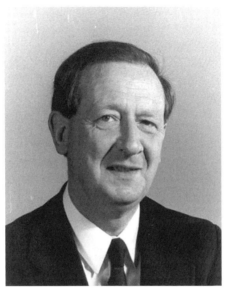

Figure 8. Sir Alan Parks (1920-1982). *Reproduced from the author's private collection.*

The era after World War II was one of great progress in surgery. A greater understanding of water and electrolyte balance, blood transfusion, advances in anaesthesia and better management of postoperative care had reduced surgical mortality and enabled surgery to be applied to more complex disorders. As a surgical pioneer, Alan Parks was gifted by his intellect, and his powers of imagination and innovation. He had always been interested in surgical craft from childhood; he understood the natural history of disease and was constantly trying to establish new strategies to help his patients. While under his tutelage, the author remembered him saying that "to define the problems, one only needed to do an outpatient clinic". He was able to combine surgical practice and intelligent thought with awareness of his patient's difficulties.

Alan Parks was born in 1920. He was a schoolboy near London and a medical student in Oxford from 1939 to 1943. During World War II, he played rugby football and captained the athletics team for Oxford University. In 1943, he was selected to continue clinical studies in the US as a Rockefeller student at Johns Hopkins Medical School, Baltimore, until 1947. As an Oxford graduate, he went to Guy's Hospital in London as an intern for Sir Heneagie Ogilvie, before doing research under Professor Hedley Atkins. During that period he graduated as a member of the Royal College of Physicians. Next he spent three years in Military Surgery before returning to Guy's Hospital in 1953 for Higher Surgical Training.

He was appointed Consultant Surgeon to the London Hospital (now the Royal London Hospital) and St. Mark's Hospital in 1959. During the next ten years he created a busy clinical practice during which he maintained a major interest in clinical research and the advancement of patient care. During his short life he gained the following honours:

- a knighthood in 1977 for his surgical work and Chairmanship of the Joint Consultants Committee;
- the Ernst Jung Prize in medicine in 1980;
- the Nessim Habif Prize from the University of Geneva;
- surgical advisor to the army;
- in 1980 he was elected President of the Royal College of Surgeons of England. Sadly, he died of a myocardial infarction before his term of office was completed.

Twenty-five years later, Sir Alan's name and opinions are still quoted and respected. He remains an inspiration to young surgeons from all countries. There are few diseases within the scope of colorectal surgery to which he has not made a contribution.

His early work on haemorrhoids while at Guy's Hospital led to the description of a new operation, the submucous haemorrhoidectomy. This, he claimed, was less painful and led to a better anatomical result than the conventional operation. While taken on by many but not all surgeons, it did not stand the test of time. Nevertheless, it highlighted the need for good surgical anal technique, which he demanded for all anal disorders.

More long-lasting was his approach to fistula-in-ano. Alongside Eisenhammer, he developed the cryptoglandular theory published in 1961, in which the source of fistula was maintained to be due to infection of an anorectal gland within the intersphincteric space. This led to a much simplified classification in 1976, which was generally accepted and remained helpful for all treating this condition.

For fissure-in-ano he advocated lateral sphincterotomy, later the main surgical treatment until the arrival of recently developed medical therapies. When surgery is still indicated, lateral sphincterotomy remains the operation of choice.

Alan Parks was the first to recognise the contribution made by surgeons in the past to the development of restorative surgery. Operations to

avoid a permanent stoma in the treatment of rectal cancer had been described and developed by Judd, Dixon, Babcock, Bacon, Goligher, Lloyd Davies and many others. Parks described the colo-anal anastomosis in 1972, in which mucosal continuity was created via an endo-anal approach between the colon above and the anal canal below. This was a significant advance on the previous colo-anal pull-through procedure.

In inflammatory bowel disease, Parks was aware of the experimental work of Ravitch and Devine. He used the latter's technique involving mucosal excision after submucosal injection of saline, in the treatment of villous adenoma of the rectum described in 1966. He was also mindful of the results of the 'straight' ileo-anal anastomosis, because of often poor reservoir capacity. When Koch in 1969 described the 'continent ileostomy' demonstrating an ileal reservoir was compatible with satisfactory health, he combined the principle with endo-anal anastomosis to create 'restorative proctocolectomy'. Described in 1978, the operation with few technical modifications has remained invaluable for ulcerative colitis and familial adenomatous polyposis.

Added to the above, Parks' contributions to functional diseases including continence and defaecation disorders were significant. In the early 1960s he developed a diagnostic service based around anal manometry, which led to the creation of the first Anorectal Physiology Unit. This is now a requirement for any credible colorectal establishment. He developed with Porter, objective measurement of pelvic floor function, and from this came the description of the descending perineal syndrome in 1966. He collaborated with Swash in the study of single-fibre electromyography, spinal stimulation, measurement of perineal descent and of terminal pudendal latency.

His work with Swash and Urich in 1977, demonstrated denervation of the pudendal nerve damaged during parturition. Immunochemical evidence of degeneration of pelvic floor musculature was compatible with denervation. These findings have influenced all academic and clinical research ever since.

Parks had discovered by radiological means, many incontinent patients with diffuse pelvic floor weakness had a widening of the anorectal angle. His operation of post-anal repair was designed to correct this. Though the early results reported in his Presidential Address to the Section of Proctology at the Royal Society of Medicine in 1975 were persuasive, the longer-term benefit did not persist. Nevertheless, this work was seminal and inspired others to develop further operations and treatments for incontinence.

As President of the Royal College of Surgeons of England, his desire for improvement of the patient's predicament was transmitted to the younger surgeons, whether they had or had not worked for him. His approach was always guided by his profound knowledge of basic medical science which he always aspired to extend. His life is an example to us all.

References

1. Sydenham T. *Observationes Medicae.* London, 1676.

2. Cruveilhier J. *Anatomie Pathologique.* Paris, 1829-42.

3. Wilks S, Moxon W. *Lectures on Pathological Anatomy,* 2nd edn. London: J & A Churchill, 1875.

4. Hale White W. On simple ulcerative colitis and other rare intestinal tumours. *Guy's Hospital Reports* 1888; 45: 131.

5. Nothnagel CW. *Beitrage zur Physiologie und Pathologie des Darmes.* Vienna, 1884.

6. Hale White W. Colitis. *Lancet* 1895; 1: 537.

7. Herschell G, Abrahams A. *Chronic colitis. Its causation diagnosis and treatment.* London, New York, Bombay and Calcutta: Longmans Green & co., 1914.

8. Cammeron H, Rippman CH. Statistics of ulcerative colitis from London Hospitals. *Proc Roy Soc Med* 1909; 2: 100.

9. Weir R. A new use for the useless appendix in surgical treatment of obstinate colitis. *Med Rec* 1902; 62: 201.

10. Lockhart-Mummery P. *Diseases of the Rectum and Anus.* London: Balliere Tindall and Cox, 1914.

11. Brown J. The value of complete physiological rest of the large bowel in the treatment of certain ulcerative and obstructive lesions of this organ. *Surg Gynecol Obstet* 1913; 16: 610.

12. Corbett R. A review of the surgical treatment of chronic ulcerative colitis. *Proc Roy Soc Med* 1945; 38: 277.

13. Bargen J. *The Modern Management of Colitis.* Springfield: Charles C Thomas, 1943.

14. Cattell R, Boehme EJ. The importance of malignant degeneration as a complication of ulcerative colitis. *Gastroenterology* 1947; 8: 695.

15. Counsell P, Dukes CE The association of chronic ulcerative colitis and carcinoma of the rectum and colon. *Br J Surg* 1952; 39: 485.

16. Estor E, Etienne E. *Les Colites: leur traitement chirurgical.* Paris: Gittler, 1914.

17. Reinhof W. The surgical treatment of ulcerative colitis by ileo-sigmoidostomy. *Ann Clin Med* 1925; 4: 430.

18. Lockhart-Mummery J, Norbury LEC, Gabriel WB, Ogilvie H, Hurst AF. Discussion on the surgical treatment of idiopathic ulcerative colitis and its sequelae. *Proc Roy Soc Med* 1940; 33: 645.

19. Bargen J. Experimental studies on the etiology of ulcerative colitis. *JAMA* 1924; 83: 332.

20. Rankin F. Surgery for ulcerative colitis. *Surg Gynecol Obstet* 1939; 68: 306.

21. Cave H, Thompson JE. Mortality factors in the surgical treatment of ulcerative colitis. *Ann Surg* 1941; 114: 46-52.

22. Cattell RD. New type of ileostomy for chronic ulcerative colitis. *Surg Clin North Am* 1939; 19: 629-35.

23. Lahey F. Indications for surgery for ulcerative colitis. *NY State J Med* 1941; 41: 475.

24. Strauss A, Strauss SF. Surgical treatment of ulcerative colitis. *Surg Clin North Am* 1944; 24: 211-24.

25. Cattell R. Discussion on the surgery of ulcerative colitis. *Proc Roy Soc Med* 1953; 46: 1021.

26. Miller C, Ripstein CB, Tabah EG. The surgical management of ucerative colitis. *Surg Gynecol Obstet* 1949; 88: 351-8.

27. Miller C, Gardner C McG, Ripstein CB. Primary resection of the colon in ulcerative colitis. *Can Med A J* 1949; 60: 584-5.

28. Ripstein C, Miller CG, Gardner C McG. Results of surgery for ulcerative colitis. *Ann Surg* 1952; 135: 13.

29. Counsell P, Goligher JC. The surgical treatment of ulcerative colitis. *Lancet* 1952; 2: 1045.

30. Crile G, Thomas CY. Treatment of acute toxic ulcerative colitis by ileostomy and simultaneous colostomy. *Gastroenterology* 1951; 19: 58.

31. Brooke B. The management of ileostomy. *Lancet* 1952; ii: 102-4.

32. Warner EC, Taylor S. Ulcerative colitis. Meeting of the Section of Proctology of the Royal Society of Medicine with the American Proctological Society, London, June 29-July 1 1959. *Proc Roy Soc Med* 1959; 52 (Supplement): 3-31.

33. Brooke B. Permanent ileostomy in ulcerative colitis. *Proc Roy Soc Med* 1959; 52 (Supplement Anglo-American Conference on Proctology): 16.

34. Ault G. Selective surgery for ulcerative colitis. *Proc Roy Soc Med* 1959; 52 (Supplement Anglo-American Conference in Proctology): 11.

35. Devine H. Method of colectomy for desperate cases of ulcerative colitis. *Surg Gynecol Obstet* 1943; 76: 136.

36. Corbett R. The early experience of ileo-rectal anastomosis. *Proc Roy Soc Med* 1959; 52 (Supplement): 21.

37. Aylett SO. Three hundred cases of diffuse ulcerative colitis treatment by total colectomy and ileorectal anastomosis. *Br Med J* 1966; 1: 1001-5.

38. Baker WNW, Glass RE, Ritchie JK, Aylett SO. Cancer of the rectum following colectomy and ileorectal anastomosis for ulcerative colitis. *Br J Surg* 1978; 65: 862-8.

39. Brown C, Turnbull RB, Diaz R. Ileorectal anastomosis in ulcerative colitis. *Am J Digest Dis* 1962; 7: 585.

40. Griffen W, Lellehei RC, Wangensteen OH. Ileoproctostomy in ulcerative colitis. *Surgery* 1963; 53: 705-10.

41. Gruner OPN, Flatmark A, Maas R, *et al.* Ileorectal anastomosis in ulcerative colitis. *Scand J Gastroenterol* 1975; 10: 641-6.

42. Adson MA, Cooperman AM, Farrow GM. Ileorectostomy for ulcerative disease of the colon. *Arch Surg* 1972; 104: 424-8.

43. Hawley PR. Ileorectal anastomosis. *Br J Surg* 1985; 72(S): 575-82.

44. Melville DM, Ritchie JK, Nicholls RJ, Hawley PR. Surgery for ulcerative colitis in the era of the pouch: the St. Mark's Hospital experience. *Gut* 1994; 35(8): 1076-80.

45. Kraske P. Zur Exstirpation hochsitzender Mastdarmkrebse. *Verhdt Chir* 1885; 14: 464.

46. Hochenegg J. Meine Operationserfolge bei Rektum Carzinom. *Wiener Klinische Wochenschrift* 1900; 13: 399-404.

47. Maunsell H. A new method of excising the two upper portions of the rectum and the lower segment of the sigmoid portion of the colon. *Lancet* 1892; 2: 473-6.

48. Weir R. An improved method of treating high seated cancers of the rectum. *Am J Surg Gynecol* 1901; 15: 134-5.

49. Nissen R. Sitzingsberichte aus Chirurgischen Gesellschaften Berliner Gesellschaft fur Chirurgie. *Zentralbl Chir* 1933; 60: 888.

50. Ravitch MM, Sabiston DC. Anal ileostomy with preservation of the sphincter; a proposed operation oin patients requiring total colectomy fro benign lesions. *Surg Gynecol Obstet* 1947; 84: 1095-9.

51. Ravitch MM. Anal ileostomy with sphincter preservation in patients requiring total colectomy for benign conditions. *Surgery* 1948; 24: 170-87.

52. Devine J, Webb R. Resection of the rectal mucosa colectomy and anal ileostomy with normal continence. *Surg Gynecol Obstet* 1951; 92: 437-42.

53. Best R. Anastomosis of the ileum to the lower part of the rectum and anus. A report on experience of ileorectostomy and ileoproctostomy with special reference to polyposis. *Arch Surg* 1948; 57: 276-85.

54. Martin L, LeCoutre C, Schubert WK. Total colectomy and mucosal proctectomy with preservation of continence in ulcerative colitis. *Ann Surg* 1977; 186: 477-9.

55. Soave F. A new surgical technique for treatment of Hirschprung's disease. *Surgery* 1964; 56: 1007-14.

56. Telander RL, Perrault J. Total colectomy with mucosectomy and ileoanal anastomosis for chronic ulcerative colitis in children and young adults. *Mayo Clin Proc* 1980; 55: 420-4.

57. Peck D, German JD, Jackson FC. Rectal resection for benign disease; a new technique. *Dis Colon Rectum* 1966; 9: 363-6.

58. Peck D. Rectal mucosal replacement. *Ann Surg* 1980; 191: 201-303.

59. Parks AG, Nicholls RJ. Proctocolectomy without ileostomy for ulcerative colitis. *Br Med J* 1978; 2(6130): 85-8.

60. Van Laarhoven CJ, et al. The ileo neorectal anastomosis: an experimental study on development of the surgical technique and theoretical background. *Colorectal Dis* 2001; 3(2): 82-94.

61. Valiente MA, Bacon HE. Construction of pouch using 'pantaloon' technique for pull through following colectomy. *Am J Surg* 1955; 90: 6621-43.

62. Kock NG. Intra-abdominal 'reservoir' in patients with permanent ileostomy. *Arch Surg* 1969; 99: 223-31.

63. Kock NG, Myrvold HE, Nilsson LO, Philipson BM. Continent ileostomy - an account of 314 patients. *Acta Chir Scand* 1981; 147: 67-72.

64. Beahrs OKK, Adson MA, Chong GC. Ileostomy with ileal reservoir rather than ileostomy alone. *Ann Surg Oncol* 1974; 179: 634.

65. Gelernt IM, Bauer JJ, Kreel I. The reservoir ileostomy: early experience with 54 patients. *Ann Surg* 1977; 185: 179.

66. Philipson B, Brandberg A, Jagenburg R, Kock NG, Lager I, Ahren C. Mucosal morphology bacteriology and absorption in intra-abdominal ileostomy reservoir. *Scand J Gastroenterol* 1975; 10: 145-53.

67. Parks AG, Nicholls RJ, Belleveau P. Proctocolectomy with ileal reservoir and anal anastomosis. *Br J Surg* 1980; 67: 533-8.

68. Utsunomiya J, Iwama T, Imago M, et al. Total colectomy mucosal proctectomy and ileo-anal anastomosis. *Dis Colon Rectum* 1980; 23: 459-66.

69. Martin L, Fischer JE. Preservation of anorectal continence following total colectomy. *Ann Surg* 1982; 196: 700-4.

70. Rothenberger DAV, Christenson FD, Balcos CE, Nemer EG, Goldberg FD, Belliveau SM, Nivatvongs P, Schottler S, Fang JL, Kennedy DT, HL. Restorative proctocolectomy with ileal reservoir and ileoanal anastomosis. *Am J Surg* 1983; 145(1): 82-8.

71. Metcalf AM, Dozois RR, Beart RW, Kelly KA, Wolff BG Jr. Ileal 'J' pouch-anal anastomosis. Clinical outcome. *Ann Surg* 1985; 202(6): 735-9.

72. Dozois RR, Goldberg SM, Rothenberger DA, Utsunomiya J, Nicholls RJ, Cohen Z, Hulten LA, Moskowitz RL, Williams NS. Restorative proctocolectomy with ileal reservoir. *Int J Colorectal Dis* 1986; 1(1): 2-19.

73. Nicholls RJ, Pezim ME. Restorative proctocolectomy with ileal reservoir for ulcerative colitis and familial adenomatous polyposis: a comparison of three reservoir designs. *Br J Surg* 1985; 72(6): 470-4.

74. Moskowitz RL, Shepherd NA, Nicholls RJ. An assessment of inflammation in the reservoir after restorative proctocolectomy with ileoanal ileal reservoir. *Int J Colorectal Dis* 1986; 1(3): 167-74.

75. Meagher AP, Farouk R, Dozois RR, Kelly KA, Pemberton JH. J ileal pouch-anal anastomosis for chronic ulcerative colitis: complications and long-term outcome in 1310 patients. *Br J Surg* 1998; 85(6): 800-3.

76. Fazio VW, Ziv Y, Church JM, Oakley JR, Lavery IC, Milsom JW, Schroeder TK. Ileal pouch-anal anastomoses complications and function in 1005 patients. *Ann Surg* 1995; 222(2): 120-7.

77. Heuschen UA, Allemeyer EH, Hinz U, Lucas M, Herfarth C, Heuschen O. Outcome after septic complications in J pouch procedures. *Br J Surg* 2002; 89: 194-200.

78. Tulchinsky H, Hawley PR, Nicholls RJ. Long-term failure after restorative proctocolectomy for ulcerative colitis. *Ann Surg* 2003; 238(2): 229-34.

79. Panis Y, Poupard B, Nemeth J, Lavergne A, Hautefeuille P, Valleur P. Ileal pouch/anal anastomosis for Crohn's disease. *Lancet* 1996; 347(9005): 854-7.

80. Olsen KO, Joelsson M, Laurberg S, Oresland T. Fertility after ileal pouch-anal anastomosis in women with ulcerative colitis. *Br J Surg* 1999; 86(4): 493-5.

81. Penna C, Dozois R, Tremaine W, Sandborn W, LaRusso N, Schleck C, Ilstrup D. Pouchitis after ileal pouch-anal

anastomosis for ulcerative colitis occurs with increased frequency in patients with associated primary sclerosing cholangitis. *Gut* 1996; 38(2): 234-9.

82. Fazio V, Tekkis PP, Remzi F, Lavery IC, Manilich IC, Connor J, Preen M, Delaney CP. Quantification for risk failure after ileal pouch anal anastomosis surgery. *Ann Surg* 2003; 238: 605-17.

83. Morgagni G. *De Sedibus et Causis Morborum.* Remondini, Ed. Venezia, 1769.

84. Coombe C, Saunders H. A singular case of stricture and thickening of ileum. *Med Transactions of Royal College of Physicians*, London 1813; 4: 16.

85. Abercrombie J. *Pathological and practical researches on disease of the stomach, the intestinal canal, the liver and other viscera of the abdomen.* Edinburgh: Waugh and Innes, 1828.

86. Dalziel T. Chronic intestinal enteritis. *Br Med J* 1913; 2: 1068-70.

87. Moynihan B. The mimicry of malignant disease in the large bowel. *Edinburgh Med J* 1907; 21: 228.

88. Robson A. Abdominal tumours simulating malignant disease and their treatment. *Br Med J* 1908; 1: 425.

89. Nuboer F. Chronische phlegmone van hit ileum. *Ned Tijdschr Geneeskd* 1932; 76: 29-89.

90. Golob M. Infectious granuloma of the intestines. *Medical J and Record* 1932; 135: 390-3.

91. Moschowitz E, Wilensky AO. Nonspecific granulomata of the intestine. *Am J Med Sci* 1923; 166: 48-66.

92. Crohn B, Ginzburg L, Oppenheimer GD. Regional ileitis: a pathologic and clinical entity. *JAMA* 1932; 99: 1323-9.

93. Ginzburg L, Oppenheimer GB. Nonspecific granulomata of the intestines, inflammatory tumors and strictures of the bowel. *Ann Surg* 1933; 27: 1046-62.

94. Colp R. Case of nonspecific granuloma of terminal ileum and cecum. *Surg Clin North Am* 1934; 14: 443-9.

95. Bargen J, Weber HM. Regional migratory chronic ulcerative colitis. *Surg Gynecol Obstet* 1930; 50: 964-72.

96. Crohn B, Rosenak BD. A combined form of ileitis and colitis. *JAMA* 1936; 106: 1.

97. Crohn B, Berg AA. Right-side (regional) colitis. *JAMA* 1938; 110: 32-8.

98. Harris F, Bell G, Brunn H. Chronic cicatrising enteritis: regional ileitis (Crohn). *Surc Gynecol Obstet* 1933; 57: 637-45.

99. Bartstra D, Kooreman PJ. Peculiar localisation of so-called regional ileitis. *Clinics in Gastroenterology* 1939; 9: 307-22.

100. Morson B, Lockhart-Mummery HE. Crohn's disease of the colon. *Gastroenterologia* 1959; 92: 168-72.

101. Lockhart Mummery H, Morson BC. Crohn's disease (regional enteritis) of the large intestine and its distinction from ulcerative colitis. *Gut* 1960; 1: 87-105.

102. Dudenay T, Todd IP. Crohn's diseaase of the mouth. *Proc Roy Soc Med* 1969; 62: 1237-8.

103. Varley E. Crohn's disease of the mouth. *Oral Surg, Oral Med, Oral Path* 1973; 33: 570.

104. Croft C, Wilkinson AR. Ulceration of the mouth, pharynx and larynx in Crohn's disease of the intestine. *Br J Surg* 1972; 59: 249-52.

105. Crohn B. In discussion on Crohn's disease. *Dis Colon Rectum* 1965; 8: 3.

106. Neuman H, Bargen JA, Judd ES. Clinical study of 201 cases of regional (segmental) colitis. *Surg Gynecol Obstet* 1954; 99: 563.

107. Manning J, Warren R, Adi AS. Segmental colitis. Results of surgery. *New Engl J Med* 1955; 252: 850.

108. Hellers GBO, Ewerth S, *et al.* Occurrence and outcome after primary treatment of anal fistulae in Crohn's disease. *Gut* 1981; 21: 525.

109. Krause U, Bergman L, Norlen BJ. Crohn's disease. A clinical study based on 186 patients. *Scand J Gastroenterol* 1971; 6: 97.

110. Van Patter W, Bargen JA, Dockerty MB, *et al.* Regional enteritis. *Gastroenterology* 1954; 26: 347-50.

111. Crohn B, Yarnis H. *Regional Ileitis*, 2nd edn. New York: Grune and Stratton, 1958.

112. Cooke W, Mallas E, Prior P, *et al.* Crohn's disease course, treatment and long-term prognosis. *Q J Med* 1980; 49: 363.

113. Burman J, Cooke WT, Williams JA. The fate of ileorectal anastomosis in Crohn's disease. *Gut* 1971; 12: 432.

114. de Dombal F, Burton IL, Goligher JC. Recurrence of Crohn's disease after primary excisional surgery. *Gut* 1971; 12: 519-27.

115. Nugent F, Viedenheimer MC, Meissner A, Haggitt RC. Prognosis after colonic resection for Crohn's disease of the colon. *Gastroenterology* 1973; 65: 398.

116. Farmer R, Hawk WA, Turnbull RB. Clinical patterns in Crohn's disease; a statistical study of 615 cases. *Gastroenterology* 1975; 68: 627-35.

117. Fasth S, Hellberg R, Hulten L, *et al.* Early complications after surgical treatment for Crohn's disease with particular reference to factors affecting their development. *Acta Chir Scand* 1980; 146: 519.

118. Muhe E, Gall FP, Hager T, *et al.* Die Chirurgie des Morbus Croh: klinische Studie an 155 Patienten mit Darmresektion. *Dtsch Med Wochenschr* 1981; 106: 165.

119. Truelove SC, Pena AS. Course and prognosis of Crohn's disease. *Gut* 1976; 17: 192.

120. Goligher JC. *Surgery of the Anus, Rectum and Colon.* London: Balliere Tindall, 1961.

121. Garlock J, Crohn BB. An appraisal of the results of surgery in treatment of regional ileitis. *JAMA* 1945; 127: 205-11.

122. Barbour K, Waugh JM, Beahrs OH, Sauer WG. Indication for and results of surgical treatment of regional enteritis. *Ann Surg* 1962; 156: 472.

123. Atwell J, Duthie HL, Goligher JC. The outcome of Crohn's disease. *Br J Surg* 1965; 52: 996.

124. Colcock B, Vansant JH. Surgical treatment of regional ileitis. *New Engl J Med* 1960; 262: 435.

125. Williams J. The place of surgery in Crohn's disease. *Gut* 1971; 12: 739.

126. Koudahl G, Kristensen Lenz K. Bypass compared with resection for ileal Crohn's disease. *Scand J Gastroenterol* 1974; 9: 203.

127. Greenstein A, Sachar D, Pucillo A. Cancer in Crohn's disease after diversionary surgery: a report of seven cancers in excluded bowel. *Am J Surg* 1978; 135: 86.

128. Savage R, Farmer RG, Hawk W. Carcinoma of the small bowel associated with transmural ileitis (Crohn's disease). *Am J Clin Path* 1975; 63: 168.

129. Bergmann JF, Krause U. Crohn's disease: a long-term study of the clinical course in 186 patients. *Scand J Gastroenterol* 1977; 12: 937.

130. Venckert G. Scandia Symposium on Regional Enteritis. Stockholm, 1971.

131. Papaionnou N, Piris J, Lee CCG, *et al.* The relationship between histological inlfammation in the cut ends after resection of Crohn's disease and recurrence. *Gut* 1979; 20: A916.

132. Pennington L, Hamilton SR, Bayless TM, *et al.* Surgical management of Crohn's disease: influence of disease at margins of resection. *Ann Surg* 1980; 192: 311.

133. Fazio V, Marchetti F, Church JM, *et al.* Effect of resection margins on the recurrence of Crohn's disease in the small bowel. A randomised controlled trial. *Ann Surg* 1996; 224: 563-73.

134. Katariya R, Sood S, Rao PG, *et al.* Strictureplasty for tuberculous strictures of the gastrointestinal tract. *Br J Surg* 1977; 64: 496-8.

135. Lee E, Papaionnou N. Minimal surgery for chronic obstruction in patients with extensive and universal Crohn's disease. *Ann Roy Coll Surg Engl* 1982; 64: 229-33.

136. Stebbing JFJD, Kettlewell MGW, Mortensen NJ McC. Long-term results of recurrence and reoperation after strictureplasty for obstructive Crohn's disease. *Br J Surg* 1995; 82: 1471-4.

137. Kumar D, Alexander Williams J. *The Surgical Management of Crohn's Disease and Ulcerative Colitis.* London: Springer Verlag, 1993.

138. Nicholls RJ, Pescatori M, Motson RW, Pezin ME. Restorative proctocolectomy with a three-loop reservoir for ulcerative colitis and familial adenomatous polyposis: clinical results in 66 patients followed for up to 6 years. *Ann Surg* 1984; 199: 383-8

Chapter 14

Evolution of surgery for colorectal cancer

Johan F Nordenstam MD, Post Doctoral Associate

Robert E Bulander MD, Surgical Resident

Anders F Mellgren MD PhD, Adjunct Associate Professor

David A Rothenberger MD, Professor and Interim Chair, Department of Surgery,

University of Minnesota School of Medicine, Minneapolis, USA

Introduction

Surgery for colorectal cancer is commonplace in today's world and can usually be performed safely. It is surprising and easily forgotten that, until recent times, such surgery was hazardous and generally avoided because of its associated morbidity and mortality. This chapter will describe the evolution of surgery for colorectal cancer by first reviewing three converging concepts and then discussing specifics of the history of surgery for colon and rectal cancer.

Three converging concepts

Concept of carcinogenesis

The development of the surgical management of colorectal carcinoma was directly influenced by the understanding of carcinogenesis and the nature of cancer. Theories dating to the time of Hippocrates suggested that cancer was predominantly a systemic condition, influenced by the humeral or chemical composition of the patient's tissues, thus obviating any hope of surgical cure by local management [1]. With the introduction of cellular theories of malignant transformation came interest in the therapeutic potential to treat tumours with surgical resection.

From the 2nd century AD to the Renaissance, the Galenic view of carcinogenesis dominated [2]. Galen's view of the origin of cancer mirrored that of Hippocrates: malignancy, he felt, arose from collections of black bile in the afflicted organs. This implied an internal imbalance as the source of disease, which would doom surgical therapy to failure. Not surprisingly, Galen favoured the use of purgatives and analgesics over surgery to rid the body of disease-causing humours, although he noted that operations could be carried out as a last resort. Paracelsus in the 16th century took a similar view, postulating that cancer reflected the influence of a fundamental mineral imbalance within the body.

The 18th century saw the first theories on local origin of cancers. John Hunter proposed extravasated blood as a potential aetiology. He postulated the tumour could excite a diseased disposition in the surrounding tissues and advocated taking normal-appearing margins in any resection of tumour in order to extirpate this potential source of recurrence. The idea that tumour may be a local process opened the possibility of surgical cure, but in the case of the colon, the limitations of abdominal surgery at the time - particularly the lack of anaesthetic or antisepsis - made wide resections of bowel for tumour unattractive [2].

The invention of light microscopy in the early 19th century led to the understanding of the cellular origins of cancer. Early investigators, such as Virchow and Rokitansky, believed connective tissues were the source of neoplasia. Billroth (Figure 17, Chapter 6), on the other hand, proposed the idea of mucosa as the origin of bowel cancer. In 1923, Lockhart-Mummery (Figure 1, Chapter 13) theorised that colonic malignancy arose from neoplastic polyps; Cuthbert Dukes suggested in 1926 that rectal tumours begin as a coalescence of abnormal epithelium that grows intraluminally and intramurally, ultimately invading deeper tissues [3]. Shortly thereafter, Karl Bauer advanced the theory that a tumour could arise from a single, mutated cell [2].

In 1927, Neil Swinton of Boston published an operative series of 156 abdominal operations for colorectal polyps and demonstrated their distribution throughout the colon in a pattern similar to that described for colorectal cancers [4]. He described the histological characteristics of colorectal adenomata, and reported a total of 121 cases in his series where malignant transformation was evident in a resected specimen. He postulated that colonic polyps "are true tumours, and that they are the results of some inherent defect in cellular growth". He therefore advocated sigmoidoscopic fulguration or excision of colorectal adenomata, and careful follow-up in all cases as a means of preventing cancer.

The following year, Dukes and Lockhart-Mummery published a report delineating their model of the adenoma-carcinoma sequence [5]. They believed an initial local hyperplastic reaction developed in susceptible areas of the colon, which Dukes described as an irregularity in the epithelium, visible under low-power microscopy. This susceptible area would go on to develop into either sessile or pedunculated adenomata, and finally, the adenoma would degenerate into carcinoma, with the capacity to invade and spread. It is only a small step to see the evolution of this work into the modern model of carcinogenesis.

Sixteen centuries of Galenic dogma delayed the advancement of surgical management of colon and rectal malignancies. Ultimately, the understanding that cancers began locally and followed an orderly progression from curable, benign lesions into invasive

tumours with metastatic potential, proved crucial in establishing belief in the possibility of curative resection, which in turn cultivated interest in advancing surgical techniques.

Concepts to improve operative techniques for intestinal surgery

The preceding millennium of a hands-off surgical approach to the abdomen left 18th and 19th-century surgeons in a largely unexplored territory in their attempts to treat large bowel cancer. Through the end of the 19th century, bowel operations were limited by the crude state of the art of surgery, plagued by problems of poor exposure, lighting, haemostasis and anaesthesia, and the challenge of postoperative sepsis. It was well understood that faecal spillage into the peritoneum was often fatal to the patient, and this reality led to the surgeon's historical aversion to operate on the intestine. Galen decried the use of intestinal sutures two thousand years ago, and Zang repeated the warning in 1818 when he stated that "every intestinal suture ... is a very dangerous undertaking" [6]. It was not until the late 1800s that operative techniques with some promise of safety evolved.

Aside from the more general problems of asepsis and haemostasis that plagued all operations, the ability to create secure bowel anastomoses remained a significant technical obstacle to the advancement of colonic surgery until modern times. Early colorectal operations were planned and carried out in often rather elaborate and complex steps to avoid creating anastomoses.

The simplest method of repairing an enterotomy or creating an anastomosis is by suture. One of the first techniques of enterorrhaphy was described by Abul-Kasim in the 2nd century AD (Figure 1). He took the heads of large ants and employed their jaw pincers in a manner not unlike modern steel surgical clips.

Another early approach is referred to as 'the glover's stitch', a through-and-through running suture that approximated the cut ends of bowel. 'The suture of the four masters' technique was described in the 16th century; it consisted of a reed stent to maintain luminal patency while the repair was effected with four interrupted sutures. Trial and error through the following years led to the use of other stent materials, such as goose trachea, elder wood, cardboard, India rubber and wax. Sutures were generally full thickness, and the whole anastomosis was often pulled up to the parietal peritoneum by the long, uncut ends of the sutures to allow the development of protective adhesions. The nature of serosal surfaces to form adhesions was used to advantage by Lembert, who in 1825, described his use of inverting sutures to reinforce a full-thickness continuous primary suture line with two layers of serosa. By the turn of the 20th century, Oscar Allis described a means of using the toothed forceps that would eventually bear his name as 'basting devices' to hold two open ends of bowel in position while a fine silk suture was used to create a full-thickness, single-layer, circumferential anastomosis.

Because hand suture techniques were not considered reliable, significant effort was spent to develop mechanical devices to improve the safety of bowel anastomoses. A strategy pursued throughout the 19th century was the use of templates, often made of metal, to speed up sutured anastomoses or eliminate sewing altogether. These devices are described in more detail in Chapter 10. In fairness, Henroz created the first successful template device

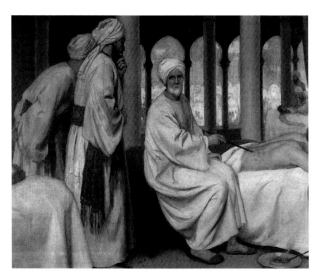

Figure 1. Abul-Kasim (936-1013). *Reproduced with permission from the Wellcome Trust Medical Photographic Library.*

in 1826. It consisted of two steel rings with interlocking pins that snapped two limbs of bowel together with an everting, end-to-end anastomosis. The most widely used anastomotic device was the Murphy button, patented in 1892 in the US [7]. It consisted of two mushroom-shaped metal pieces placed into cut ends of bowel or lateral enterotomies, secured with purse-string sutures, and then snapped together. Pressure necrosis and adhesion formation would seal the anastomosis, and the button sloughed and passed with the stool (Figure 8, Chapter 10).

The risks associated with man-made anastomoses led many surgeons to forego their use, opting instead for a controlled-fistula technique. Sutures were used to bring the open loops of bowel up to a laparotomy wound where it would adhere as the wound healed. As postoperative ileus resolved, fistula output tapered off and the wound then closed. Dupuytren, in the early 19th century, developed a crushing clamp known as an enterotome (Figure 2, Chapter 10), which he used to create side-to-side anastomoses through externalised loops of bowel. The jaws of the clamp were fed through the fistula opening into the proximal and distal loops of bowel, trapping the two lengths of bowel parallel to one another. The clamp was then closed and sequentially tightened over several days. Serosal adhesions formed to hold the two limbs together, and pressure necrosis created a widely patent anastomosis between them. The fistula was then allowed to close spontaneously. This technique would find use for more than a century, culminating in the Mikulicz colostomy, in which a primary anastomosis was formed with the enterotome in a 'double-barrelled' stoma of bowel, proximal and distal to a resection. This approach still found wide use in the 1950s.

The enterotome can be considered a direct ancestor of the intestinal stapling devices, which are described in Chapter 11. The subsequent evolution of transanal circular stapling devices ultimately offered surgeons the ability to perform low rectal anastomoses that otherwise would have required proctectomy and formation of a permanent stoma [7-9].

Concepts of early detection of colorectal cancer

It is today well recognised that early diagnosis of cancer leads to a more favourable outcome of therapy. This fact was understood by the early 20th century. Lockhart-Mummery noted in 1927: "It is to earlier diagnosis that we must look for any material improvement in our cancer cures from operation." The ability to diagnose cancer of the colon before the era of roentgenography and endoscopy was limited to identifying masses palpable through the abdomen or in the rectum, and by clinical recognition of what proved to be the late signs of illness: bowel obstruction, tenesmus, cachexia and anaemia. The ability to identify tumours at a curable stage was a crucial step in advancing cancer operations from palliative to curative in intent.

The 14th-century English surgeon, John Arderne, described his diagnostic approach to anorectal problems as follows: "The doctor should put his finger into the anus of this patient and if he finds within something as hard as a stone ... this is certainly a bubo (tumour)." He gave the less-than-reassuring prognosis that "often it erodes and consumes the whole circumference of [the anus, and] it may never be cured with human treatment"[10].

The first gastroenterologic radiographic studies were performed by Walter Cannon in 1898, using contrast medium made of gruel and bismuth [11]. The barium enema and air-contrast barium enema became standard diagnostic studies by the middle of the 20th century [12].

Guaiac, a natural substance derived from trees, was discovered in 1864 to react with heme and thus provided a means to detect occult blood in a specimen. A century elapsed, however, before this finding found clinical use in the detection of asymptomatic colon cancers [13].

Rigid proctoscopy was initially described in 1853, but was not practised widely until after 1900. This technique brought the rectum and distal sigmoid into diagnostic and therapeutic reach, but the remainder of the bowel remained inaccessible until the development of fiber-optic endoscopes in the 1960s.

Endoscopic evaluation of the entire colon, colonoscopy, was introduced in 1969 [11]. True to Lockhart-Mummery's prediction, this ability to systematically screen the entire colon for polyps and tumours proved a major advance in reducing mortality from colorectal cancer.

Evolution of surgery for colon cancer

Early days (1700-1950)

Diversion and the lumbar colostomy

Given the aforementioned limitations in understanding malignant disease, diagnosing intra-abdominal pathology, and operating in the pre-anaesthetic, pre-antiseptic era, the earliest operations for colon cancer were not oncologic operations at all. Rather, surgeons addressed the problem of malignant bowel obstruction, the so-called 'iliac passion', and the first procedures were all operations for faecal diversion.

The first recorded description of how a colostomy operation can be performed was reported in the French Royal Academy of Sciences in 1710 [14]. Alexis Littré reported his findings after examining a boy who had died from bowel obstruction caused by imperforate anus [15]. The events around that time are described in Chapter 16. This idea was put into practice when a French surgeon, Pillore, performed the first known caecostomy in 1776 on a patient suffering from bowel obstruction caused by a rectal cancer. The patient lived for 28 days after the operation. His death was not attributable to the operation, but to the two pounds of mercury that he had taken to cure his bowel obstruction a month earlier. The weight of the quicksilver had pulled a distal part of the jejunum down into the pelvis, behind the bladder, where the jejunum became gangrenous [15].

Another French surgeon, Duret, performed a successful left iliac colostomy in a three-day-old child with imperforate anus in 1793 [15]. This patient lived until the age of 45. Not all patients fared so well before anaesthesia and antisepsis. Operations on the colon carried a terrible toll. Amussat's 'extraperitoneal operation' described and illustrated in Figure 6, Chapter 9, became the procedure of choice for bowel obstruction and rectal cancer in Europe and the US [16]. As surgical technique improved toward the beginning of the 20th century, and survival of transperitoneal operations improved, the left iliac colostomy gained in popularity [17].

Resection and anastomosis

Lack of confidence in bowel anastomosis limited early operations for cancer to diversion and stoma creation. Nonetheless, attempts were made by 19th-century surgeons to resect and re-establish continuity. Reybard of Lyon submitted a paper in 1844, reporting that in 1833, he had excised a tumour the size of an orange from the sigmoid flexure and reunited the bowel ends by sutures. The patient was reported to have lived for ten months postoperatively before succumbing to recurrence of his disease. The paper lacked in scientific validity and it was never accepted for presentation [18].

Several attempts at colon resection were made in the latter half of the 1800s. In 1879, Billroth successfully performed a sigmoid resection, closing the distal stump and bringing the proximal end out as an end-colostomy [19]. A similar success was reported by Martini of Hamburg the same year, who performed an end-colostomy and oversewed the rectal stump after resecting a sigmoid tumour and finding himself unable to complete the anastomosis. This operation is often associated with the procedure called Hartmann's operation which he published in 1909. The following year, Czerny of Heidelberg performed a two-and-a-half-hour operation to resect a colon tumour involving both the transverse and the sigmoid colon. After removing bowel from both parts of the colon, an anastomosis was constructed and the patient lived more than seven months before recurrent cancer killed him [18].

Rates of postoperative intra-abdominal sepsis were high, and much thought and discussion focused on how to establish an 'aseptic anastomosis'. The initial approach would be exteriorisation of the bowel; later, major additional contributions were made by Halsted, Mall, and Wangensteen [20, 21].

Exteriorisation

Debate over the safety of operating in the peritoneal cavity led to the development of exteriorisation, or extracorporeal bowel resection. The tumour-bearing loop of bowel was mobilised at laparotomy, brought out through the incision, and then resected, often in a staged procedure after adhesions had formed to seal the peritoneum.

Bloch, practising in Copenhagen, described this ingenious technique in a Danish journal in 1894, when he resected a left colon cancer via an extraperitoneal approach [22]. He first externalised the sigmoid colon through the abdominal wall and drained the proximal loop through a tube. A few days later, when the bowel had adhered to the abdominal wall, the externalised sigmoid and part of the transverse colon were resected and a 'double-barrel' type of colostomy resulted. At a yet later stage, Bloch was able to close the colostomy, having performed the entire bowel resection and anastomosis without risk of intra-peritoneal soiling.

Johann Mikulicz from Breslau and Frank T. Paul from Liverpool, both independently developed their own techniques of exteriorising the colon before performing the resection. Mikulicz performed an operation almost identical to Bloch's, whereas Paul resected the bowel at the time of the original operation. In 1903, Mikulicz reported a major decrease in operative mortality after he started to perform the exteriorisation operation for obstruction, a finding which gained great influence over the practice of colon surgery at the time [23].

Intraperitoneal resection

Many surgeons still preferred an intraperitoneal resection and most of them used a pre-operative caecostomy as an adjunct to the colon resection [24]. In 1931, Devine suggested that a protective transverse colostomy should be performed two to three weeks prior to a colon resection. He recommended placing the colostomy as far to the proximal side of the transverse colon as possible in order to keep the stoma out of the way of the resection. The construction of a defunctioning transverse colostomy prior to colon resection became the method of choice in the 1930s and 1940s.

Modern times (since 1950)

The addition of antibiotics and antiseptic bowel preparation

The arrival of systemic antibiotics and antiseptic pre-operative bowel preparations enabled new intra-abdominal techniques performed in one stage. There was also a movement away from externalisation operations with the increasing knowledge of how colon cancer spreads through the lymphatic system. Many surgeons felt that the externalisation operation did not offer the possibility to remove all tissue necessary to achieve a satisfactory rate of cancer recurrence. At the same time, improved anaesthesia granted surgeons better working conditions, and the increased overall understanding of peri-operative physiology made the postoperative period less hazardous for patients. These improvements allowed surgeons to perform one-stage colon resections with intraperitoneal primary anastomosis. Surgeons at St. Mark's Hospital in London reported a series of 109 patients in 1953 with only three postoperative deaths [25]. Colonic surgery could now enter a new era. Cancer recurrence, and not postoperative sepsis, had become the main threat to the colorectal cancer patient after surgery.

Colon obstruction

Colon obstruction was traditionally treated with a three-stage procedure (transverse colostomy, resection, colostomy takedown) during the first decades of the 20th century. Since the 1950s, there has been a gradual movement from this three-stage procedure for managing colon obstruction; initially to a two-stage procedure and finally, to one-stage surgery with simultaneous resection and anastomosis. Today, three-stage procedures are almost never used.

The push to single-stage resection and anastomosis has been promoted by advocates who use subtotal colectomy for acute obstruction. The advantage of subtotal colectomy compared to

segmental resection and the use of on-table lavage have been debated. The SCOTIA (Subtotal Colectomy versus On-Table Irrigation and Anastomosis) study group could find no difference in operative time, complications or hospital stay, but the authors still recommended lavage because of the reputed change in bowel habits after subtotal colectomy. The two-stage approach is still generally recommended when diffuse peritonitis is encountered. Today, if a two-stage operation is used, many surgeons prefer a resection, anastomosis and proximal diverting ileostomy to the classic Hartmann operation. Advocates of this approach state it is equally safe in the acute setting to the Hartmann operation, and it offers the advantage that takedown of a loop ileostomy is easier and less morbid than takedown of a Hartmann pouch. There are, however, insufficient data to dictate the best approach, leaving surgeons to their own judgment to decide which operation to perform in specific circumstances of acute malignant colonic obstruction [26-28].

Stenting is a newer development for managing malignant colonic obstruction. Stenting may be used as palliative treatment to relieve symptoms of colon obstruction, or it may be used to decompress an obstructed colon to allow a mechanical bowel preparation and single-stage resection, thus converting an emergency procedure to an elective one [29].

Lymphadenectomy and mesenteric resection

The increased understanding of malignant spread via the lymphatic system inspired Miles to recommend wider margins and resection of the regional lymphatics draining the affected area when operating for large bowel carcinoma. The exteriorioation operation did not allow for this type of extensive dissection, and by the mid-20th century most surgeons performed a primary resection with anastomosis protected by a transverse colostomy.

At an international cancer meeting in Norway, 1964, Owen Wangensteen (Figure 15, Chapter 9) presented data from the University of Minnesota where total or near-total colectomies were performed for all cancers located at or distal to the splenic flexure. The five-year survival rate was 40% for all cases operated and 52% for the cases deemed as cured during surgery. These results represented a 10% improvement when compared with earlier results at the same institution [30]. Even though Wangensteen explained the importance of excising the lymphatic drainage of the tumour with the specimen, he did not attempt to compare the results of the operations with respect to the stage of the cancer (other than whether the surgeon had operated with intent to cure).

The second-look program

Patients with malignant lymph node involvement in their surgical specimen were found to have a worse prognosis than those without nodal involvement. It was also known from experience with gastric cancer that there is a 20-month silent interval between histological evidence of cancer and the onset of symptoms of the disease. This knowledge prompted what became known as the 'second-look program' at the University of Minnesota in 1948.

In this program, patients operated for colorectal cancer, as well as other abdominal malignancies, were followed-up with sequential explorations if the pathological specimen demonstrated lymph node involvement. The patient was then taken back for a second-look operation six to 12 months after the original surgery. If histological evidence of cancer was present, the patient would be taken back again after another six months, and so on. When following this protocol Wangensteen noted that right-sided cancers often recurred in the paracaval lymph nodes and left-sided tumours in the para-aortic nodes in addition to the regional lymph nodes. Consequently, he recommended including these nodes with the specimen when performing the original operation for colon cancer. In a report from 1964, a salvage rate of 9% was presented [31].

Early detection

With improved understanding of the paths of cancer spread, and knowledge of the poor prognosis of late-stage tumours, efforts were made to improve early detection of colon tumours in order to improve

patient overall survival. So-called cancer detection centres were established at several institutions in the 1940s. During a 15-year period starting in 1948, 11,963 patients came to the University of Minnesota centre for annual or biannual examinations which included proctosigmoidoscopy and sometimes guaiac stool examination. This regimen was referred to as 'screening tests' [32].

Technical tools of early detection

When searching for an asymptomatic colon lesion in the 1950s, a surgeon could perform a guaiac test for blood in the stool, but this test was non-specific. Rigid proctosigmoidoscopy offered examination of the rectum and sometimes the most distal part of the sigmoid colon, but in order to examine the more proximal colon the surgeon had to rely on barium enemas. This technique was dependable for large, perhaps circumferential tumours, but lacked in sensitivity when searching for small cancers and polyps. In 1955, Andren, Frieberg and Welin published a paper that described using the double-contrast technique for the diagnosis of polyps as small as 5mm [12]. This method of diagnosing colon lesions was the gold standard until colonoscopy became widely available in the late 1970s. Virtual colonoscopy using spiral CT technology is now being evaluated in clinical trials to determine if it can replace traditional colonoscopy for screening purposes.

Polyps

The concept of endoscopic polypectomy was initially developed at the Beth Israel Medical Center in New York in the early 1970s. By 1979, over 5,000 polypectomies had been performed without mortality at this institution [11].

Simultaneously with the development of the polypectomy technique using the colonoscope, Morson published several articles on the evolution of colorectal cancer. He postulated that there is a polyp-cancer sequence that starts with the formation of an adenoma that grows larger and eventually transforms into invasive cancer [33]. This association between polyps and colorectal cancer had been suggested much earlier by Dukes and other researchers, but general acceptance of the polyp-cancer sequence came after Morson had published his article.

Laparoscopic surgery for colon cancer

After the first laparoscopic cholecystectomy in the mid-1980s, the technique has been adopted for an increasing range of indications. Laparoscopic approaches to the colon began with appendectomy in the late 1980s, and in 1991, Moises Jacobs of Miami published the first case series of laparoscopic-assisted colonic resections for colon cancer. Both right colectomy and sigmoid resection were described, and Jacobs concluded that "although laparoscope-assisted colonic surgery may still be considered a technique in evolution, we feel that this procedure will become as accepted as laparoscopic cholecystectomy" [34]. The initial enthusiasm was effectively quenched by reports describing long operating times and somewhat alarming oncological outcomes, including port-site recurrences. Current prospective studies are evaluating whether colorectal cancer patients treated with laparoscopic or laparoscopy-assisted resections have worse, the same or better long-term outcome compared to patients treated with 'open procedures' [35, 36]. Laparoscopy in colorectal surgery has come to stay, but surgeons have to wait for the evidence to arrive before cancer patients can be recommended laparoscopy outside the research setting.

Evolution of surgery for rectal cancer

Early days (1700-1950)

Surgical management of rectal cancer was developed much earlier than operations on the more proximal colon. The rectum had three features that bolstered the ambition of early surgeons and led to more aggressive approaches. First, unlike the abdominal colon, the anorectum is readily accessible to visual and digital examination, allowing much earlier diagnosis of tumours. Second, all but the most proximal portion of the rectum lies below the peritoneal reflection, where wounds predictably heal and soiling of the abdomen is not a concern. Finally, even the ancients felt comfortable operating on the

anus and rectum, thus 19th-century surgeons did not have to overcome centuries of dogma-induced aversion in order to work on this region.

Early perineal approaches

The first record of a rectal resection was performed by Faget in 1737. He resected the lower part of the rectum, leaving a permanent sacral stoma.

In 1826, Lisfranc performed the first known successful resection of a rectal tumour. Five years later he published a series of nine cases, six of them successful. His operation was limited and intended for palpable tumours. Lisfranc described a perineal incision and subsequent blunt mobilisation of the rectum, ultimately amputating it proximal to the tumour [37]. The whole operation was carried out extraperitoneally, but despite this, operative mortality was common, and the surviving patient was likely to succumb to cancer recurrence.

In the 1830s, Herbert Mayo, of the Middlesex Hospital, reported a case of rectal resection for rectal cancer. The patient had, according to Mayo, good bowel control postoperatively, despite the fact that the entire anal sphincter was removed by Mayo through a perineal approach used to perform Lisfranc's operation. The patient, a 40-year-old woman, survived for two years after the operation [38].

In order to resect more proximal rectal tumours, Verneuil suggested a modified Lisfranc approach in 1873. He added a routine coccygectomy to the procedure to allow better exposure. The operative mortality rates from cellulitis and peritonitis remained high, prompting Pollosson and Madelung, independent of each other, to suggest a preliminary diverting colostomy before rectal resection. This offered the possibility of an aseptic second operation for rectal resection, with later takedown of the stoma [18].

The importance of aseptic operations was becoming increasingly clear. In 1875, Kocher suggested a new technique in order to prevent spillage of faecal matter during the procedure. Kocher closed the anus by means of a purse-string suture and thereafter performed an intersphincteric dissection, thus preserving the external sphincter. The pouch of

Douglas was opened through a perineal approach, allowing mobilisation of the distal colon. After division of the rectum about an inch above the upper margin of the tumour a colo-anal anastomosis could be created. Kocher had a low operative mortality rate of 'only' 20%. The recurrence rate, however, remained high.

The British surgeon Cripps made modest modifications to Lisfranc's original operation. In 1878, Cripps described making an incision extending from the tip of the coccyx to the anal verge, transecting skin, subcutaneous tissue and the posterior rectal wall. A circular incision around the anus ensured that both sphincters were included with the specimen. The levators were divided close to the bowel wall. The peritoneum was never incised; instead it was dissected loose from the anterior wall of the rectum to the extent needed to mobilise the tumour. The rectum was divided an inch above the tumour and the wound left open to heal by granulation. No reconstruction or anastomosis was made, and the patients were left with an artificial anus without faecal control. In a series of 85 patients, Cripps had a three-year survival rate of 38%.

Access and sacrectomy

Cancers located in the proximal rectum or recto-sigmoid junction proved difficult to adequately manage with Lisfranc's operation. As Paul Kraske (Figure 2) summarised in 1886, these tumours were "too deep for an operation through laparotomy and too high for an extirpation from the outside". A last resort procedure at the time was abdominal compression under deep anaesthesia, in an attempt to push the tumour deep enough into the pelvis to allow perineal resection. Kraske described two incidences where he was persuaded to undertake such operations, noting "the difficulties were tremendous". The poor exposure required him to work "in the dark, and under control of the fingers", creating inadvertent rents in the peritoneum and encountering significant haemorrhage. Both patients died postoperatively, one of pneumonia and the other of peritonitis.

Frustrated, Kraske developed an alternative operation. Recalling the earlier work of Kocher, which advocated sacral resection as a possible means of accessing the posterior rectum, Kraske decided to explore the feasibility of reaching the rectosigmoid junction from this direction. Reasoning that the sigmoid colon and rectosigmoid junction lay to the left of the midline, he proposed removal of the left wing of the sacral bone as his approach.

Kraske recounts perfecting his technique through cadaver studies: "I made an incision with the cadaver lying on the right side in the midline from the middle portion of the sacral bone to the anus. I detached the gluteal muscles at their insertion at the lowest portion of the left wing of the sacral bone, cut and excised the sacral bone, and separated the lowest part after expanding the outer margin of the wound, the ligaments tuberosacral and the underneath ligament, the spino-sacral close to the attachment of the sacral bone."

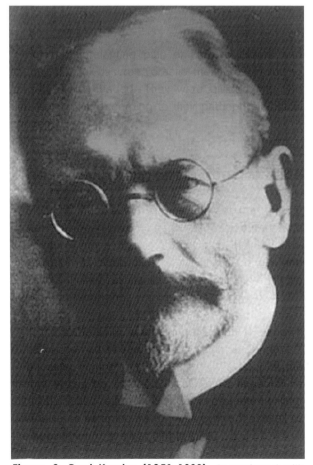

Figure 2. Paul Kraske (1851-1930). *Reproduced with permission from Dr. Marvin Corman, New York, USA.*

With refinement of this technique, Kraske noted with pleasant surprise "how easy it was to mobilise the large bowel" following division of the pelvic ligaments and removal of the lower left sacral ala. He regarded sacrifice of the fourth and fifth sacral nerves as harmless, and reasoned that any disturbance in sitting or gait caused by taking down the inferior gluteal attachments would be far outweighed by the benefit of tumour resection.

Kraske's first attempt at the operation on a live patient came in December 1884. The patient was a thin, scoliotic, 47-year-old woman with a carcinomatous stricture of the rectum starting 5cm from the orifice and extending proximally an indeterminate distance. He completed the left sacrectomy without difficulty, then placed the patient in the lithotomy position to open the perineum and mobilise the distal rectum. He opened the peritoneum at the pouch of Douglas, allowing delivery of the tumour into the pelvis and exposing the presence of ascites and intra-abdominal tumour implants. The bowel was transected proximally and distally, and a primary colo-anal anastomosis was performed with catgut suture. According to Kraske's notes, the patient's postoperative course was unremarkable; she was able to return to her pre-operative activities and diet, and passed stool without difficulty. Her chance at cure was nil, given the peritoneal carcinomatosis and the ominous postoperative clinic finding of firm nodules in the neorectal mucosa, but the technical success of the operation led Kraske to entreat his colleagues to take up the procedure.

Several other surgeons were inspired by Kraske and modified his exposure by removing more bone to achieve an even better exposure for lesions located more proximally in the rectum. Bardenhauer, for example, described a modification where the sacrum below the third sacral foramina was removed, and others recommended even larger sacral resections. These operations had higher rates of complications, including septic osteitis of the sacrum and disturbances of pelvic floor function. Further modifications of Kraske's operation were devised to alleviate these problems. Heinecke described a soft tissue and bone flap to allow the sacrum to be united again after the specimen had been resected. Problems with a high postoperative mortality rate

(around 20%) and recurrence rates of 80% to 90% remained, despite these technical advancements.

The pull-through operation

Maunsell criticised the Kraske approach for "mutilating important structures" and in 1892 he described a laparotomy approach. The abdomen was opened by a low midline incision, followed by mobilisation of the rectosigmoid and upper rectum. The tumour was then invaginated out through the anus and resected. Finally, a primary anastomosis was constructed. This procedure later became known as the 'pull-through' [39].

The abdominoperineal resection (APR)

The local recurrence rates remained depressingly high at the turn of the century. Convinced that the high recurrence rates were the outcome of insufficient removal of malignant tissue, Miles (Figure 3) gradually increased his margins when performing rectal resections using the perineal approach. In 1906, Miles presented in his book *Rectal Surgery* his disappointing results using this approach. Of 55 patients operated, one died and 51 experienced recurrent disease.

Miles noted that the recurrent tumours appeared in the lymphatic drainage of the rectum and he defined three routes of local spread of rectal cancer. The downward route consisted of spread to the peri-anal skin, ischiorectal fat and the external sphincter. The lateral route consisted of spread to the area between the levators and the pelvic fascia. The upward route included local metastases to retrorectal nodes and nodes in the pelvic mesocolon.

Having exhausted the extent of resection possible through the perineal approach, Miles logically searched for an alternative method. His solution, presented in 1908, was the single-stage abdominoperineal resection [40]. In the procedure's first part, the colon was divided just distal to its descending part, with the sigmoid and rectum mobilised down to the upper part of the prostate anteriorly, the levators laterally and the

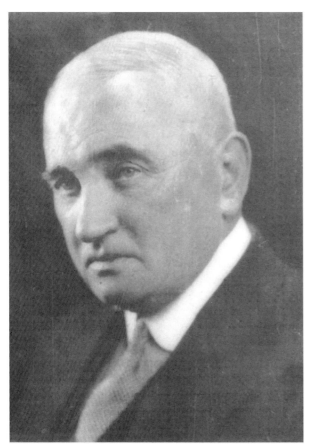

Figure 3. Sir William Ernest Miles (1869-1947).

sacrococcygeal joint posteriorly. The pelvic colon was thereafter pushed into the pelvis and the pelvic floor reperitonealised before a colostomy was prepared. The second part of the operation was the perineal portion, in which Miles advocated a wide excision including the coccyx, the coccygeus muscles and as much as possible of the ischiorectal fat and the levators. After the rectum was removed, the perineal defect was left to heal by granulation.

Incidentally, the same procedure had been unintentionally performed by Czerny (Figure 16, Chapter 4) in 1883. He had attempted to perform a resection of the rectum using a perineal approach but realised that he was unable to bring the tumour, located in the rectosigmoid junction, down enough for resection. Czerny proceeded to laparotomy to remove the rectum and lower part of the sigmoid after ligating the blood supply of the lower sigmoid.

According to Miles, the abdominal part of the operation should not take longer than 45 minutes to complete, and the perineal part a mere 15. The five-year survival rate after operation for rectal cancer increased from 6% to 69% at the Royal Cancer Hospital after the introduction of the abdomino-perineal operation [41].

Coffey presented a two-stage version of the abdominoperineal operation in 1917. The operation was identical to Miles', but performed in two stages with a 10- to 14-day interval between the abdominal procedure and the perineal excision. Because of the ligation of the blood supply to the rectum during the first stage, the specimen was at an advanced stage of decomposition at the second procedure. Coffey argued that the two-stage procedure, in his hands, had a lower mortality rate than the original operation.

The humble beginnings of adjuvant radiation therapy for rectal cancer

The first reference in literature to radiation therapy for rectal cancer was Symonds' short description of pre-operative radiation therapy in 1913 [42]. A typical annular growth 1.5 inches proximal to the anus was treated with 100mg of radium bromide and screened with 2mm of lead and 3mm of rubber. The treatment was applied daily, during a six-hour period for five consecutive days. Ten days after initiation of the treatment there were no visible or palpable signs of the growth, only a complete, stricturing ring of cicatricial tissue remained. Three months later the patient required a colostomy because of symptoms from the stricture, and after an additional two months the rectum was resected using the pull-through technique. The pathological report did not show any remnant malignant growth and the colostomy could be closed a month after the resection.

A combined modality treatment for rectal cancer with radiation and surgery, was described in the tenth Mackenzie Davidson Memorial Lecture in 1929 by Forssell of Radiumhemmet in Sweden [43]. He described the theoretical advantages of tumour shrinkage and decreased vitality of the tumour treated with pre-operative radiotherapy. Gordon-Watson, in an article from 1930, came to similar conclusions as

Forssell when describing three different approaches to pre-operative radiation therapy for rectal cancer [44]. Miles, however, presented a different view in the second edition of his textbook *Rectal Surgery*. He described the treatment of cancerous growths in the rectum by radium as "extremely unsatisfactory" because of the "widespread dissemination" that takes place in the surrounding tissues, even though "local improvements sometimes take place" [41].

Many others have described pre- and postoperative radiation for rectal cancer, but it wasn't until Stearns and colleagues in 1959 published a non-randomised comparison between a group of patients treated with radiation prior to surgery and a group treated with surgery alone, that the interest in combined modality treatment for rectal cancer finally accelerated [45].

Modern times (since 1950)

Dixon and the anterior resection

Miles based his rationale for the abdominoperineal resection on studies of lymphatic spread in patients dying from rectal cancer. However, others subsequently demonstrated that the primary spread of rectal cancer was upward along the inferior mesenteric artery and that distal spread was a late phenomenon, generally occurring when extensive nodal metastases were present and cure was unlikely. This understanding set the stage for the development and acceptance of the anterior resection approach to many rectal cancers.

Dixon (Figure 4) performed his first low anterior resection for a malignant lesion in 1930 [46] and in 1948 he presented a series of 426 patients operated between 1930 and 1947 [47]. He reported an operative mortality rate of 6% and a five-year survival rate of 68% among the 272 patients operated at least five years earlier. Patients whose tumour lacked lymph node involvement did better than patients with positive nodes. Low tumours, located 6-10cm from the dentate line, had a lower five-year survival rate than patients with more proximal disease.

With the obvious advantage of avoiding a colostomy, anterior resection became the operation of choice for high cancers of the rectum. It has remained the only universally accepted operation for sphincter-preserving treatment for rectal cancer [48].

Goligher's 5cm rule for low anterior resection

Dixon and others showed that the anterior resection with anastomosis was an alternative to the abdominoperineal resection, but it was unclear when sphincter sacrifice was needed to effect cure or when an anastomosis could be done safely without increasing local recurrence. Understandably, since the proximal and lateral margins could be identical with both operations, attention was devoted to the extent of distal margin of resection needed to effect

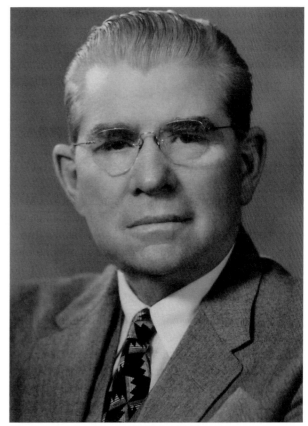

Figure 4. C. Dixon (1893-1968). *Reproduced with permission from The Mayo Foundation for Medical Education and Research. All rights reserved.*

cure. Goligher reported a series of 105 patients operated with anterior resection and anastomosis in 1951 [49]. In the article he recommends a 5cm distal resection margin. Despite the lack of firm data to support this recommendation, the so called '5cm rule' soon became accepted dogma. Over time, this dogma was challenged and studies showed that distal intramural spread greater than 1cm was exceedingly rare unless extensive proximal lymph node spread had already developed. Thus, surgeons began accepting a 2cm distal margin of clearance as adequate to achieve cure.

Heald and the total mesorectal excision

In 1982, the English surgeon Bill Heald (Figure 5) described a new dissection technique he claimed would lower local recurrence rates after low anterior resection. Heald reported that viable cancer cells left in the mesorectum may result in local recurrence and that mesorectal tumour deposits can be found up to 4cm distal to the primary tumour [50]. Heald therefore advocated that the entire mesorectum, without violation of its external envelope, should be excised at anterior resection. This technique has been coined 'total mesorectal excision' (TME).

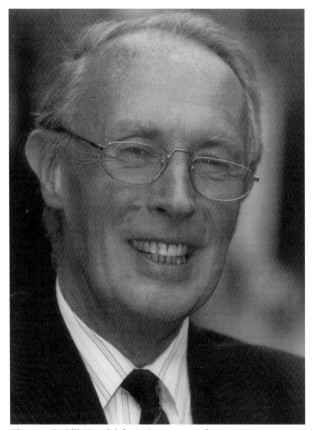

Figure 5. Bill Heald (contemporary). *Reproduced with permission from Mr. R.J. Heald.*

At TME, the dissection is carried out sharply in "the holy plane" of the endopelvic fascia, preserving the entire mesorectum and meticulously sparing the autonomic pelvic nerves. The mesorectum ends just above the levators, and the rectum is divided at this level. An anastomosis is constructed between the descending colon and the remaining anal cuff using a circular stapler. In a series of 50 patients, Heald reported no recurrences after up to two years [50]. Heald initially suggested that this technique would obviate the need for pelvic radiation recommended by others to decrease local recurrences.

The current frontier

Randomised studies in the 1980s demonstrated that rectal cancer patients treated with postoperative chemoradiation had improved survival and fewer local recurrences than patients receiving no or single modality adjuvant treatment [51]. These patients were not operated by Heald's TME concept, but the studies still led to the current NIH recommendations for treatment of patients with rectal cancer [52].

In 1997, the Swedish Rectal Cancer Trial demonstrated that pre-operative adjuvant radiotherapy reduced local recurrence rates and improved survival among patients with resectable rectal cancer [54]. This study was conducted prior to the introduction of the TME technique in Sweden. A subsequent Dutch study, reported in 2001, has reconfirmed a benefit of pre-operative radiation also in patients operated with the TME technique [53]. However, an increased overall survival after neoadjuvant radiotherapy was found in only the Swedish Rectal Cancer Trial.

Controversy has remained between advocates for postoperative chemoradiation vs. supporters of neoadjuvant therapy. A recent German study indicated that pre-operative long-course chemoradiation may be superior to postoperative treatment for local control of the tumour [55]. However, there was no difference in survival between the two groups.

Several studies have demonstrated that adjuvant therapies decrease local recurrence rates; but long-term survival does not appear to be affected. Controversy persists surrounding the length and dosage of pre-operative radiation and if pre-operative chemoradiation is better than radiation alone. Experience of short-course neoadjuvant radiotherapy is limited in the US and critics are concerned with possible increased late onset toxicity [56, 57]. Pre-operative therapy does allow for down-staging of a percentage of tumours and North American treatment centres are now also increasingly using neoadjuvant therapy before APR or low anterior resection [58]. However, it is difficult to predict which tumours ultimately will respond to various neoadjuvant treatment options and new pioneers will likely evolve to address this and other issues.

Conclusions

Modern surgery for colon and rectal cancer has gradually evolved during the past 200 years. From humble beginnings - where palliation of malignant rectal obstruction was the surgeon's only option and operations were as deadly to patients as their tumours - came much of the modern practice of colorectal surgery.

As a result of two centuries of innovation and experiment, the mortality of surgery for colorectal cancer is now around 2% in most large series. Morbidity has decreased as surgeons have developed techniques to minimise bowel, urinary and sexual disturbances. Cure is more often achieved, and modern surgeons use a variety of staging techniques to pick a treatment regimen ideal for a specific cancer. Treatments vary from local to radical surgery and may incorporate radiation, chemotherapy and the newer biological agents.

Sadly, despite overwhelming evidence that screening and surveillance programs are beneficial, the majority of populations are not offered such tests. Even in affluent Western societies, surgeons continue to see patients presenting with advanced cancers of the colon and rectum. Prevention and early detection will hopefully have an increasing place in the management of colorectal cancer in the coming decades.

References

1. Hajdu SI. Greco-Roman thought about cancer. *Cancer* 2004; 100 (10): 2048-51.
2. Ballantyne GH. Theories of carcinogenesis and their impact on surgical treatment of colorectal cancer. A historical review. *Dis Colon Rectum* 1988; 31 (7): 513-7.
3. Dukes C. Simple tumours of the large intestine and their relation to cancer. *Br J Surg* 1926; 13: 720.
4. Swinton NW, Warren S. Polyps of the colon and rectum and their relation to malignancy, 1939. *Dis Colon Rectum* 1989; 32 (9): 807-16.
5. Lockhart-Mummery J, Dukes C. The precancerous changes in the rectum and colon. *Surg Gynecol Obstet* 1928; 46 (5): 591-6.
6. Senn N. Enterorrhaphy: its history, technique, and present status. *JAMA* 1893; 21: 275-83.
7. Ravitch MM. Development of intestinal anastomotic devices. *South Med J* 1982; 75 (12): 1520-4.
8. Fraser I. An historical perspective on mechanical aids in intestinal anastomosis. *Surg Gynecol Obstet* 1982; 155 (4): 566-74.
9. Moran BJ. Stapling instruments for intestinal anastomosis in colorectal surgery. *Br J Surg* 1996; 83 (7): 902-9.
10. Arderne J. A fourteenth-century description of rectal cancer. *World J Surg* 1983; 7 (2): 304-7.
11. Wolff WI. Colonoscopy updated. *Adv Surg* 1979; 13: 145-68.
12. Andren L, Frieberg S, Welin S. Roentgen diagnosis of small polyps in the colon and rectum. *Acta Radiol* 1955; 43 (3): 201-8.
13. Moeller DD. The odyssey of guaiac. *Am J Gastroenterol* 1984; 79 (3): 236-7.
14. Littré. *L'Histoire de l'Académie de Science*, 1710: 37.
15. Dinnick T. The origins and evolution of colostomy. *Br J Surg* 1934; 22: 142-54.
16. Curling TB. Observations on the treatment of painful cancer of the rectum, without obstruction, by establishing an anus in the left loin: with cases, 1811-1888. *Dis Colon Rectum* 1998; 41 (4): 506-11.
17. Paul FT, Frank T. Paul - his life. *Br J Surg* 1951; 39 (155): 195-8.
18. Cromar CD. The evolution of colostomy. *Dis Colon Rectum* 1968; 11 (5): 367-90.
19. Rankin FW. How surgery of the colon and rectum developed. *Surg Gynecol Obstet* 1937; 64: 705-10.

20. Halsted WS. Circular suture of the intestine. *Am J Med Sci* 1887; 94: 436-61.

21. Hardy KJ. A view of the development of intestinal suture. Part II. Principles and techniques. *ANZ J Surg* 1990; 60 (5): 377-84.

22. Bloch O. Extra-abdominal resektion af hele colon descendens og et stykke af colon transversum for cancer. *Hosp Tid Kjöbenh* 1894; 4: 1053.

23. Mikulicz Jv. Small contributions to the surgery of the intestinal tract. *Boston Med Surg J* 1903; 148: 608-11.

24. Whipple AO. Advantages of cecostomy preliminary to resections of colon and rectum. *JAMA* 1931; 97: 1962.

25. Lloyd-Davies O, Morgan C, Goligher J. The treatment of carcinoma of the colon. In: *British Surgical Practice* 1953: 71-86.

26. Anonymous. Single-stage treatment for malignant left-sided colonic obstruction: a prospective randomized clinical trial comparing subtotal colectomy with segmental resection following intraoperative irrigation. The SCOTIA Study Group. Subtotal Colectomy versus On-table Irrigation and Anastomosis. *Br J Surg* 1995; 82 (12): 1622-7.

27. Deans GT, Krukowski ZH, Irwin ST. Malignant obstruction of the left colon. *Br J Surg* 1994; 81 (9): 1270-6.

28. Lau PW, Lo CY, Law WL. The role of one-stage surgery in acute left-sided colonic obstruction. *Am J Surg* 1995; 169 (4): 406-9.

29. Sebastian S, Johnston S, Geoghegan T, Torreggiani W, Buckley M. Pooled analysis of the efficacy and safety of self-expanding metal stenting in malignant colorectal obstruction. *Am J Gastroenterol* 2004; 99 (10): 2051-7.

30. Wangensteen OH, Gilbertsen VA. Results of surgery for cancer of the colon and rectum at the University of Minnesota Medical Center, 1940-1954. *Natl Cancer Inst Monogr* 1964; 15: 325-37.

31. Griffen WO, Jr., Gilbertsen VA, Wangensteen OH. The second-look operation for abdominal malignancies, 1948-1963. *Natl Cancer Inst Monogr* 1964; 15: 267-76.

32. Gilbertsen VA, Wangensteen OH. Cancer detection studies of the rectum. *Natl Cancer Inst Monogr* 1964; 15: 321-4.

33. Morson B. President's address. The polyp-cancer sequence in the large bowel. *Proc Roy Soc Med* 1974; 67 (6): 451-7.

34. Jacobs M, Verdeja JC, Goldstein HS. Minimally invasive colon resection (laparoscopic colectomy). *Surgical Laparoscopy & Endoscopy* 1991; 1: 144-50.

35. Greene FL. Laparoscopic management of colorectal cancer. *CA Cancer J Clin* 1999; 49 (4): 221-8.

36. Kieran JA, Curet MJ. Laparoscopic colon resection for colon cancer. *J Surg Res* 2004; 117: 79-91.

37. Tuttle JP. *A treatise on diseases of the anus, rectum, and pelvic colon*, 2nd edition, rev. edn. New York, London: D. Appleton and Company, 1905.

38. Mayo H. *Observations on injuries and diseases of the rectum.* Washington: D. Green, 1834.

39. Corman ML. Classic articles in colonic and rectal surgery. A new method of excising the two upper portions of the rectum and the lower segment of the sigmoid flexure of the colon - by H. Widenham Maunsell. *Dis Colon Rectum* 1981; 24 (8): 649-54.

40. Miles WE. A method of performing abdomino-perineal excision for carcinoma of the rectum and of the terminal portion of the pelvic colon (1908). *CA Cancer J Clin* 1971; 21 (6): 361-4.

41. Miles WE. *Rectal Surgery*, 2nd edition. London: Cassell and Company Ltd, 1944.

42. Symonds CJ. Cancer of Rectum; Excision after application of Radium. *Royal Society of Medicine Proceedings* 1913-1914; 7: 152.

43. Forssell G. Radiotherapy of malignant tumours in Sweden. *Br J Radiol* 1930; 3: 198-234.

44. Gordon-Watson C. The radium problem: the treatment of carcinoma of the rectum with radium. *Br J Surg* 1930; 17: 649-69.

45. Stearns MW, Jr., Deddish MR, Quan SH. Preoperative roentgen therapy for cancer of the rectum. *Surg Gynecol Obstet* 1959; 109 (2): 225-9.

46. Dixon C. Surgical removal of lesions occuring in the sigmoid and rectosigmoid. *Am J Surg* 1939; 46: 12-7.

47. Dixon C. Anterior resection for malignant lesions of the upper part of the rectum and the lower part of the sigmoid. *Trans Am Surg Assoc* 1948; 66: 175.

48. Goligher JC. Recent trends in the practice of sphincter-saving excision for carcinoma of the rectum. *Adv Surg* 1979; 13: 1-31.

49. Goligher JC, Dukes CE, Bussey HJ. Local recurrences after sphincter-saving excisions for carcinoma of the rectum and rectosigmoid. *Br J Surg* 1951; 39 (155): 199-211.

50. Heald RJ, Husband EM, Ryall RD. The mesorectum in rectal cancer surgery - the clue to pelvic recurrence? *Br J Surg* 1982; 69 (10): 613-6.

51. Prolongation of the disease-free interval in surgically treated rectal carcinoma. Gastrointestinal Tumor Study Group. *N Engl J Med* 1985; 312 (23): 1465-72.

52. NIH consensus conference. Adjuvant therapy for patients with colon and rectal cancer. *JAMA* 1990; 264(11): 1444-50.

53. Kapiteijn E, Marijnen CA, Nagtegaal ID, *et al.* Preoperative radiotherapy combined with total mesorectal excision for resectable rectal cancer. *N Engl J Med* 2001; 345 (9): 638-46.

54. Improved survival with preoperative radiotherapy in resectable rectal cancer. Swedish Rectal Cancer Trial. *N Engl J Med* 1997; 336 (14): 980-7.

55. Sauer R, Becker H, Hohenberger W, *et al.* Preoperative versus postoperative chemo-radiotherapy for rectal cancer. *N Engl J Med* 2004; 351 (17): 1731-40.

56. Tankel K, Hay J, Ma R, Toy E, Larsson S, MacFarlane J. Short-course preoperative radiation therapy for operable rectal cancer. *Am J Surg* 2002; 183 (5): 509-11.

57. Holm T, Singnomklao T, Rutqvist LE, Cedermark B. Adjuvant preoperative radiotherapy in patients with rectal carcinoma. Adverse effects during long-term follow-up of two randomized trials. *Cancer* 1996; 78 (5): 968-76.

58. Rothenberger DA. Commentary on Cecil, *et al.* Total mesorectal excision results in low local recurrence rates in lymph node-positive rectal cancer. *Dis Colon Rectum* 2004; 47: 1149-50.

Pioneers in Surgical Gastroenterology

Chapter 15

The anus and peri-anal conditions

Paul Benfredj MD
Médecin adjoint de l'hôpital Bellan, Paris, France
Praticien attaché du Centre Hospitalier de Versailles, France

Introduction

Anal disease has always been a subject of interest since antiquity. In ancient China, 'Yin' was considered to escape from the genital organs and from the anus [1]. So, examination of the anus, urine and faeces became mandatory. In ancient India, haemorrhoids and fistula were mentioned, at least from 500 BC, and were regarded as lesions caused either by ingested bones or by bites from insects [2].

It was from ancient Egypt that first records of proctology as an independent discipline appeared. Several medical papyri discovered approximately 100 years ago, but written about 1200 BC, described anal symptoms, and provided general counselling and remedies for anal disease [3]. On tablets of stone near the pyramids were lists of distinguished physicians. An eminent physician proctologist was referred to as 'Shepherd of the Anus' [4].

It took a long time to see the birth of the independent profession of coloproctology, and for science to emerge from magic and divinations.

Knowledge of the anorectal region

Progress in anal and peri-anal disease would not have been possible without the advances of pioneers, then and now, who found the way to understand the structure of the region, to examine and explore it and to know how it worked. Progress can roughly be divided into three sections according to history and technical advances.

The pathfinders

Anatomy is naturally the first gateway of medical knowledge. Galen [5] (130-200 AD) is said to have been the first to use the term 'rectum', and correctly distinguished between the internal sphincter, external sphincter and levator ani muscle. It was not until the beginning of the 18th century that the description of the anal valves, crypts and columns attributed to Giovanni Battista Morgagni [6] (Figure 1), became essential landmarks.

In the 19th century, came the descriptions of the pudendal nerve and canal by Alcock [7], the rectal valves by Houston [8], and the alleged white line, corresponding to the lower end of the internal sphincter by the anatomist and surgeon, John Hilton [9].

HEROES OF MEDICINE.

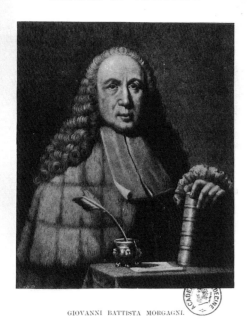

GIOVANNI BATTISTA MORGAGNI.

Figure 1. Giovanni Battista Morgagni (1682-1771).
Reproduced with permission from the Académie de Médecine, Paris, France.

Thanks to histological advances, our knowledge was further increased by Straud [10] in 1896, with his description of the mucosa lying just below the dentate line, called the 'Pecten'. Also, came the crucial discovery of the anal glands arising from deep in the mucosa and submucosa, which open at the base of Morgagni's valves, often crossing through the internal sphincter (see page 264, Abscess and fistula). Their discovery was made and published in Germany in 1878 by Hans Chiari [11] and independently in France in 1880 by Hermann and Desfosses [12]. In France, they are still called 'Hermann and Desfosses' glands, and the squamous non-keratinised mucosa of the anal canal is called 'Hermann's mucosa'.

Clinical examination was traditionally in the knee-elbow position until 1883. James Marion Sims advised the left lateral position, favoured in Anglo-Saxon countries. Anal specula have been used since the period of Hippocrates, but they are properly mentioned for the first time in Guy de Chauliac's treatise *Grande Chirurgie* published in Montpellier in 1363. The proctoscope seems to have been discovered by Gustave Trouvé [13] in 1873, and

improved in 1895, when it was able to reach the sigmoid colon, and introduced as a routine examination in 1903 by the American, Howard Atwood Kelly [14].

Few were ready to share their scientific knowledge of proctology; however, Hippocrates around 430 BC wrote several treatises on haemorrhoids and fistulas. Later, John of Arderne around 1380 with his *Treatise of the fistulae in the fundament and other places* [15], and the first treatise on colon and rectal surgery in the US by George MacArtney Bushe [16] in 1837, both spread information in this field.

The theorists and the builders

Anatomy drew attention around the middle of the 20th century to the complex local anal muscular systems. In particular, the work of Milligan (Figure 10) and Naunton-Morgan [17] in 1934 clarified much of the anatomy, which was increased further by Courtney in 1950 [18], and by Naunton-Morgan and Henry Thompson in 1956 [19]. They elaborated further on the intermuscular and peri-anal fascias, the posterior inter-sphincteric space and the transitional mucosa. This work led to a clear classification of fistula-in-ano (see later) and had implications on surgery for fistula and haemorrhoids.

In the same spirit, the anatomical studies of Sir Alan Parks [20] (Figure 8, Chapter 13) between 1955 and 1966, not only allowed for the description of the mucosal suspensory ligament, an important landmark in haemorrhoidectomy, but also led to a comprehensive physiopathological explanation, especially on anal incontinence and rectal static disorders.

Less academic pioneers understood the need to establish highly specialised independent institutions. Frederick Salmon (Figure 2), inspired on the subject of anorectal disease, founded in London the "Infirmary for the relief of the poor afflicted with fistula and other diseases of the rectum" in 1835 [21].

This institution flourished and became known as St. Mark's Hospital (Figure 3), noted for its high workload, post-graduate teaching and research in coloproctology.

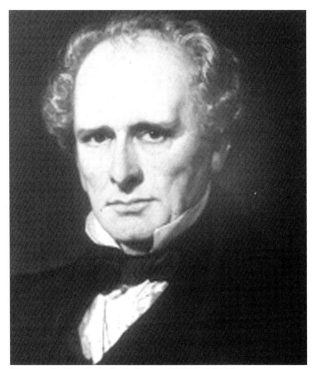

Figure 2. Frederick Salmon (1796-1868). *Reproduced with permission from St. Mark's Hospital, Harrow.*

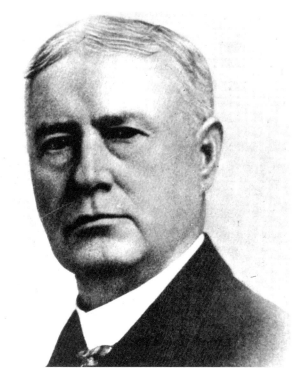

Figure 4. Joseph Mathews (1847-1928). *Reproduced with permission from AMS Press, New York, USA.*

In the US, Joseph Mathews (Figure 4), who was the first President of the American Proctologic Society in 1899, was often named the 'father of proctology'[22].

Charles Kelsey founded the 'Saint Paul's Clinic for haemorrhoids, fistula and other diseases of the rectum' at the end of the 19th century in New York.

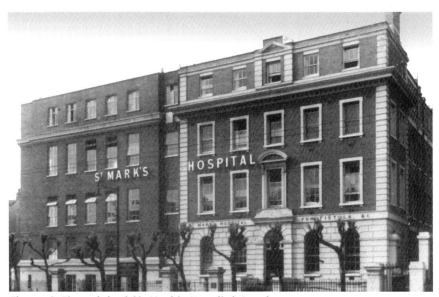

Figure 3. The original St. Mark's Hospital, London. *Reproduced with permission from St. Mark's Hospital, Harrow.*

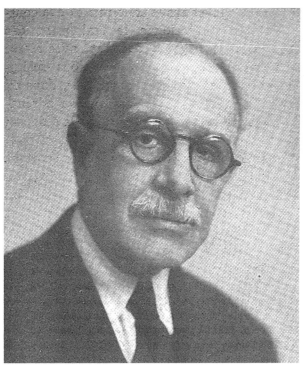

Figure 5. Raoul Bensaude (1866-1938). *Reproduced with permission from the Bibliothèque Inter-Universitaire de Médecine, Paris, France.*

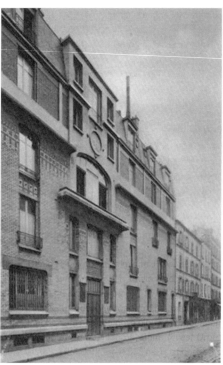

Figure 7. Hôpital Bellan, Paris, France. *Reproduced with permission from Hôpital Bellan, Paris, France.*

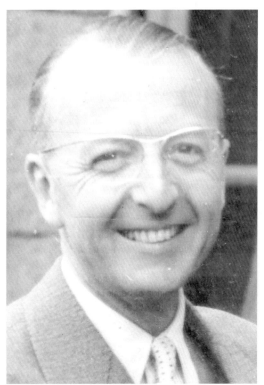

Figure 6. Jean Arnous (1908-1981). *Reproduced with permission from Dr. Noëlle Dubois Arnous, daughter to Jean Arnous.*

In France, modern proctology was introduced by Raoul Bensaude (Figure 5), physician at the Hôpital Saint-Antoine in Paris, between 1920 and 1930.

However, it was Jean Arnous [23] (Figure 6) who created the first Department of Proctology in 1961, in the Hôpital Léopold Bellan in Paris (Figure 7). Apart from his other clinical and surgical achievements (see later), he was a gastroenterologist, devoted to anorectal surgery. Hôpital Bellan has trained and continues to train French physicians and other nationalities in medical and surgical proctology. Some emerging graduates have founded similar institutions elsewhere.

The explosion of scientific advances

Advances in physiology after 1950 accelerated our knowledge of this region. Space permits mention of only some of the main contributors. These include:

- Kerremans from Belgium [24] in 1969, and Ihre [25] from Scandinavia in 1974, on continence and defaecation;

- Pierre Arhan [26, 27] in Paris in 1972 and Philippe Denis [28] in Rouen in 1979, on visco-elasticity of the rectum;
- Shafik [29] from Cairo on the correlation of muscular anatomy and physiology in 1975;
- Duthie and Bennett [30, 31] in Britain, who described the relationship between rectal sensitivity and innervation, as well as the recto-anal inhibitory and contractory reflexes, in 1963;
- Thompson [32] (from London) who in 1975 described the anal cushions; others have wrongly confused them with symptomatic haemorrhoids.

The advent of manometry, computed tomography (CT) and magnetic resonance imaging (MRI), in addition to improved office endoscopes, have much increased our knowledge and benefited patients. Examples of progress by technology are:

- fistulography was developed as early as 1929 by Delherm [33];
- the determination of colonic transit time has slowly evolved from the use of colouring materials, such as carmine red, radioactive chromium isotopes, or radio-opaque substances. Hinton and Lennard-Jones [34], in 1969, were able to calculate transit times counting the number of radio-opaque markers in stools, and Arhan [35], in 1981, on plain radiographs of the abdomen. The procedure that used to require radiographs during seven days was successively simplified to two or three films by Chaussade [36] in 1986. Bouchoucha and Devroede [37] and Danquechin-Dorval [38] managed to reduce this test to one film;
- defecography was presented in 1984 by Mahieu [39] in Belgium and later improved by combined opacification of the bladder, genital tract in women, and colon;
- electrophysiology has been developed by different teams, in particular those of Henry, Swash and Snooks [40, 41] in Britain from 1978, and later, Steven Wexner [42] in the US;
- Sultan, Kamm, Bartram and Nicholls [43] made progress with mapping of sphincter lesions after 1985;
- anorectal manometry, developed after urological manometry, was researched by people such as Hancock, Matheson and Keighley [44] from Birmingham, UK. Intrarectal saline infusion manometry was introduced by Read, Read and Bartolo [45] from Sheffield in 1984.

Haemorrhoids (piles)

It is well known that the word comes from the ancient Greek 'hoema' for blood and 'rheo' for flood, making it clear that it has no specificity for the anal region. In fact, although Hippocrates described the term for this condition, it has long been applied to any other anal swelling capable of bleeding. Since the 11th century, its use has been slowly restricted to those structures until the 19th century, when a consensus was finally reached. The definition given by Celsus was fairly precise: "Haemorrhoids are swellings of the orifice of the anal veins, forming granulations, and frequently letting blood flow out." At the beginning of the 11th century, Abu Ali ibn Sina, better known as Avicenna (Figure 8), seems to have been the first to differentiate between external and internal haemorrhoids. Although the name is Greek, the condition has been appreciated for a long time in history. There may not be a clear account in Mesopotamian records, but the Egyptians at their zenith were very knowledgeable, and even described thrombosed piles. (The word 'piles' is derived from the Latin word 'pila' meaning a ball).

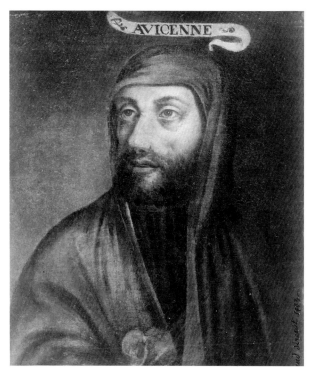

Figure 8. Avicenna (980-1037). *Reproduced with permission from the Bibliothèque Inter-Universitaire de Médecine, Paris, France.*

In the Bible, the reference to haemorrhoids is explicit in Deuteronomy (Chapter 27, verse 27) as punishment of God's enemies: "Jehovah will strike you with ulcers, as He once stroke Egypt and He will also strike you with emerods, with mange, and with an intractable itching of the part of the body through which Nature throws out what is left of its food." In the book of Samuel, this particular punishment was inflicted on the Philistines several times, because they dared to steal the Ark of the Covenant.

Although piles had been regarded by some as stigmata of a shameful disease, physicians appear to have long wondered if treatment were really necessary. Hippocrates, and after him Galen, affirmed that bleeding from the anus could have a beneficial effect on several conditions, including arthritis and gout. As recently as 1729, Georg Ernst Stahl [46] supposed that to arrest haemorrhoidal bleeding could worsen illnesses such as melancholy, and spoke of piles as 'golden veins'. Some even advocated provoking such a bleed, and proved very imaginative in this exercise employing very hot baths, irritating clysters (enemata), inserting of an entire clove of garlic, or producing friction by chafing the piles with fig leaves!

It was only since the second half of the 18th century that haemorrhoids were regarded clearly as abnormal, producing several theories to explain their cause. Robert James [47] from the UK suspected some degree of obstruction to the venous drainage of the portal system. Almost a century later, the French surgeon, Edouard Quenu [48], underlined the role of inflammatory changes to the venous wall from infection.

Conservative treatment

Until the beginning of the 20th century, diverse opinions were given about the patients' lIfestyle. many authors condemned anger, wine, spirits, sitting on a sun-heated stone or on humid soil, eating a variety of food, not excluding Roquefort cheese (Daniel Mollière 1877)! Horse-riding and sex drew adverse opinions: Dominique Larrey [49] believed riding beneficial unlike Baldinger [50]. Heterosexual relations with women were approved, but not in excess! Pornographic literature was firmly discouraged!

Some amazing oral preparations were advertised. One exotic example is that of Hildebrandt [51] in 1804

who still recommended a 17th century recipe: "Boil a pint of beer, add two well mixed yolks and some sugar, and let roasted bread cut into small pieces soak in it."

Topical applications have also been described since medical literature began. Egyptians have recorded all sorts of preparations. Hippocrates used some suppositories coated with honey, alum-impregnated plasters, or even cuttlefish shells.

Ambroise Paré during the 16th century favoured a preparation made with an onion first cooked under ashes, then pounded and mixed with ox bile. Two centuries later, de Montègre firmly applied a whole clove of garlic. Charles V, Emperor of Austria, was said only to be relieved by local applications of 'painters' varnish', a material made of flax oil, Venetian turpentine and juniper resin.

Instrumental treatment

Lancing

Many earlier clinicians, including Ambroise Paré, advocated incision with a knife or lancet (still justifiable for peri-anal haematoma), to produce bleeding. Keen competition came from leeches, because the bleeding was better controlled and the wounds healed more quickly. One leech could be placed on each primary pile, until empty, before its removal. In 1460, a Doctor Ferrari wrote to King Louis XIth of France recommending leeches, and even Napoleon spoke emphatically to his brother Jérôme in 1797 about his relief from them.

Injections

This technique has been used since the 19th century. According to Keighley and Williams [52], Morgan from Ireland used ferrous sulphate in 1869, and Colles used iron perchloride in 1874. Knowing how many patients wanted to avoid surgery, the American Mitchell [53] obtained some success with a solution of phenol in the order of 25%-30% in 1871. Mitchell got into trouble with his surgical peers not just because he jealously guarded his recipe by only letting a few assistants into the secret, but because he allowed non-medical practitioners to use his method.

In 1876, Professor Andrews [54] of Chicago made the first serious study on the subject, experimenting with solutions varying from 20%-95% concentration. Injections were introduced in Britain by Edwards [52] in 1888. In 1938, Albright and Blanchard [55] popularised a submucosal injection technique, as we still know it, using phenol in vegetable oil, or quinine and urea hydrochloride. In 1922, Raoul Bensaude [56] introduced injection sclerotherapy into France.

Ligatures

Blaisdell [57] devised an instrument for ligation of internal haemorrhoids, using a silk thread in 1954. Barron [58] replaced the silk ligature with rubber bands, which diminished the risk of haemorrhage in 1963. Soullard [59] introduced banding into France in 1966. The technique, now known as rubber band ligation, was used to strangulate part of the haemorrhoidal and mucosal prolapse. Several varieties of banding equipment, including suction to avoid the need of an assistant, are now used.

Freezing (cryotherapy)

A contrasting approach was by freezing. Fraser and Gill [60] in 1967 introduced cryosurgery using nitrous oxide down to -70°C, or liquid nitrogen to -190°C, to produce controlled destruction of a single pile. Lloyd-Williams [61] augmented freezing with rubber band ligation.

Surgical treatment

Cautery

Cautery as a treatment appears to have been widely used. It has been reported in medieval Arabic medicine and in the Veda texts of Hinduism, and was available in the early 19th century in Europe. Hippocrates in one of his treaties advised the surgeon to "force out the anus as much as possible with the fingers and make the irons red hot, burn the pile until it be dried up and so that no part may be left behind". To facilitate the exteriorisation of the piles, he advised to make the patient yell; the mere sight of the red-hot irons no doubt helped! Until modern photocoagulation was available, stricture was a frequent sequel after cautery.

Neiger [62] modified Nath's photocoagulation [63] for haemostasis for the purpose of reducing the symptoms of piles. The coagulation was limited to the mucosa and submucosa, as in injection sclerotherapy. It was also used for small benign tumours, especially condyloma acuminata.

Anal dilatation

It is believed anal dilatation was practised in ancient Greece, either as a treatment or as a punishment, but it lapsed for centuries. Treatment was reinstated at the beginning of the 19th century for both fissure and piles, following some evidence of increased sphincter tone in some patients. Miles [64] described in 1919 a 'Pecten band' of circular fibrosis lying under Hilton's line in the anal canal. He considered 'pectenotomy' as a treatment. Eisenhammer's [65] (1951) radical sphincterotomy and Lord's [66] (1968) anal dilatation for fissure have been performed for piles.

Surgical excision

Hippocrates' account [67] on extracting condylomas appeared to be the first report on thrombectomy. He advised: "do as if your finger made its way between skin and flesh of a sheep that is being spayed ... operate while chatting, without warning of what you are doing." This approach is unlikely to satisfy ethics committees or defence lawyers today!

Piles have been surgically removed for centuries. Hippocrates recommended a woollen thread; Galen [68] used a flax ligature combined with an incision of the mucosa above. Apart from pain, the main anxieties were haemorrhage and stenosis. Excision of piles reported by the Byzantine Aetius of Amida, then by Paul of Egina in the 6th and 7th centuries, respectively, remained unchanged until in 1774, when Jean-Louis Petit [69] (Figure 9) improved it by incising the insensitive mucosa at the base of the pile first, making the procedure much less painful.

Before the Whitehead procedure, haemorrhoidectomy was highly dangerous. It is probable that both the famous Polish scientist, Copernicus, and Don Juan of Austria (victor of the battle of Lepante), died from haemorrhage after haemorrhoidectomy, in 1543 and 1578, respectively.

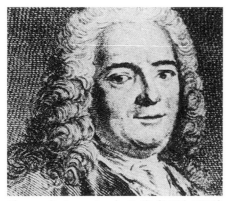

Figure 9. Jean-Louis Petit (1674-1750).
Reproduced with permission from the Musée de L'histoire de la Médecine, Paris, France.

In 1882, Whitehead [70] excised the whole pile-bearing area including much of the transitional epithelium by a circumferential incision followed by immediate anorectal suture, which aimed at permanent cure and reduced the chances of postoperative bleeding. Unhappily, it had some complications: stenosis, loss of anal sensitivity and the occasional everted suture line caused excessive mucus spillage known by his antagonists as 'Whitehead's anus'.

Pedicular haemorrhoidectomy was a major advance. Salmon [71], founder of St. Mark's Hospital, devised a radical version too frequently complicated by stricture. The standard operation described by Milligan (Figure 10) and Morgan [72] in 1937 has stood a long test of time, especially in Europe. Each of the three main haemorrhoidal plexuses was, in turn, carefully dissected, its vascular pedicle then ligated before the complete resection, the wounds being laid wide open (Figure 11).

Modifications to the above include sphincterotomy [73], and popular in France, the addition of anoplasty [74] to reduce discomfort and accelerate the healing of the raw areas, and to be able to excise any additional secondary pile.

Further attempts to reduce postoperative pain, are closed haemorrhoidectomy techniques, such as Parks' submucosal removal of piles [75]. The mucosal flaps are replaced and the appearance has a resemblance to Petit's operation two centuries earlier. Ferguson's closed haemorrhoidectomy [76] required each haemorrhoidal plexus to be totally excised and the rectal mucosa being fixed to the muscle beneath.

Finally, a new concept for prolapsing piles was presented by Antonio Longo [77] in Italy in 1995. He modified the cylindrical cartridge used for anterior resection. After creating a mucosal and submucosal ridge, including the apex of each primary pile with a purse-string suture, partial resection of the pedicles and immediate stapling closes the defect. Stapled haemorrhoidectomy is a very recent treatment; it requires less local care and allows a speedier return to normal activities. Time is needed to judge if it is to replace other surgical treatments.

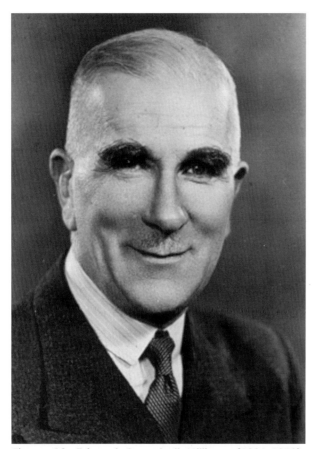

Figure 10. Edward Campbell Milligan (1886-1972).
Reproduced from the editor's private collection.

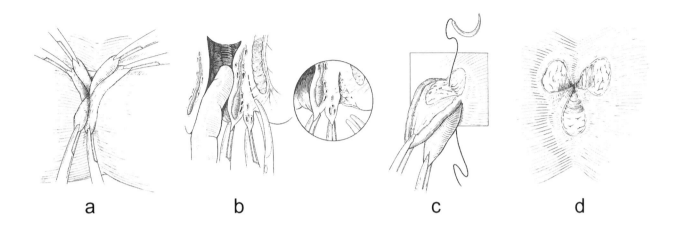

a   b   c   d

Figure 11. Morgan and Milligan haemorrhoidectomy. Final appearance: "If it looks like a dahlia the 'op' is a failure; if it looks like a clover, your troubles are over!" [52] *Reproduced with permission from Elsevier Scientific Inc.*

Anal fissure

Anal fissure seems to have been known since antiquity and is mentioned in the works of Avicenna and Aetius of Amida. Nevertheless, no clear distinction generally appeared between all types of anorectal ulcerations. During the 19th century, since the discovery of infection by organisms, tuberculosis and syphilis were considered suspect causes. This made it a difficult situation for patients, especially if suspected of having venereal disease. Frenchman, Lemonnier [78], was the first to clearly differentiate fissure from other ulcerations in 1689. His description was prophetically accurate: "Fissures are small and painful ulcers, following the whole length of the bottom wrinkles, resembling chilblains of the lips or hands; they are caused sometimes by the hardening of faeces …"

Just as in treating piles, topical measures to make fissures heal or relieve the pain were attempted universally. The role of constipation was rightly recognised, and treated with diet and purgatives. As we know today, recent fissures can and did heal with simple measures.

For the unrelenting pain of chronic fissure and acutely painful fissures, drastic measures including surgery were needed. They were divided into two different types, according to their pathophysiological concept.

Procedures acting on the ulceration itself

Most of them acted on the floor of the fissure; cautery has been used for centuries to try to transform the fissure into a fibrotic scar. Since then electro-coagulation replaced cautery with the same aim and the same limited results, the scar being generally so fragile that recurrence was common.

In the same spirit, a scraping procedure is known to have been advocated by Abul Kasim al-Zahrawi [79] (Albucasis; Figure 1, Chapter 14). The floor of the fissure would be scraped initially by a fingernail to stimulate tissue regrowth in order to promote healing; later, diverse scraping instruments evolved, as well as the application of a silver nitrate stick.

In the second half of the 19th century, injections used in the treatment of piles were used to provoke fibrosis of the fissure floor.

It is hard to determine when the removal of the fissure itself was first attempted, but it has been much employed during the 20th century [80], and is still the choice procedure in France. Wounds have sometimes had difficulty in healing or have been left with a depressed zone or fossa as a sequel.

Several techniques have been imagined to improve the results of fissurectomy; some have employed an anoplasty technique, derived from plastic surgery, using cutaneous flaps. In France, in 1968, Jean Arnous and Ernest Parnaud [81] described a mucosal anoplasty, an easier procedure in which a mucosal flap dissected from the rectal mucosa was lowered and sutured on the inner part of the wound, not only to facilitate healing but also to prevent a relapse. It is still a favoured technique among French proctologists today.

Procedures acting on the anal sphincter

All these procedures are designed to counteract the abnormally high sphincter tone commonly associated with fissure.

Enemata with local anaesthetic properties were frequently used at the end of the 18th century. They were later replaced in the middle of the 19th century by local anaesthetic injections. Meshes of lint of increasing size constituted the first attempt to stretch the anal sphincter [82].

In 1829, Joseph Claude Anthelme Récamier [83] advocated anal dilatation at the French Academy of Medicine, gently introducing both thumbs into the anal canal and stretching the sphincter in directions at right angles to each other. This method had little acceptance, until Jacques Gilles Thomas Maisonneuve [84] publicised it in 1849 and developed it in the following decade.

Dilatation was steadily replaced by sphincterotomy, until it was rediscovered by Peter Lord [66] in Britain in 1968. The procedure was quite similar to the one by Récamier, with the successive introduction of one, two, three and then four fingers from both hands. It was of course brief, easy to do, and although often effective, full anal continence afterwards could not always be guaranteed.

In 1818, Parisian Alexis Boyer [85] (Figure 12) declared division of the internal sphincter to be a great success. He first advocated a thorough division, but his followers, among them Dupuytren, advised a more limited one. The division was applied to the fissure if posterior, or laterally if anterior, to prevent complications especially in women. It was quickly recognised as a great revolution and widely adopted by many contemporaries.

In 1951, Eisenhammer [86] of South Africa resected the fissure and combined posterior sphincterotomy simultaneously. The French sphincterotomy was accepted by more conservative British counterparts, who left the fissure to heal untouched after lateral sphincterotomy. Parks [87] described an open lateral internal sphincterotomy in 1967; Notaras [88] described a less invasive closed subcutaneous procedure in 1969, dividing the sphincter from the submucosal plane. Hoffman and Goligher [89] in 1970 stressed the importance of the division starting from the inter-sphincteric plane. Nevertheless, more recent

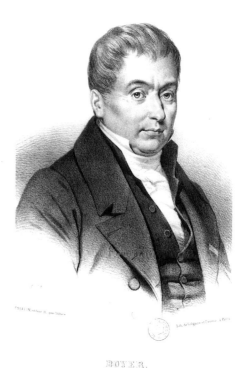

BOYER.

Figure 12. Alexis Boyer (1757-1833).
Reproduced with permission from the Académie de Médecine, Paris, France.

publications, in the 1990s, have still cautioned against the continued risk of lateral sphincterotomy and anal continence.

More recently, diltiazem or botulinic toxin has been tried to produce a temporary sphincterotomy, but after initial enthusiasm, long-term results appeared to be disappointing.

Tumours of the anal region

Peri-anal warts

Peri-anal warts have been identified since Greek and Roman antiquity, to be associated with sexual, especially homosexual relations. Additionally, they have even been the subject of satirical texts of Juvenal, Martial and other Roman authors [90].

The terminology has been varied and erratic. Aetious of Amida used to call them 'thymes', in reference to the shape of this plant's flowers. Throughout the Middle Ages up to the beginning of the 19th century, classification led to subtle distinctions, between tumours, vegetations and excrescences on the one hand, and varieties of fruit and vegetables on the other, such as strawberries, raspberries, leeks, figs, cock's combs, or cauliflowers [91]. Celsus used to distinguish between tubercules and condylomas, the latter referring at that time to older and harder warts, and is of course still in use.

If the venereal origin had long been suspected, syphilis was suspected around 1550 by physicians such as Fallopius and Petronius. This hypothesis seems to have remained in force until the middle of the 19th century, when inflammatory causes were added to the aetiology, including those associated with diabetes mellitus and pregnancy. Hebra and Kaposi [92] later refuted their contagious character.

Treatment has been largely based on the destruction or removal of warts. Diverse conservative treatments have been tried such as silver nitrate, phenic acid, acetic acid and arsenic. In the second half of the 20th century, chloroquine, colchicines, anti-mitotic drugs, like bleomycin and 5-fluorouracil, have been tried. Nowadays, podophyllin, a caustic resin used since 1942, and cryotherapy, generally with liquid nitrogen used since 1960, are often applied by dermatologists [93].

The only exception among all these destructive treatments is imiquimod, available since the mid-1990s, implementing local immuno-stimulation.

Nevertheless, surgery was, and still remains, the most effective treatment. From cautery, advocated by Hippocrates, to destruction by laser, photocoagulation in the anal canal, electrocoagulation, simple scraping, thread ligation, excision using scalpel or scissors, no dramatic progress has been made. Hoped-for antiviral drugs or vaccination may win the argument eventually.

Some rare peri-anal diseases

New conditions were discovered at the end of the 19th and the beginning of the 20th centuries. In 1874, Sir James Paget [94] described in London a cutaneous disease of the mammary areola, a precursor of breast cancer. Other manifestations of the disease were later discovered, the peri-anal manifestation in 1893 in France, by Darier [95]. It is an intra-epithelial cancer, which can slowly become invasive, and become a florid cancer.

In 1912, James Templeton Bowen [96] presented in Boston, a precancerous cutaneous disease occurring anywhere, which changed to obvious cancer later. Vickers [97] described it in the anal region in 1939, with its association with the Human Papilloma Virus.

In 1925, Abraham Buschke and Ludwig Löwenstein [98] described in Berlin a giant tumour of the penis, and clearly stressed its relation with condyloma acuminata. The Buschke-Löwenstein tumour of the anal region can, like the urogenital variety, be very invasive and requires extensive surgical resection.

Benign tumours of the anal canal and of the rectum

Improved proctoscopes enabled clinicians to reach and remove some of the lower adenomatous polyps. The main concern was postoperative bleeding. Controlled diathermy reduced the risk but not completely. From the 1960s, flexible endoscopes prolonged the range of endoscopy, and polyps could be routinely removed either by snare, forceps or diathermy.

In 1966, Parks [99, 100] published a transanal excision technique, with the aid of a retractor, followed by saline infiltration and dissection of the submucosal plane starting from the lower edge. In 1983, he extended this technique to large, almost circumferential tumours, and insisted on closure of the defect to avoid stenosis.

In 1970, York Mason [101] revived a trans-sphincteric technique originally described in 1917 by Bevan [102], dividing the sphincters and the rectal wall on their posterior side. It offered a better access to higher or anterior tumours, but required meticulous sphincter reconstruction to avoid complications.

From Lyon in France, Francillon [103] presented in 1974 what he called the 'parachute technique', in which the tumour was surrounded by thread loops which could be pulled down to enable excision. In 1977, in Bordeaux, Jacques Faivre carefully fashioned a mucosal flap to follow the tumour down before excision of the polyp. It was named 'the tractor flap' technique [104]. Both techniques today are still used to remove large sessile polyps, villous adenomas, or even small cancers.

Anal cancer

For a long period of time no clear distinction was made between cancers of the anus and of the rectum. Apart from local excision of small cutaneous cancers, the treatment of anal cancer followed the path of that of rectal cancer. Until the beginning of the 19th century, palliative treatments which included dilatation, cautery or partial excision were applied. In 1826, Lisfranc had published his method of excision of the lower half of the rectum. And for much of the 20th century, the standard treatment was abdominoperineal excision of the rectum, whenever possible.

Since then marked changes occurred in three consecutive stages.

During the late 1960s and early 1970s, Basil Morson [105, 106] classified malignant tumours of the anal region more clearly. Adenocarcinoma from the

rectum and colloid anal adenocarcinoma were distinguished from epidermoid cancers of the anal margin and of the anal canal. The latter were divided into three varieties:

- squamous cell;
- basaloid or cloacogenic; and
- muco-epidermoid carcinomas.

In 1974, Papillon [107], at the Institut Léon Bérard in Lyon, rationalised radiotherapy which had been used since the 1940s. He advised an initial high dose of approximately 30 Grays, and after a rest period of two months, complementary interstitial irradiation, using Iridium[192]. He was the first to show that radiation therapy could be as effective as resection, and could also treat lymph nodes.

Also in 1974, Nigro and his colleagues [108] in the US used an association of chemotherapy (mitomycin plus 5-fluorouracil) and external radiotherapy, prior to excision. Having noticed that no tumour was generally left on the resection specimens, he was the first to advise in 1981 a combined chemoradiotherapy procedure without surgery, achieving encouraging results.

Abscess and fistula

Fistula-in-ano before the 19th century

Most of the means at our disposal today to treat fistula-in-ano have been known since antiquity. The word 'fistula' is derived from Latin, and means flute in reference to its structure, but the essential knowledge on the disease was known in 4th century Greece since Hippocrates.

Hippocrates [109] knew the relationship between abscess and fistula; he advised the early drainage of abscess, "even if not yet totally mature". He insisted on the exploration of the fistula track and used a stalk of fresh garlic for that purpose. He proposed to lay it open whenever the track was superficial, and otherwise to use a strip of linen or horse-hair, often with an addition of a caustic substance, and to tighten it day after day until all tissues were cut open. In addition, Hippocrates knew the risk of incontinence afterwards. Furthermore, he discovered fistulotomy using a cutting seton, a technique still used today. In fact, he had introduced the three techniques which would be discussed during the following centuries:

- cautery, which applied a caustic substance through a strip of material to try to provoke a slow erosion or at least fibrosis;
- ligature otherwise called 'apolinosis', which consisted of the progressive tightening of a seton; and
- direct excision.

His successors more or less resorted to the same methods, and sometimes brought in some improvements. Celsus [110], a Greek physician living in Rome in the first century AD, used a probe to explore the fistula track, and sometimes attached the threads introduced into the track, to the patient's thigh, which progressively laid the track open by movement. He also advocated complete resection of the fistula, which often turned out both bloody and painful. Galen [110] (Figure 1, Chapter 1), another Greek physician living in the Roman Empire during the 2nd century, insisted on the need for early surgery and used a syringotome, a sort of curved knife, for fistulotomy. During the 7th century in the Byzantine Empire, Paulus of Aegineta [110] underlined the importance of palpation of the fistula track, before curetting the track from its base using an implement resembling a carpenter's nail.

At the beginning of the 11th century in the Abbasid Empire, Avicenna [110] used setons even in superficial tracks, and cautery up to the muscular plane in deeper ones, followed by the introduction of a silken thread, as direct excision had been largely forgotten. It was John of Arderne [111] (Figure 13), in Europe's Middle Ages in the 14th century, who revived excision, stressed the need to perform clean surgery and to look for fistula in the case of an abscess. He was famous for accurate fistulotomies aided by his skilful use of probes.

The famous Girolamo Fabrizio d'Acquapendente [110], an Italian anatomist of the 16th century, designed a large variety of surgical instruments for fistula.

In 1765, the British surgeon, Percival Pott [112] (Figure 2, Chapter 9), recommended in a treatise, simple opening of a fistula and simple care of the wound.

About that time, King Louis XIV of France happened to be suffering from a fistula. After having tried some useless remedies proposed by the Court's physicians, Charles François Félix [113], Surgeon to the King, operated on his royal patient on November 18th, 1686. He resorted to fistulotomy, as advocated by Arderne, although still controversial in France. He modified Acquapendente's lancet, later known as the 'royal lancet' for the operation. The King allegedly did not even sigh during the operation (so history relates!) and finally recovered after three other smaller interventions during December. The operation was

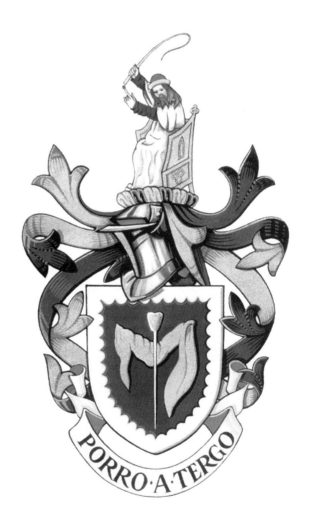

Figure 13. Caricature of John of Arderne, father of British coloproctology shown on the badge of the Association of Coloproctologists of Great Britain and Ireland. *Reproduced with permission from the Association of ColoProctology of Great Britain and Ireland.*

declared a success, to the relief of the people of France as well as to the King. No doubt the surgeon was more relieved than any of them!

Fistula was so prevalent and important which is why, in 1835, Frederick Salmon [114] (Figure 2) devoted his energies to the treatment of fistula when he founded St. Mark's Hospital in London, the first specialised hospital of its type in the world (Figure 3).

Fistula-in-ano after the third quarter of the 19th century

From that period, progress came from four main directions.

Anal crypts and glands

The discovery of the anal glands opening into the anal crypts by Chiari [11] in 1878 was most important. This was confirmed by the 'pathfinders', Hermann and Desfosses [12], in 1880. It then became clear that anal fistulas almost always originated from them.

Prediction of fistula direction

In 1900, Goodsall [115] (associated with 'Goodsall's rule') stated that a fistula, whose external opening lies anterior to the anus, has a direct track and usually an anterolateral internal opening. A fistula with a posterior external opening has a curved track and an internal opening at or very near to the midline. He suggested exceptions to this rule required further investigation.

Fistulography developed in 1929, and other non-interventional techniques, such as intra-anal ultrasonography from the end of the 1980s and magnetic resonance imaging (MRI) from the end of the 1990s made a huge difference in management.

Classifications of fistula

Classifications of fistula constituted an important breakthrough, allowing both a better spatial vision of the disease and rationalisation of its treatment.

The classification of fistula had been established by Milligan and Morgan [17] in 1934 and was based primarily on the trans-sphincteric track; it separated high and low fistulas, depending on the crossing point in the external sphincter, the crucial level being the dentate line. Low fistulas were classified as submucous, subcutaneous and trans-sphincteric according to the same principle.

Thompson [116] presented a similar classification in 1962, distinguishing between simple and complex fistulae, according not only to the height of the crossing point through the external sphincter, but also to the proportion of the anal circumference involved.

John Goligher [117], in 1975, modified slightly the Milligan and Morgan classification, differentiating between trans-sphincteric and inter-sphincteric fistulae.

The most widely accepted current classification was presented by Parks [118] in 1976, and later completed by Hardcastle [119] in 1985. It was derived from the classification by Stelzner [120] in 1959 in Germany, based on the importance of a primary inter-sphincteric track starting from the anal crypts. In Parks' classification, the primary track may be solely inter-sphincteric if it crosses the internal sphincter only, trans-sphincteric if it goes on through the external sphincter, supra-sphincteric if it goes up in the inter-sphincteric plane to cross over the sphincter, or less frequently, extra-sphincteric if it goes back over the whole sphincter into the rectum. Added to those four main categories, possible correlated abscess or secondary tracks has led to a total of 14 categories.

In 1980, in Paris, Jean Arnous and Jean Denis [121] published their classification, adapted from Milligan and Morgan's. Widely used in France, it separated simple and complex fistulae, the former having one track (low, medium or high trans-sphincteric, supra-sphincteric, or inter-sphincteric), the latter associating with a secondary track, or having a complex single track. It also classified all the types of fistulas of the anal region into supra-anal, anal, and extra-anal, according to the origin of the infection.

On reflection, complex disorders are bound to have complex classifications.

The final progress

The final progress was the avoidance of mutilating interventions by trying to close the tracks. The mucosal advancement flap procedure already known in the beginning of the 20th century in Britain (in France under the name of the 'curtain procedure' [122]) had been revived in the US in 1985 by Aguilar [123]. This involved resection of the lower part of the fistula and of the internal opening; the emergence of the track in the internal sphincter is then sutured and covered by a rectal mucosal flap.

Other causes of abscess

Tuberculosis has been responsible for many abscesses of the region, particularly in the 19th century, and it was considered at that time that surgery was contraindicated.

Crohn's disease was earlier recognised as being able to provoke peri-anal lesions. Hughes [124] was the first to establish a classification of these lesions in 1992. Treatment is usually conservative and results with new drugs are still on trial.

Rectovaginal fistulas are difficult, especially when the fistula is high in the rectovaginal wall. In France, René Musset [125] published his personal technique in 1975; it started with laying open the track by perineotomy, later followed by reconstruction of the sphincter and perineum. Mucosal advancement flap is another possibility for high fistulas since the work of David Rothenberger and Stanley Goldberg [126].

Alfred Velpeau [127] discovered in 1839 a curious chronic infection of the skin; Aristide Verneuil [128] proved it to be an infection of apocrine sudoral glands in 1854. Peri-anal localisations are frequent, but the disease may also extend beyond the perineum, to the groin, or arm-pit. Not much progress has been made on its aetiology since then, and the lesions require generally wide excision. Generally known as hidradenitis suppurativa, it is called Verneuil's disease in France.

Anatomical and functional conditions

Rectal prolapse

Rectal prolapse has been described since antiquity, but it has often been considered and treated like a form of tumour. It was only in 1831 that Frederick Salmon in London made the first comprehensive description of the disease [21]. Yet during most of the 19th century, it was still treated by cautery or ligature, later replaced by a lineal crushing method. It is easy to imagine how many patients experienced haemorrhage, peritonitis or stenosis afterwards. To counter those complications and perhaps avoid surgery, many contentious devices were designed, such as the application of gum, air-filled or ivory balls, and since the advent of electricity, various needles were linked to an electric battery to stimulate the anal sphincter.

The application of anatomical and physiological principles came only during the 20th century. In the US, Alexis Moschcowitz in 1912 [129] underlined the role of an elongated pouch of Douglas acting as a hernia through the anal sphincter. In the UK, Pemberton and Stalker in 1939 related the prolapse to a loose attachment of the rectum, and Parks [130] in 1977, to pelvic floor deficiency. In 1980, Keighley [131] established that incontinence was more often a consequence than a cause of prolapse.

Another approach was to create an anal stricture. Dupuytren [132] had tried to narrow the anus by excising radial mucosal flaps, but it was Thiersch in 1891 [133], who imagined the first encirclement procedure of the anus, using a silver wire. Other materials were experimented with in the 20th century, including collars, but the main problem remained the risk of faecal impaction. This mechanical approach has been used in severe faecal incontinence with only moderate success. In 1937, Sarafoff [134] described a circular incision of the peri-anal skin, sometimes with a partial skin resection. This very simple procedure may still be used to control small prolapses, and for stenosis of the lower anal canal.

Other perineal procedures became more aggressive, trying to suppress the prolapse. Johann von Mikulicz-Radecki was the first in 1888, in the

Prussian part of Poland, to dare to perform a perineal rectosigmoidectomy [135]. The procedure presented by Altemeier [136] in 1952 was merely an adaptation of this operation; it allowed dissection and division of the rectum and of the pouch of Douglas, the closure being often followed by a sphincter repair. It is still used thanks to a low morbidity rate even in the very elderly, but it has two main drawbacks: a medium high recurrence rate and a risk of incontinence due to the loss of the rectal reservoir.

In 1900, Edmond Delorme [137] described in Paris a procedure which required resection of the redundant prolapsed mucosa and plication of the denuded muscular wall. After a long period of oblivion, it was revived mainly by Nay and Blair [138] in 1972 in the US and by Lechaux [139] in France in the 1980s. Although minimally invasive, it is still applicable to minor prolapses or high risk patients, but its recurrence rate is far from negligible.

Abdominal procedures were developed later and were mainly represented by rectopexy. In 1947, Thomas Orr [140], in Kansas City in the US, devised a suspension of the posterior and lateral walls of the rectum to the promontory of the sacrum through strips of the fascia lata.

Many other varieties of rectopexy have been described since then. For example, a posterior suspension using a polyvinyl alcohol sponge by Wells [141] in 1959 has been widely used in the UK, but carried an excessive risk of infection. Ripstein [142] devised an anterior suspension using a nylon sling which has been widely used in the US, but sometimes provoked stenosis. In 1971, Loygue, Huguier and Malafosse [143] adapted the Orr procedure, using either simple sutures or strips of nylon, and this is still in use, especially in France. It has been shown since then that if rectopexy - whatever the technique - is highly effective, its main complication is the development or aggravation of constipation. Prevention is believed to come from the preservation of the lateral ligaments of the rectum, or by combining rectopexy with sigmoidectomy, as advocated by Frykman and Goldberg [144] in the US in 1969.

Anal incontinence

Although anciently known, surprisingly, anal incontinence has drawn very little attention until recently. It is only from the mid-1970s onwards that epidemiological studies have shown the importance of the problem, and pathophysiological studies have understood its mechanisms, especially the frequency of obstetric damage and the notion of descending perineum, described in the works of Parks [145], Henry [40] and others. Simultaneously, the use of bulking agents, enemas or anti-diarrhoeal agents has become more effective. Treatment of anal incontinence has often gone hand-in-hand with treatment of urinary incontinence. These treatments can be summarised into three main categories.

Attempts to improve the function of the anal sphincter

Biofeedback training has been developed from combined urological and gynaecological experience in the 1960s, following the works of Cerulli and Schuster [146] in Baltimore, and Penninckx [147] in Belgium. This approach can improve external sphincter contractions as well as rectal sensitivity.

Radiofrequency energy has been delivered to the anal sphincter in the first years of this century in order to obtain a tightening of tissue by heating, following its use in benign prostatic hyperplasia or gastro-oesophageal reflux

The first attempts at electrostimulation have been used as early as the end of the 19th century, either as a form of physiotherapy to augment biofeedback using contact electrodes or from the urological experience, as a means of permanent electrical stimulation using implanted needles, first in the perineum and more recently near the sacral nerve. This work followed the publications of Matzel [148] in Germany and Vaizey, Nicholls and Kamm [149] in the UK around 1995.

One unfortunate episode occurred in the middle of the 20th century in the UK, when the radio signal to a rescue lifeboat stimulated some implanted electrodes in elderly nursing home residents, causing impressive synchronous defaecations! Needless to say this has been abandoned in favour of methods described below.

Direct surgical repair of the sphincter

This has been developed mainly in the 1920s in Germany, Austria and the US, treating local damage of the external sphincter, by suturing either end-to-end or overlapping flaps [150]. Parks presented his post-anal repair in 1974 [151], a technique designed to treat incontinence in the descending perineum syndrome by suturing together the three different components of the levator ani muscle and the external sphincter. A total floor repair, associating posterior and anterior sphincter repair, was later described [152]. Sadly, results have worsened with time.

Treatments trying to replace the sphincter

In 1925, Harvey Stone [153] had imagined a transposition of a preserved fascia through a subcutaneous tunnel around the anus; the technique was improved by the same author in 1929 by using two fascia loops and attaching their ends to the opposite gluteus maximus [154]. In 1952, in Durham (North Carolina), Kenneth Pickrell described his gracioplasty [155], which we now know only survives if electrically stimulated. He transposed the whole gracilis muscle in the same way as the fascia. It was not then realised that the muscle, which is a type 2 skeletal muscle, was unfit for continuous use because it slowly degenerated.

In 1995, gracioplasty was modified by implanting at the same time a neuro-stimulatory device, providing continuous low-frequency stimulation which enabled the transformation of type 2 into type 1 musculature. This mainly successful electro-stimulated gracioplasty, complicated by occasional infections, was studied by many teams, for example Baeten and Konsten [156] in the Netherlands, Wexner [157] in the US and Williams and George [158] in the UK.

In 1989, Christiansen and Lorentzen [159] reported their first experience with an artificial implantable sphincter, similar to those used in urology, which comprises a cuff encircling the anus, and a balloon which may fill or empty the cuff that is serviced by a pump. The procedure is under study by several teams at the time of this publication.

Solitary ulcer of the rectum

Chronic ulcer of the rectum was first described in France in 1829 by Cruveilhier [160] (Figure 4, Chapter 6), who compared it with gastroduodenal incompetence and considered it to be a local equivalent of a gastroduodenal ulcer. It is only in 1937 that its specificity was recognised in London by Lloyd-Davies [161], who coined the phrase 'solitary ulcer of the rectum'.

Madigan and Morson [162] attempted in 1969 to correlate a histological diagnosis with a series of previously different pathological entities. For example:

- Goodall and Sinclair [163] in 1957 described a 'colitis cystica profunda';
- Shannon Allen [164] in 1966 described a 'hamartomatous inverted polyp';
- Talerman [165] in 1971 described an 'enterogenous cyst'.

Madigan and Morson believed these were all different aspects of the same disease.

With more physiological explanations by Rutter and Riddell [166] in 1975, it became clear that this affliction was generally the result of an anterior or total intussusception or even overt prolapse of the rectum, associated with inappropriate pelvic floor contraction. Although controversial with some experts, it did clear the way for rational treatment for the remainder.

Constipation

Constipation has certainly been a preoccupation since the origins of mankind. Evacuation enemas have been used in ancient Egypt, Greece and Rome. During the Middle-Ages, Avicenna was said to be the first to devise a clyster (enema) syringe, and North American, as well as pre-Colombian South American Indian civilisations, have resorted to periodical purifying purgatives or enemas. In Europe, the 17th century had seen the climax of this 'clysteromania', two of the main works on this topic being *De clysteribus et colica liber* published in 1530 attributed to Galen, and *De clysteribus* published in Leyden (Netherlands) in 1668 by Reinier de Graaf. In the 19th century, new worries about auto-intoxication emerged and led to the conclusion that several illnesses, mainly nervous and psychiatric, could be attributed to constipation.

It was in that spirit that Sir William Arbuthnot Lane [167], until then a highly respected British surgeon, advocated subtotal colectomy with ileorectal anastomosis not only for constipation, but being so obsessed with the idea of toxin retention he even treated breast cancer by colectomy!

Only from the late 1960s until the early 1980s, the physiological studies of distinguished pioneers such as Hinton [168], Preston and Lennard-Jones [169] from the UK, Patrick Meunier [170] from Lyon, Hélène Martelli and Pierre Arhan [27] from Paris, Ghislain Devroede [171] from Québec, and Kerremans [172] from Belgium, all pointed out that constipation needed to be differentiated between slow colonic transit and outlet obstruction. In the former case, a severe variety of colonic inertia was isolated and allowed a come-back of the Arbuthnot-Lane procedure, seemingly with excessive enthusiasm. In 1990, Malone [173] proposed an ante-grade enema via an appendicostomy, or caecostomy if previous appendicectomy had been performed. It being fairly benign and reversible, it is still of value for intractable incontinence.

In the case of outlet obstruction, biofeedback was proved to be effective in anismus - a term coined by Preston and Lennard-Jones [174] in 1985 comparable with vaginismus. Biofeedback was also applied to some rectal sensitivity abnormalities, especially by Philippe Denis and his team in Rouen [175] in the late 1080o. The same authors later in 1995 established with Ghislain Devroede, a link between anismus and sexual abuse [176].

Anorectal myotomy was proposed by Bentley [177] in 1966, followed by the suggestion of myectomy as had previously been proposed for outlet obstruction for conditions other than that of Hirschsprung's disease. Despite its initial enthusiasm for the treatment of constipation, it later proved disappointing. The same occurred with experimentation with botulinum toxin in the 1990s.

There has been a proposal to modify Longo's stapled anopexy procedure for haemorrhoids, in order to perform a stapled transanal rectal resection, as an attempt to cure rectal intussusception associated with outlet obstruction [178]. It had been hoped by some, that this could be a promising comprehensive solution to many related problems, including solitary ulcer of the rectum and rectocoele. Such a hope, like so many others in history, requires the unrelenting test of time.

Conclusions

Apart form the achievements of this chapter's pioneers, what alternative treatments have been tried? In certain churches, especially in Latin America as well as in Europe, candles or tapers have been purchased and applied to the afflicted part of the body in the hope of cure [179]. Similarly, in Brittany, one of the big toes of the statue of Saint Guénolé can be unscrewed and applied to the symptomatic part [180].

The Irish Saint, Fiacre, came to live as a hermit in the French region of Brie, about 660 AD. After accusations of witchcraft, he went to see the bishop of Meaux, where he had to sit on a stone in front of the church for several days before gaining an audience. His innocence was finally accepted, and the stone on which he had been seated, was said to be transformed to the shape of his posterior anatomy like a mould. Since then, the stone, and later the Saint's relics, have been considered able to relieve anal disorders, resulting in pilgrimages with claims of relief [181]!

Anal disease has had an immense role in history and has not spared the elite. Musicians like Giacomo Meyerbeer, authors and philosophers like René Descartes or Wilhelm Gottfried Leibniz, have been affected by haemorrhoids; so also King Louis XI of France and Emperor Charles V of Austria [179].

Franz Liszt had been obliged to cancel concerts because of acute crises, and Johannes Brahms had his piles removed by Billroth. It has been suggested that his Tragic Overture was named in memory of the operation [180]! François Marie Arouet better known as Voltaire, suffered all his life from constipation. His contemporaries believed his temper reflected his bowel function of the day [182].

Charles Maurice, Marquis of Talleyrand, who loyally served successive regimes from Louis XVI until the 1830 Revolution, suffered from typical outlet obstruction, and had instructed a servant how to make the best use of a boxwood spoon he had devised for stool evacuation [182].

Can one imagine what direction history might have taken if Queen Eleanor of Aquitaine, so pivotal in Anglo-French affairs, had not succumbed to frequent episodes of haemorrhoidal thrombosis [180], or if Hitler and Göring had been less affected by severe constipation [182]?

The Protestant reformer Martin Luther was alleged to have had an anal fissure. He was desperate enough to try a recommended treatment based on eating birds' faeces; perhaps, the course of Reformation could have been different had he a better health and temper [182]. Perhaps King Charles IX of France, whose outbursts of anger were often triggered by episodes of constipation and anal bleeding, might not have precipitated the Massacre of Protestants on St. Bartholomew's Day, had he been given effective treatment [180]!

According to some of his close aids and relatives, if Napoleon Bonaparte had not abandoned the control of the Battle of Waterloo at a very crucial stage because of haemorrhoidal pain, the outcome might have been different [183]!

A strange quirk of fate took place following the cure of the French King Louis XIV's fistula. An anthem ('God save the King') was composed to celebrate that event, but it was later adopted by Britain for its own National Anthem. Had it not been for the fistula another anthem would have been required [184]!

There is no doubt pioneers have achieved as much in proctology as in other branches of surgical gastroenterology. However, so much remains to be accomplished, for example, simpler techniques of prediction and prevention of rectal and anal cancer, determining the aetiology of anal fistula, clear management of anal incontinence and managing peri-anal Crohn's disease. Added to these, the understanding of the pathogenesis and prevention of pelvic floor disorders are all tasks that lie ahead of us. No doubt, new pioneers will emerge in the coming decades, who will overcome the new frontiers.

References

1. Cocheton J-J, Guerre J, Péquignot H, Pallardy G. *Histoire illustrée de l'Hépato-Gastroentérologie de l'Antiquité à nos jours.* Paris: éditions Roger Dacosta, 1987: 14.

2. Cocheton J-J, Guerre J, Péquignot H, Pallardy G. *Histoire illustrée de l'Hépato-Gastroentérologie de l'Antiquité à nos jours.* Paris: éditions Roger Dacosta, 1987: 25.

3. de Jonckheere F. *Le Papyrus Médical.* Chester Beatty, Bruxelles: Fondation égyptologique de la Reine Elisabeth, 1947.

4. Denis J. La Proctologie à l'ombre des Pyramides. *Gastro à la une.* Laboratoires Beaufour, 1997: 29-32

5. Galen. Des facultés naturelles. In: *Oeuvres anatomiques, physiologiques et médicales.* Paris: J-B Baillière, édition de Charles Daremberg, 1854-56; vol. 2: chapter 6.

6. Morgagni G-B. *De sedibus et causis morborum per anatomen indagatis.* Naples, 1766, french translation by Désormeaux and Destouet. Paris: A. Delahays, 1855.

7. Alcock B. Account of some particulars in the anatomys of the fifth nerve in the human subject and in fish not hitherto observed. *Dublin Journal Med Chem Sci* 1836; 323-7.

8. Houston J. Observations on the mucous membrane of the rectum. *Dublin Hospital Reports* 1830; 5: 158

9. Hilton J. *On rest and pain*, 2nd edition. London: W.H.A. Jacobson, 1877.

10. Straud BB. On the anatomy of the anus. *Ann Surg* 1896; 24: 1.

11. Chiari H. Über nalen Divertikel der rectum schteim hant und ihre Beziehung zu den anal fisteln. *Wien Med Presse* 1878; 19: 1482-3.

12. Hermann G, Desfosses L. *Sur la muqueuse du rectum. Comptes-rendus hebdomadaires de l'Académie des Sciences* 1880; 90: 1301-2.

13. Trouvé G. *Manuel d'Electrologie Médicale.* Paris: Octave Doin, 1893.

14. Kelly HA. Instruments for use through cylindrical rectal specula, with the patients in the knee-chest posture. *Ann Surg* 1903; 37: 924-7.

15. Arderne J. *Treatise of the fistulae in the fundament and other places.* London: Thomas East, 1588.

16. Bushe JM. *A treatise on the malformations, injuries and diseases of the rectum and anus.* New York: French and Adlard, 1837.

17. Milligan ETO, Morgan CN. Surgical anatomy of the anal canal with special reference to ano-rectum fistulae. *Lancet* 1934; 2: 1150-6.

18. Courtney H. Anatomy of the pelvic diaphragm and ano-rectal musculature as related to sphincter preservation in ano-rectal surgery. *Am J Surg* 1950; 79: 155-73.

19. Morgan CN, Thomson HR. Surgical anatomy of the anal canal with special reference to the surgical importance of the internal sphincter and conjoint longitudinal muscle. *Ann Roy Coll Surg Engl* 1956; 19: 88.

20. Parks AG. The surgical treatment of haemorrhoids. *Br J Surg* 1955; 43: 337.

21. Salmon F. A practical treatise on stricture of the rectum. *Lancet* 1832.

22. Mathews JM. *Treatise on Diseases of the Rectum.* New York: Appleton, 1893.

23. Arnous J, Parnaud E, Denis J. Une hémorroïdectomie de sécurité, à propos de 5000 observations. *Presse Méd* 1971; 3: 87-90

24. Kerremans R. *Morphological and physiological aspects of anal continence and defecation.* Bruxelles: Arscia, 1969.

25. Ihre T. Studies on anal function in continent and incontinent patients. *Scand J Gastroenterol* 1974; 9 suppl.25: 1-80.

26. Arhan P, Devroede G, Danis K. Visco-elastic properties of the rectal wall in Hirschsprung's disease. *J Clin Invest* 1978; 62: 82-7.

27. Martelli H, Devroede G, Arhan P, *et al.* Some parameters of large bowel motility in normal man. *Gastroenterology* 1978; 76: 612-8.

28. Denis P, Colin R, Galmiche JP, *et al.* Elastic properties of the rectal wall in normal adults and in patients with ulcerative colitis. *Gastroenterology* 1979; 77: 45-8.

29. Shafik A. A new concept of the anatomy of the anal sphincter mechanism and the physiology of defecation; the external anal sphincter: a triple loop system. *Invest Urol* 1975; 12: 412-9.

30. Duthie HL, Bennett RC. The relation of the sensation in the anal canal to the functional anal sphincter: a possible factor in anal continence. *Gut* 1963; 4: 179-82.

31. Duthie HL, Bennett RC. The functional importance of the internal sphincter. *Br J Surg* 1964; 51: 355-7.

32. Thompson WHF. The nature of haemorrhoids. *Br J Surg* 1975; 62: 542-52.

33. Delherm L. Le collothor (dioxyde de thorium) dans l'exploration des fistules anales. *J Radiol et électrol* 1935; 19: 122-3.

34. Hinton JM, Lennard-Jones JE, Young C. A new method for studying gut transit times using radio-opaque markers. *Gut* 1969; 10: 842-7.

35. Arhan P, Devroede G, Jehannin B, *et al.* Segmental colonic transit time. *Dis Colon Rectum* 1981; 24: 625-9.

36. Chaussade S, Roche H, Khyari A, Couturier D, Guerre J. Mesure du temps de transit colique: description et validation d'une nouvelle technique. *Gastroentérol Clin Biol* 1986; 10: 385-9.

37. Bouchoucha M, Devroede G, Arhan P, *et al.* What is the meaning of colorectal transit time measurement? *Dis Colon Rectum* 1992; 35: 773-82.

38. Danquechin-Dorval E, Barbieux JP, Picon L, *et al.* Mesure simplifiée du temps de transit colique par une seule radiographie de l'abdomen et un seul type de marqueur. *Gastro-entérol Clin Biol* 1994; 18: 141-4.

39. Mahieu P, Pringot J, Bodart P. Defecography: description of a new procedure and results in normal patients. *Gastrointest Radiol* 1984; 9: 247-51.

40. Henry MM, Swash M. Assessment of pelvic floor disorders and incontinence by electrophysiological recording of the anal reflex. *Lancet* 1978; 17: 1290-1.

41. Swash M, Snooks SJ. Electromyography in pelvic floor disorders. In: *Coloproctology and the pelvic floor.* Henry MM, Swash M. London: Butterworth, 1985: 86-103.

42. Wexner SD, Marchetti F, Salanga VD, Corredor C, Jagelman DG. Neurophysiologic assessment of the anal sphincters. *Dis Colon Rectum* 1991; 34: 606-11.

43. Bartram C, Sultan AH. Anal endosonography in faecal incontinence. *Gut* 1995; 37: 4-6.

44. Matheson DM, Keighley MRB. Manometric evaluation of rectal prolapse and faecal incontinence. *Gut* 1981; 22: 126-9.

45. Read NW, Bartolo DCC, Read MG. Differences in anal function in patients with incontinence to solids and in patients with incontinence to liquids. *Br J Surg* 1984; 71: 39-42.

46. Stahl GE. *Dissertatio de motu sanguinis haemorrhoidali et haemorrhoidibus externis.* Halle, 1698-1705.

47. James R. *A medicinal dictionary with a history of drugs.* London: Roberts, 1743.

48. Quenu E, Hartmann H. *Chirurgie du rectum.* Paris: Steinheil, 1895; chapter 7: 367-73.

49. Larrey D. *Recueil de mémoires de chirurgie.* Paris: Compère le Jeune, 1821.

50. Baldinger EG. *Von den Krankenheiten einer Armee, aus eigenen wahrnehmungen.* Langensalz, 1765.

51. Hildebrandt GF. *Über die blinden Haemorrhoiden.* Erlangen, 1795.

52. Keighley M, Williams N. *Surgery of the anus, rectum and colon.* London: WB Saunders, 1993; chapter 13: 311.

53. Blanchard CE. *The Romance of Proctology.* Youngstown: Medical Success Press, 1938; chapter 5: 107-18.

54. Andrews E. The treatment of haemorrhoids by injection. *Med Rec* 1879; 15: 451.

55. Blanchard CE. *The Romance of Proctology.* Youngstown: Medical Success Press, 1938; chapter 6: 130-43.

56. Bensaude R. *Maladies de l'intestin.* Paris: Masson, 1939. chapter 4.

57. Blaisdell PC. Office ligation of internal haemorrhoids. *Am J Surg* 1958; 96: 401.

58. Barron J. Office ligation of internal haemorrhoids. *Am J Surg* 1963; 105: 563.

59. Soullard J. La ligature élastique: indications comparées avec les injections sclérosantes et la chirurgie. *Concours Médical* 1966; 88(43): 6339-43.

60. Fraser J, Gill W. Observations on ultrafrozen tissue. *Br J Surg* 1967; 54: 770.

61. Lloyd-Williams K, Haq IU, Elem B. Cryodestruction of haemorrhoids. *Br Med J* 1973; 1: 666.

62. Neiger A. Haemorrhoids in every day practice. *Proctology* 1979; 2: 22-8.

63. Nath G, Kreitmayer A, Kiefhaber F, Moritz K. Neue infrarot Koagulation Methode, Verhand lungeband des 9. Kongress der deutschen Gesellschaft für Gastro-enterologie, 1976. Permied Verlag, Erlangen, 17, 1977.

64. Miles WE. Observations upon internal piles. *Surg Gynecol Obstet* 1919; 29: 496.

65. Eisenhammer S. The surgical correction of internal anal (sphincteric) contracture. *S Afr Med J* 1951; 25: 486-7.

66. Lord PH. A new regime for the treatment of haemorrhoids. *Proc Roy Soc Med* 1968; 61: 935.

67. Hippocrates. *The Genuine Works.* Translation by Francis Adams. London: Sydenham Society, 1929.

68. Galen. Des lieux affectés. In: *Oeuvres anatomiques, physiologiques et médicales.* Paris: J.-B. Baillière, édition de Charles Daremberg, 1854-56; vol. 2: chapter 10.

69. Petit JL. *Traité des Maladies Chirurgicales et des Opérations qui leur conviennent.* Paris: TF Didot, 1774; vol. 2: 137.

70. Whitehead W. Surgical treatment of haemorrhoids. *Br Med J* 1882; 1: 149.

71. Allingham W, Allingham HW. *The diagnosis and treatment of diseases of the rectum*, 7th ed. London: Baillière, 1901.

72. Milligan ETC, Morgan C, Nauton LE, Officer R. Surgical anatomy of the anal canal and the operative treatment of haemorrhoids. *Lancet* 1937; 11: 1119-24.

73. Eisenhammer S. Proper principles and practices in the surgical management of haemorrhoids. *Dis Colon Rectum* 1969; 12: 288.

74. Arnous J, Parnaud E, Denis J. Une hémorroïdectomie de sécurité, à propos de 5000 observations. *Presse Méd* 1971; 3: 87-90.

75. Parks AG. The surgical treatment of haemorrhoids. *Br J Surg* 1956; 43: 337-51.

76. Ferguson JA, Mazier WP, Gretchen MJ, Friend WG. The closed technique of haemorrhoidectomy. *Surgery* 1971; 70: 480-4.

77. Longo A. Treatment of haemorrhoid disease by reduction of mucosa and haemorrhoidal prolapse with a circular suturing device: a new procedure. Proceedings of the 6th World Congress of Endoscopic Surgery, Mundozzi, Rome, 1998.

78. Lemonnier LG. *Traité de la fistule de l'anus ou du fondement.* Paris, 1689.

79. Valensi R. *Un chirurgien arabe au Moyen-Age: Abulcassis, Thèse.* Montpellier, 1908.

80. Gabriel WB. Anal fissure. *Br Med J* 1929; 1: 1070-2.

81. Parnaud E, Arnous J. La léïomyotomie avec anoplastie dans le traitement des fissures anales. *Presse Méd* 1968; 76(34): 1661-3.

82. Fabre A, *et al. Rectum, in Dictionnaires des dictionnaires de Médecine français et étrangers.* Paris: Germer-Baillière, 1850; vol. 7.

83. Récamier JCA. *Essai sur les hémorroïdes.* Paris: Brosson, 1799.

84. Maisonneuve JG. Du traitement de la fissure à l'anus par la dilatation forcée. *Gazette des hôpitaux* 1849; 1: 220.

85. Boyer A. Sur quelques maladies de l'anus. *Journal Comp des Sc Méd* 1818; 2: 24-44.

86. Eisenhammer S. The evaluation of the internal anal sphincterotomy operation with special reference to anal fissure. *Surg Gynecol Obstet* 1959; 109: 583-90.

87. Parks AG. The management of fissure in ano. *Hosp Med* 1967; 1: 737-9.

88. Notaras M. Lateral subcutaneous sphincterotomy for anal fissure: a new technique. *Proc Roy Soc Med* 1969; 62: 713.

89. Hoffman DC, Goligher JC. Lateral subcutaneous internal sphincterotomy in the treatment of anal fissure. *Br Med J* 1970; 3: 673-5.

90. Soullard J, Contou JF. Condylomes acuminés. In: *Colo-Proctologie.* Paris: Masson, 1984: 263.

91. Lagneau L. Excroissances syphilitiques. In: *Dictionnaire de Médecine ou Répertoire général des Sciences médicales,*

2nd ed. Adelon, Béclard, Bérard, *et al*. Paris: Béchet jeune, 1835; vol. 12: 443-57.

92. Mauriac C. Végétations. In: *Nouveau Dictionnaire de Médecine et de Chirurgie pratiques sous la direction du Dr. Jaccoud*. Paris: J-B. Baillière, 1886; vol. 39: 564-615.

93. Culp OS, Kaplan IW. Condylomata acuminata: two hundred cases treated with podophyllin. *Ann Surg* 1944; 120: 251-6.

94. Paget J. On diseases of the mammary areola preceding cancer of the mammary gland. *Saint Bartholomew Hospital Reports* 1874; 10: 87-9.

95. Darier J. *Précis de Dermatologie*. Paris: Masson, 1923.

96. Bowen JT. Precancerous dermatoses: a study of 2 cases of chronic atypical proliferation. *The Journal of Cutaneous Diseases including Syphilis* 1912; 30: 241-55.

97. Vickers PM, Jackman RJ, MacDonald JR. Anal carcinoma *in situ*: report of three cases. *South Surg* 1939; 8: 503-7.

98. Buschke A., Löwenstein L. Über carcinomähnliche Condylomata acuminata des Penis. *Berliner klinische Wochenschrift* 1925; 4: 1726-8.

99. Parks AG. Benign tumours of the rectum. In: *Abdomen, Rectum and Clinical Surgery*. Rob C, Smith R, Morgan CN. London: Butterworth, 1966; vol.10.

100. Parks AG, Stuart AE. The management of villous tumours of the large bowel. *Br Med J* 1973; 60: 688-95.

101. York Mason A. Transsphincteric surgery of the rectum. *Prog Surg* 1974; 13: 66-9.

102. Bevan AD. Carcinoma of the rectum - treatment by local excision. *Surg Clin North Am* 1917; 1: 1233.

103. Francillon J, Moulay A, Vignal J, Tissot E. L'exérèse par voie basse des cancers de l'ampoule rectale. *Nouv Pressé Méd* 1974; 3: 1365-6.

104. Faivre J, Weber F. La place de l'électrorésection dans le traitement du cancer du rectum. *Bordeaux Méd* 1977; 10: 2131-4.

105. Morson BC. The pathology and results of treatment of squamous cell carcinoma of the anal canal and anal margin. *Proc Roy Soc Med* 1960; 53: 416-20.

106. Morson BC, Sobin LH. *Histological typing of intestinal tumours*. Geneva: World Health Organisation, 1976: 62-5.

107. Papillon J. Radiation therapy in the management of epidermoidal carcinoma of the anal region. *Dis Colon Rectum* 1974; 17: 184-7.

108. Nigro ND, Vaitkevicius VK, Bukoker T, Bradley GT, Considine B. Combined therapy for cancer of the anal canal. *Dis Colon Rectum* 1981; 24: 73-5.

109. Hillemand P. Histoire de la Gastro-enterologie. In: *Histoire de la Médecine, de la Pharmacie, de l'Art dentaire et de l'Art vétérinaire*. Poulet J, Sournia JC, Martiny M. Paris: Albin Michel / Laffont / Tchou, 1978; vol. 5.

110. Giordano M, Blanco G. *Le fistole anali*. Roma: Mediprint, 2003: 8-10.

111. Ellis H. *A History of Surgery*. London: Greenwich Medical Media, 2001: 36-7.

112. Pott P. *Remarks on the disease commonly called fistula in ano*. London, 1765.

113. Ellis H. *A History of Surgery*. London: Greenwich Medical Media, 2001: 50.

114. Blanchard CE. *The Romance of Proctology*. Youngstown: Medical Success Press, 1938: 75-8.

115. Goodsall DH, Miles WE. *Diseases of the Anus and Rectum*, part 1. London: Longmans, 1900.

116. Thompson HR. The orthodox conception of fistula in ano and its treatment. *Proc Roy Soc Med* 1962; 55: 754-6.

117. Goligher JC. *Surgery of the Anus, Rectum and Colon*, 3rd ed. London: Baillière Tindall, 1975: 210.

118. Parks AG, Gordon PH, Hardcastle JD. A classification of fistula in ano. *Br J Surg* 1976; 63: 1-12.

119. Hardcastle JD. The classification of fistula in ano. *Ann Roy Coll Surg Engl* (suppl.) 1985; 58: 6-9.

120. Stelzner F. *Die anorectalen Fisteln*. Berlin: Springer-Verlag, 1959; chapter 8: 87-155.

121. Arnous J, Denis J, du Puy-Montbrun T. Les suppurations anales et péri-anales. A propos de 6500 cas. *Concours Méd* 1980; 102: 1715-29.

122. Elting DW. The treatment of fistula in ano with special reference to the Whitehead operation. *Ann Surg* 1912; 56: 744-52.

123. Aguilar PS, Plasencia G, Hardy TG, Hartmann RF, Stewart WR. Mucosal advancement in the treatment of anal fistula. *Dis Colon Rectum* 1985; 28: 496-8.

124. Hughes LE. Clinical classification of perianal Crohn's disease. *Dis Colon Rectum* 1992; 35: 928-32.

125. Musset R, Arnous J, Poitout P, Parnaud E, Truc JB, Paniel BJ. Notre expérience du traitement chirurgical selon un procédé personnel de 105 incontinences anales féminines et 77 fistules recto-vaginales. In: *Actualités gynécologiques* (6è série). Paris: Masson, 1975.

126. Rothenberger DA, Christenson CE, Balcos EG, Schottler JL, Nemer FD, Nivatvong S, Goldberg SM. Endorectal advancement flap for treatment of simple rectovaginal fistula. *Dis Colon Rectum* 1982; 25: 297-300.

127. Velpeau A. *Dictionnaire de Médecine ou Répertoire général des Sciences médicales sous le rapport théorique et pratique*. Paris: Béchet Jeune, 1839; vol. 2: 91; vol. 3: 304; vol. 19: 1.

128. Verneuil A. Etude sur les tumeurs de la peau: de quelques maladies des glandes sudoripares. *Arch gén Méd* 1859; 94: 447-8, 693-703.

129. Moschcowitz AV. The pathogenesis and anatomy and care of prolapse of the rectum. *Surg Gynecol Obstet* 1912; 15: 7-21.

130. Parks AG. Sphincter denervation in anorectal incontinence and rectal prolapse. *Gut* 1977; 18: 656-9.

131. Keighley MRB, Makuria T, Alexander-Williams J, Arabi Y. Clinical and manometric evaluation of rectal prolapse and incontinence. *Br J Surg* 1980; 67: 54-6.

132. Dupuytren G. *Leçons orales de clinique chirurgicale faites à l'Hôtel-Dieu de Paris*. Bruxelles: Ode et Wodon, 1832.

133. Thiersch (1891, Halle) quoted by Gabriel WB. *The principles and practice of rectal surgery*. London: HK Lewis, 1963: 179-90.

134. Sarafoff D. Ein einfaches ungefährliches verfahren zur operativen behandlung des Mastdamvorfalles. *Arch Klin Chir* 1937; 190: 219-32.

135. von Mikulicz-Radecki J. Zur operativen Behandlung des Prolapsus recti et coli invaginati. *Verh Dtsch Ges Chir* 1888; 17: 294-317.

136. Altemeier WA, Guiseffi J, Hoxworth PI. Treatment of extensive prolapse of the rectum in aged or debilitated patients. *Arch Surg* 1952; 65: 72-80.

137. Delorme E. Sur le traitement des prolapsus du rectum totaux par l'excision de la muqueuse rectale ou recto-colique. *Bull Mém Soc Chir Paris* 1900; 26: 498-9.

138. Nay HR, Blair CR. Perineal surgical repair of rectal prolapse, *Am J Surg* 1972; 123: 577-9.

139. Lechaux JP, Lechaux D, Perez M. Results of Delorme's procedure for rectal prolapse. *Dis Colon Rectum* 1995; 38: 301-7.

140. Orr T. A suspension operation for prolapse of the rectum. *Ann Surg* 1947; 126: 833.

141. Wells C. New operation for rectal prolapse. *Proc Roy Soc Med* 1959; 52I: 602-4.

142. Ripstein CB. Surgical care of massive rectal prolapse. *Dis Colon Rectum* 1965; 8: 34-8.

143. Loygue J, Huguier M, Malafosse M, Biotois H. Complete prolapse of the rectum: a report on 140 cases treated by rectopexy. *Br J Surg* 1971; 58: 847-8.

144. Frykman HM, Goldberg SM. The surgical treatment of rectal procidentia. *Surg Gynecol Obstet* 1969; 129: 1225-30.

145. Parks AG, Porter NH, Hardcastle J. The syndrome of the descending perineum. *Proc Roy Soc Med* 1966; 59: 477-82.

146. Cerulli MA, Nikoomanesh P, Schuster MM. Progress in biofeedback conditioning for fecal incontinence. *Gastroenterology* 1979; 76: 742-6.

147. Penninckx F, Lestar B, Kerremans R. A new balloon-retaining test for evaluation of anorectal function in incontinent patients. *Dis Colon Rectum* 1989; 32: 202-5.

148. Matzel KE, Stadelmaier U, Hohenfeller M, *et al*. Electrical stimulation of spinal nerves for treatment of fecal incontinence. *Lancet* 1995; 346: 1124-7.

149. Vaizey CJ, Kamm MA, Turner IC, *et al*. Effects of short term sacral nerve stimulation on anal and rectal function in patients with anal incontinence. *Gut* 1999; 44: 407-12.

150. Blaisdell PC. Repair of the incontinent sphincter ani. *Surg Gynecol Obstet* 1940; 70: 692-7.

151. Parks AG. Anorectal incontinence. *Proc Roy Soc Med* 1975; 68: 681-90.

152. Deen KI, Oya M, Oritz J, Keighley MRB. Randomised trial comparing three forms of pelvic floor repair for neuropathic faecal incontinence. *Br J Surg* 1993; 80: 794-8.

153. Stone HB. Plastic operation for anal incontinence. *Tr South Surg Ass* 1926; 41: 235.

154. Stone HB. Plastic operation for anal incontinence. *Arch Surg* 1929; 18: 845.

155. Pickrell KL, Broadbent TR, Masters FW, Metzger JT. Construction of a rectal sphincter and restoration of anal continence by transplanting the gracilis muscle. *Ann Surg* 1952; 135: 853-62.

156. Baeten CGM, Konsten J, Spaans F. Dynamic graciloplasty for treatment of faecal incontinence. *Lancet* 1991; 338: 1163-5.

157. Wexner SD, Marchetti F, Jagelman DG. The role of sphincteroplasty for fecal incontinence re-evaluated: a prospective physiologic and functional review. *Dis Colon Rectum* 1991; 34: 22-30.

158. Williams NS, Patel J, George BD, Hallan RI, Watkins ES. Development of an electrically stimulated neo-anal sphincter. *Lancet* 1991; 338: 1166-9.

159. Christiansen J, Lorentzen M. Implantation of artificial sphincter for anal incontinence. *Lancet* 1987; 1: 244-5.

160. Cruveilhier J. *Ulcère chronique du rectum. In: Anatomie pathologique du corps humain*. Paris: Baillière, 1829; vol. 2: 4.

161. Lloyd-Davies OV. Quoted by Rutter KPR. Solitary rectal ulcer syndrome. *J Roy Soc Med* 1975; 68; 22-6.

162. Madigan MR, Morson BC. Solitary ulcer of the rectum. *Gut* 1969; 10: 871-81.

163. Goodall HB, Sinclair ISR. Colitis cystica profunda. *J Pathol Bacteriol* 1973; 73: 33-42.

164. Shannon Allen M. Hamartomatous inverted polyps of the rectum. *Cancer* 1966; 19: 257-65.

165. Talerman A. Enterogenous cysts of the rectum. *Br J Surg* 1971; 58: 643-7.

166. Rutter KPR, Riddell RH. The solitary ulcer syndrome of the rectum. *Clin Gastroenterol* 1975; 4: 505-30.

167. Arbuthnot Lane WA. The operative treatment of chronic constipation. *Br Med J* (Clin Res) 1908; 1: 126-30.

168. Hinton JM, Lennard-Jones JE. Constipation: definition and classification. *Postgrad Med J* 1968; 44: 720-3.

169. Preston DM, Lennard-Jones JE, Parks AG. Balloon proctogram: a new technique for the study of disorders of defaecation. *Gut* 1982; 23I: 437.

170. Meunier P, Rochas A, Lambert R. Motor activity of the sigmoid colon in chronic constipation: comparative study with normal subjects. *Gut* 1979; 20: 1095-101.

171. Martelli H, Devroede G, Arhan P, Duguay C. Mechanisms of idiopathic constipation: outlet obstruction. *Gastroenterology* 1978; 75: 623-31.

172. Kerremans R. Radio-cinematographic examination of the rectum and anal canal in cases of rectal constipation. *Acta Gastroenterol Belg* 1968; 31: 561-70.

173. Malone PS, Ransley PG, Kiely EM. Preliminary report: the antegrade continence enema. *Lancet* 1990; 336: 1217-8.

174. Preston DM, Lennard-Jones JE. Anismus in chronic constipation. *Dig Dis Sci* 1985; 30: 413.

175. Weber J, Ducrotté P, Touchais JY, Rossignol C, Denis P. Biofeedback training for constipation in adults and children. *Dis Colon Rectum* 1987; 30: 844-6.

176. Leroi AM, Berkelmans I, Denis P, Hémond M, Devroede G. Anismus as a marker of sexual abuse. Consequences of abuse on anorectal motility. *Dig Dis Sci* 1995; 40: 1411-6.

177. Bentley JFR. Posterior excisional anorectal myotomy in management of chronic faecal accumulation. *Arch Dis Child* 1966; 41: 144-7.

178. Pescatori M, Favetta U, Dedola S, Orsini S. Trans-anal stapled excision of rectal mucosal prolapse. *Tech Coloproctol* 1997; 1: 96-8.

179. Bensaude R, Bensaude A. Les hémorroïdes et leur traitement-historique. In: *Maladies de l'intestin*. Bensaude R. Paris: Masson, 1939: 17-21.

180. Denis J. Histoire d'hémorroïdes, hémorroïdes de l'Histoire. *Gastro à la une* (Laboratoires Beaufour) 1998: 31-6.

181. Racouchot JE, Petouraud C, Rivoir J. Saint Fiacre: the healer of haemorrhoids. *Am J Proctol* 1971; 22: 175-9.

182. Frexinos J. *Les ventres serrés, Histoire naturelle et sociale de la constipation et des constipés.* Paris: Louis Parienté, 1992.

183. Welling D, Wolff B, Dozois R. Piles of defeat, Napoleon at Waterloo. *Dis Colon Rectum* 1988; 31: 303-5.

184. Haeger K. *The illustrated history of surgery.* Jon van Leuven ed. London: Harold Stark (Medical), 1989.

Chapter 16

Alimentary tract disorders in infants and children

Jay L Grosfeld MD, Emeritus Lafayette Page Professor of Surgery

Indiana University School of Medicine, Indianapolis, USA

Introduction

The early history of surgery in infancy is characterised by sporadic reports documenting the first observations of specific surface anomalies. In the 2nd and 3rd century, treatment was not offered to most infants with visible abnormalities. High infant mortality and maternal death rates noted at birth, often no doubt related to sepsis, played a role in the scarcity of information concerning alimentary tract abnormalities in the newly born. The lack of available diagnostic modalities to study the alimentary tract until the turn of the 20th century limited insight into these conditions. Most information was derived from autopsy studies following the demise of an infant from some otherwise unknown cause. The advent of antisepsis, the development of anaesthesia and Roentgen's discovery of X-ray would subsequently open windows of opportunity to recognise and eventually treat disorders affecting the alimentary tract. The following chapter attempts to highlight developments and recognise those individuals that pioneered the treatment of selected major alimentary tract disorders in children.

Oesophageal atresia (OeA)

In 1670, William Durston described a blind-ending upper oesophageal pouch in an infant of a set of female thoracopagus conjoined twins [1]. In 1697, Thomas Gibson published the first description of the most common form of proximal oesophageal atresia and distal tracheo-oesophageal fistula (OeA-TOeF) [2, 3]. Sporadic case reports concerning oesophageal atresia appeared in the 19th century by Hill in 1840, Hirschsprung in 1861, and McKenzie in 1880 [4]. In 1919, a survey of the literature by Plass noted 136 instances of atresia, including 92 with a TOeF [5].

In 1888, Charles Steele attempted to repair oesophageal atresia by passing a probe superiorly through a gastrotomy into the lower oesophagus while the upper blind pouch was pushed distally. This effort was unsuccessful and autopsy demonstrated the two blind-ending oesophageal segments and no fistula [6]. Hoffman performed the first gastrostomy in an infant with OeA in 1889 [7]. In 1913, Richter of Chicago described two infants with OeA-TOeF, on whom he performed transpleural ligation of the fistula and gastrostomy without success [8]. The mortality rate for OeA remained 100%. In 1925, Lilienthal proposed division of the tracheo-oesophageal fistula and 'anastomosis' of the atretic oesophagus by tying each blind pouch over a rubber tube stent [9]. In 1936, Gage and Ochsner, proposed early transabdominal ligation of the distal end of the oesophagus and gastrostomy with secondary cervical oesophagostomy, suggesting that attempts at an extensive intrathoracic procedure was not justified in a newborn infant [10]. In 1938, Shaw performed an extrapleural ligation of the TOeF and primary oesophageal anastomosis [11]. The baby died on the 12th postoperative day of an anastomotic disruption and transfusion reaction. Lanman performed primary oesophageal repair for OeA-TOeF between 1936 and 1937, using an extrapleural approach in four infants that were unsuccessful [12]. These cases were included in a November 1940 report by Lanman regarding five cases of primary oesophageal repair and 27 other cases of OeA seen at Boston Children's Hospital during an 11-year period from 1929 to 1940 [12]. All 32 patients in the series died. Despite these fatal outcomes, Lanman was convinced that "successful operative treatment of a patient with this anomaly is only a question of time".

Humphreys and Ferrer noted that the first survivor of OeA without a TOeF was born in New York and initially treated by gastrostomy in 1935 with a thoracic operation performed 11 years later in 1946 [13]. Leven of Minneapolis described a staged approach by performing a gastrostomy on a 2500-gram male infant with OeA-TOeF on November 29th, 1939, extrapleural ligation of the TOeF on January 5th 1940 and a cervical oesophagostomy on March 27th 1940 when the infant weighed 4630 grams [14]. Similarly, William E. Ladd of Boston performed a gastrostomy on a female infant on November 28th 1939 and ligated the TOeF as well as creating a cervical oesophagostomy on March 15th 1940 [15]. Both of these patients survived, and oesophagogastric continuity was achieved using an anterior subcutaneously placed skin-tube requiring multiple operations [14, 15].

Cameron Haight was born in San Francisco, California, on September 2nd 1901, the son of a general practitioner. He attended undergraduate school at the University of California graduating with a BA degree in 1923. He attended Harvard Medical School from 1923-1926. He was an intern at Peter Bent Brigham Hospital for two years and completed surgical training at Yale from 1928-1931 [16]. Dr. Haight joined the Faculty at the University of Michigan in Ann Arbor in 1932 and was influenced by his mentor, a Dr. John Alexander. In 1935, Cameron Haight began caring for infants with OeA. His first patient was managed unsuccessfully by a gastrostomy alone. In 1939, Haight attempted five primary repairs of OeA, which were all unsuccessful. However, on March 15th 1941, the first successful primary repair of an oesophageal atresia was performed. The infant girl was described as an "unusually robust" baby who weighed 8lbs, 4oz and had been transferred from Marquette, Michigan at age 12 days [4].

The first successful primary repair of oesophageal atresia with TOeF was accomplished using a left extrapleural thoracotomy with fistula ligation and a single-layered oesophageal anastomosis using silk sutures. The patient developed an anastomotic leak on the sixth postoperative day that was managed conservatively. She later developed a stricture at the anastomosis which responded to a single dilatation. Dr. Haight presented this case in February 1942 at the Central Surgical Association meeting in Chicago, Ilinois, and published the report in 1943 [17]. In 1943, Haight revised his procedure to a right extrapleural approach because he believed that better exposure of the distal segment was obtained from this side. He also modified the anastomosis changing to a two-layer, 'telescoping' anastomosis to decrease the risk of a leak. Between 1939 and 1969, Dr. Haight (Figure 1) cared for more than 284 infants with OeA and reported a 52% overall survival rate [4]. After Haight's first success in 1941, reports of survival after direct oesophageal anastomosis were sporadic; however, many centres soon began reporting series of successes. Dr. Haight died on September 25th 1970 just after his 69th birthday.

Following Dr. Haight's historic case, efforts to further refine the classification of oesophageal anomalies was advocated by Gross [18] (who modified Vogt's classification [4]), and Waterston and colleagues [19] developed a system of risk categorisation. Attention in recent years has been focused on evaluating new risk classifications [4, 20], the timing of surgical intervention in premature babies and those with multiple associated anomalies [4]. Attention went towards the care of postoperative complications including leak, stricture, tracheomalacia, recurrent fistula [21], gastro-oesophageal reflux, and oesophageal dysfunction [4].

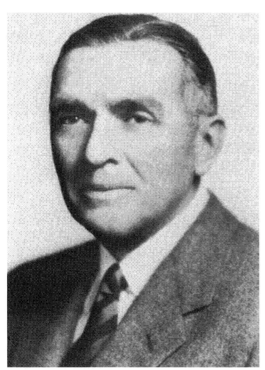

Figure 1. Cameron Haight (1901-1970).
Reproduced from the author's private collection.

Attention was also given to managing instances of long gap atresia, including proximal oesophago-myotomy [22], stretching procedures, and oesophageal replacement procedures requiring isolated colon interposition, jejunal replacement, gastric tube or total gastric transposition [4, 23]. In recent years, repair of oesophageal atresia and TOeF has been performed successfully using minimally invasive thoracoscopic techniques [24].

Oesophageal dysfunction may be a problem extending into adulthood, indicating that long-term follow-up in these patients is essential [25]. Despite the many complexities surrounding the care of patients with variants of this anomaly, the current overall survival for patients with oesophageal atresia approaches 90% at most major paediatric surgical centres [4].

Pyloric stenosis

In 1627, Hildanus provided a description of an infant that likely had pyloric stenosis who eventually survived following treatment with broth, sugar and egg yolk enemas [26]. In 1717, Blair wrote of an emaciated five-month-old infant, despite an apparent eager appetite, who had ongoing vomiting that began at one month of age. At autopsy when the baby died, the pylorus was described as cartilagenous consistent with hypertrophic pyloric stenosis [27]. In 1788, Hezekiah Beardsley of New Haven, Connecticut, provided clinical and autopsy findings in a boy that began vomiting after feeds at one week, and continued to do so until first seen at the age of two [28]. The child died at the age of five and at his post mortem examination on April 2nd 1788, he had an enlarged stomach with a hard enlarged pyloric outlet that was almost completely obstructed [28].

In 1841, Thomas Williamson of Edinburgh described a similar case [28]. In 1887, Harald Hirschsprung (Figure 7), a Danish paediatrician from Copenhagen, presented the post mortem findings on two infant girls with proof of pyloric stenosis at the German Paediatric Congress in Wiesbaden, Germany. This represented the first complete description of this condition. His treatise was published in 1888 [29]. He suggested that this entity was congenital in nature and represented failure of involution of the foetal pylorus and named it "angeborener pylorusstenose" ("congenital pyloric stenosis") [29]. Hirschsprung was convinced that this condition would be amenable to subsequent surgical treatment. In 1898, Löbker reported the first survival following performance of a gastroenterostomy [30]. He performed the procedure on two occasions; one of the infants died but the other survived. The mortality at that time for this procedure in babies was greater than 60% [28]. In 1900, Nicoll attempted to forcefully dilate the pylorus through a gastrotomy (divulsion of the pylorus) [31]. The procedure was successful in five of six patients but one was complicated by haemorrhage and perforation, and the patient died [31]. Nicoll considered the best method of treatment a gastroenterostomy with either a pyloroplasty or divulsion through a gastrotomy [28]. In 1907, Dufour and Fredet suggested that surgical correction could be accomplished by splitting the hypertrophied pyloric muscle to the submucosa and closing the muscle transversely [32]. Mack's review on the subject, noted that pyloroplasty or submucous transverse pylorotomy became the procedure of choice at the turn of the

20th century and was employed by Dent, Nicoll, Fredet, Guillemot and Weber [26, 30]. Pyloroplasty was associated with a 40% mortality [26, 30].

In 1911, Conrad Ramstedt (Figure 2) suggested that closure of the pyloric muscle was not necessary and a simple longitudinal myotomy would suffice. This observation followed an unsuccessful attempt at closing the muscle transversely on a case in which the sutures cut through the smooth muscle. The muscular defect was covered by omentum and left unsewn. The infant survived after a protracted eight-day course during which he continued to vomit. In 1912, on his next operation for pyloric stenosis, he did not attempt to suture the incised smooth muscle at all and the baby did extremely well [33]. Hence, the procedure became known as Ramstedt's pyloromyotomy [33]. Fredet continued to employ gastroenterostomy or modified pyloroplasty until the 1920s when he too adopted Ramstedt's technique [28]. The procedure has stood the test of time and continues to be the standard of care for infants with hypertrophic pyloric stenosis.

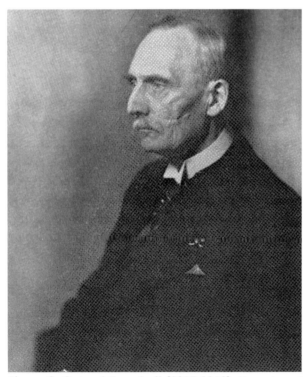

Figure 2. Conrad Ramstedt (1867-1962). *Reproduced with permission from Elsevier Science* [28].

Conrad Ramstedt was born in 1867 in Hamersleben, a small village in central Prussia. His father was the town physician. He obtained his medical education in Heidelberg and Berlin and graduated from the medical school in Halle, Germany, in 1894. After six years as a surgical assistant in Halle, Ramstedt joined the German Army medical corps. Following World War I he was discharged from the Army and in 1919, was appointed Chief of Surgery at the Rafaelklinik in Munster, Germany. He remained in Munster for the remainder of his career. Ramstedt described his early experience with pyloric stenosis at a medical congress in Munster in 1912. His observations described above were published in the October 20th 1912 issue of *Medizinische Klinik* [33]. Ramstedt was described as a quiet and humble man. His 1912 report was the only manuscript he ever published on the subject and although the condition is quite common, he performed pyloromyotomy in only 70 babies throughout his entire career. Conrad Ramstedt died in 1962 at the age of 95.

Pyloromyotomy is one of the most common operations performed in infancy. Survival was uncommon prior to 1904. However, ten years after the introduction of pyloromyotomy, the survival improved significantly. Early on, because of the significant morbidity and mortality, paediatricians would shy away from referring their patients and often attempted non-operative management of pyloric stenosis. However, they were forced to refer the baby for operative intervention when more than 30% weight loss was observed. The affected infant was often three to five months of age and appeared as a dehydrated, malnourished, shrunken, little old man with severe metabolic derangements such as hypochloraemic, hypokalaemic metabolic alkalosis. On physical examination, the hypertrophied stomach would be often visible on the abdominal wall as peristalsis proceeded from left to right across the epigastrium ('gastric waves') towards the area of pyloric obstruction. For many years an upper gastrointestinal contrast study was the mainstay of diagnosis in cases in which the hypertrophied pyloric muscle assuming an 'olive shape' was not palpated. However, in 1977, Teele and Smith described five infants in whom the diagnosis of pyloric stenosis was achieved with B-mode ultrasound [34]. In the current era, early diagnosis is facilitated by palpation of the pyloric olive on physical examination at the time of a standard well baby consultation and frequent use of ultrasonography (US) (with new generation real-time advancement in resolution and linear transducers) in babies that present with non-bilious projectile vomiting when the olive is not palpable.

In the author's opinion, a contrast barium swallow is usually reserved for those infants in whom the pyloric olive is either not palpable or the US scan is equivocal, in case the vomiting might be related to another cause. This avoids radiation exposure in most cases. Endoscopy has been suggested as an accurate method of diagnosis; however, this is an invasive procedure and should be reserved for infants with vomiting due to other causes than pyloric stenosis and is not routinely recommended. At present, the diagnosis is usually achieved early when the infant is in good condition. Pyloromyotomy is performed routinely as the first line of therapy by either a traditional open technique, using a small right upper quadrant or umbilical incison or, laparoscopically, using minimally invasive techniques [34]. Hospitalisation is usually short (one to two days) and the mortality is less than 0.5%. Despite considerable research, the exact aetiology of this condition has yet to be elucidated [30, 34].

Biliary atresia

In 1892, a thesis by John Thomson of Edinburgh titled "On so-called congenital obliteration of the bile ducts (clinical and pathological)" was the first report to clarify the findings in biliary atresia [35, 36]. In 1916, Holmes reviewed the literature and introduced the concept of 'correctable' and 'non-correctable' forms of the disease [37]. Ladd described the results of surgery in 11 infants with obstructive jaundice and documented the first successful operation for a correctable case of biliary atresia in 1928 [38]. In 1953, in his textbook *Surgery of Infancy and Childhood*, Gross reported that biliary atresia was the most common cause of obstructive jaundice in infants having non-correctable disease [18]. He noted that only 27 of 146 babies had correctable findings that permitted an anastomosis of a biliary structure to the duodenum. Fifteen of the 27 died, as did all 119 infants with uncorrectable biliary atresia [18]. A number

of procedures were developed attempting to achieve bile drainage including: partial hepatectomy with intrahepatic cholangiojejunostomy by Longmire in 1949, insertion of artificial bile ducts into the liver by Sterling in 1961, and the establishment of lymphatic drainage from the liver hilum into the jejunum by Fonkalsrud *et al* in 1966 [39]. None of these techniques proved successful. During the 1960s, early surgery for persistent jaundice was controversial, as most cases of biliary atresia could not be differentiated from 'neonatal hepatitis' or other cholestatic syndromes [36, 39]. In 1968, Thaler and Gellis suggested that neonatal hepatitis was made worse by an operation, and recommended that surgery be postponed until four months of age [36].

In 1955, Morio Kasai of Sendai, Japan, pioneered the modern day treatment of infants traditionally considered to have non-correctable biliary atresia with the introduction of hepatic porto-enterostomy. His initial reports were published in Japanese with few in the Western World becoming familiar with his findings until the next decade [40, 41]. Although there were sceptics, Kasai's results were confirmed by other Japanese and American paediatric surgeons, including Bill, and Lilly and Altman [39, 42]. Kasai's hepatic porto-enterostomy with Roux-en-Y reconstruction is now the standard surgical treatment for biliary atresia. Primary biliary drainage is achieved in over two thirds, although nearly one half of these patients had progressive liver failure [42]. Those that are less than three months of age at the time of the operation do better than older infants and have an improved chance of becoming free of jaundice [36, 43]. Since the Kasai operation is not uniformly successful, early diagnosis and intervention is the key to success [36]. The initial procedure by Kasai (and modifications by others) employed a temporary biliary stoma in the hope of reducing the risk of postoperative cholangitis [44]. Stomas have subsequently been abandoned [39, 42]. Steroids are employed to improve the flow of bile and reduce the risk of postoperative ascending cholangitis [45]. However, the results of this have been controversial [46]. Similarly, the efficacy of creating an antireflux jejunal valve in the hepatic porto-enterostomy to achieve this goal has not been sustained [47, 48]. Attempts to restore bile drainage in patients that initially drained bile with a second hepatoporto-enterostomy have for the most part been abandoned [36, 39]. In the long term, approximately 20% of patients remain free of jaundice. The remaining patients will eventually require liver transplantation [39].

Liver transplantation has been the cornerstone of salvage therapy for the initial failed hepatic porto-enterostomy and for those who later developed end-stage liver disease [37, 49]. With the availability of reduced-size and living-related donor organs, the outlook for patients with biliary atresia has improved [47, 50]. The Kasai procedure and liver transplantation have changed the survival for a disease that at one time was uniformly fatal, to greater than 85% [51]. Recently, the hepatic porto-enterostomy procedure has been successfully performed using minimally invasive laparoscopic techniques, resulting in fewer intestinal adhesions and perhaps the benefit of reducing potential blood loss at the time of future liver transplantation [52]. Biliary atresia registries of patients in the US and Japan continue to follow the long-term outcomes of these patients [53, 54].

Morio Kasai was born on September 29nd 1922 in the Aomori prefecture. He was schooled at Tohoku University in Sendai graduating from the Medical School in 1947. He became a member of the Faculty at Tohoku in 1949. Dr. Kasai spent time in research in Los Angeles in 1950 investigating the pathology of the intra and extrahepatic bile ducts in infants with biliary atresia. He continued his work with vigour upon his return to Japan. He demonstrated that there was progressive destruction of intralobular bile ducts between two months and one year of age and noted microscopic bile ductules in the fibrous remnant at the porta hepatis. He also noted that if the obliterated extrahepatic bile ducts were removed while there was still some continuity between the porta hepatis and intrahepatic biliary system that the progression of biliary atresia could be arrested. He addressed these findings by performing the first hepatic porto-enterostomy procedure in 1955. Dr. Kasai was also recognised for his expertise in the surgical management of adult patients with oesophageal cancer. He was appointed Chairman of the Department of Surgery at Tohoku University, Sendai, in 1963 and remained in that post until he retired in 1986 (Figure 3). He was awarded the Ladd Medal from the American Academy of Pediatrics for his outstanding contributions to the field of paediatric

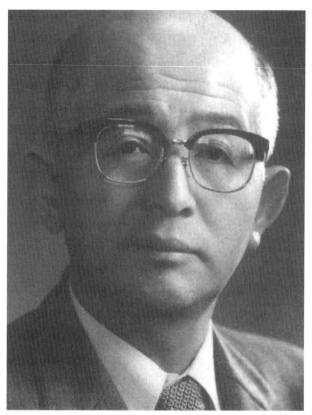

Figure 3. Morio Kasai (born 1922). Presented to the author by Professor Kasai. *Reproduced from the author's private collection.*

surgery. He is now 83 years of age and is in the rehabilitation phase following a stroke [55]. His pioneering procedure dramatically changed the care and outcomes of thousands of babies throughout the world with biliary atresia.

Intestinal atresia

Goeller is credited with the first description of ileal atresia in 1684 [56]. Other early observations concerning intestinal atresia were recorded by Calder in 1773 [57] and Osiander in 1779 [57]. Voisin performed an enterostomy for intestinal atresia in 1804, and Meckel published a review of the topic and speculated on its cause in 1812 [57]. In 1889, Bland-Sutton [57] proposed a classification of the types of atresia and postulated that intestinal atresia occurred at the sites of obliterative embryologic events, such as atrophy of the vitelline duct. In 1894, Wanitschek attempted the first resection and anastomosis for intestinal atresia unsuccessfully [57]. In 1900, Tandler [58] proposed the theory that atresia was related to failure of recanalisation (vacuolisation) of the solid-cord stage of bowel development. In 1911, Fockens [59] performed the first successful anastomosis for intestinal atresia. In 1912, Spriggs [57] suggested that mechanical accidents, including vascular occlusions, might be responsible for these occurrences. This concept was supported by clinical observations on atresia by Davis and Poynter in 1922 and Webb and Wangensteen in 1931 [57]. Evans' extensive review in 1951 [56] concerning 1498 instances of gastrointestinal atresia documented a successful result that was achieved in only 139 infants. Although mucosal atresia was frequently noted in instances of duodenal atresia, jejuno-ileal atresia as a result of epithelial plugging was uncommon. Most jejuno-ileal atresias are separated by a cordlike segment or a V-shaped mesenteric gap defect. Clinical observations by Louw and Barnard [60], Santulli and Blanc [61], and Nixon [62] that bile pigments, squames, and lanugo hairs were often found distal to atretic segments strongly suggested that factors other than epithelial plugging were involved. Foetal bile secretion and swallowing of amniotic fluid are known to take place in the eleventh and twelfth week of intra-uterine life, well after revacuolisation of the solid-cord stage.

In 1955, Louw and Barnard [60] subjected dog foetuses to ligation of mesenteric vessels and strangulation obstruction late in the course of gestation. Ten to 14 days later, examination of affected foetal intestine demonstrated a variety of atretic conditions similar to those observed clinically in human neonates. These findings strongly suggested that most jejuno-ileal atresias are the result of a late intra-uterine mesenteric vascular catastrophe.

Jan Hendrik Louw (Figure 4) was born in 1915 in Middleberg, the Central Karoo region of South Africa. His father was a school teacher and he grew up in a rural environment in Graaff-Reinet, and became an avid reader from early life. He attended school at Rondebosch Boy's School graduating in 1932, followed by attending Cape Town Medical School graduating in 1938. After an internship at Groote Schuur Hospital in 1939, he went off to military training in World War I, serving as a captain in the South African Medical Corps assigned to the British

8th Army. At that time he met David Waterston, a surgeon from London, who stimulated his interest in caring for children. Following the War he completed postgraduate surgical studies that led to an MCh (Master of Surgery) with honours. He went into general surgical private practice in Cape Town and was a part-time Lecturer and Assistant Surgeon at Groote Schuur Hospital and at the University of Cape Town. In 1951, Louw received a Nuffield Travelling Fellowship and visited children's centres in Europe (Sweden, Denmark, Scotland and England). Most of his time was spent at the Hospital for Sick Children, Great Ormond Street, London, under the direction of Denis Browne characterised as the father of paediatric surgery in the UK. He returned to Cape Town and was appointed Director of the Department of Paediatric Surgery in 1952 and subsequently,

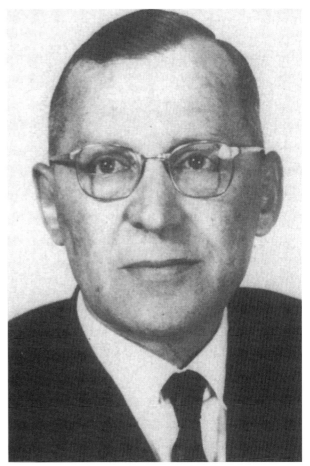

Figure 4. Jan H. Louw (1915-1992). *Courtesy of Professor Sidney Cywes.*

Professor and Chairman of Surgery at the University of Cape Town in 1955 [63]. In 1956, the Red Cross Memorial Children's Hospital was opened, serving as the first comprehensive paediatric facility in Southern Africa. Christian Barnard, his research associate, became well recognised for performing the first cardiac transplantation procedure. Professor Louw implemented his understanding of the aetiology of bowel atresia and developed a classification of these anomalies, performing numerous corrective operations at the Red Cross Memorial Children's Hospital with excellent results. Ironically, his interest in this condition was kindled by the fact that his first born son had a bowel atresia and died. Under his direction, Cape Town became a training centre for many future paediatric surgeons. Professor Louw retired in 1980. That same year he was awarded the Denis Browne Gold Medal from the British Association of Paediatric Surgeons for his numerous contributions to children's surgery. He served as President of the Surgical Research Society of South Africa and the South African Association of Paediatric Surgeons. He was awarded the Silver Medal from the Medical Association of South Africa and died at the age of 77 years in 1992. The classic experimental observations of Louw and Barnard in 1955 [60], confirming the role of late intra-uterine mesenteric vascular accidents as the cause of most jejuno-ileal atresias, laid the foundations for the modern day understanding and care of these interesting anomalies.

Following the studies performed by Louw and Barnard, others examined the origins of bowel atresia. Courtois [57] demonstrated that after foetal operations in rabbits, intra-uterine intestinal perforation can heal without a trace (with or without evidence of meconium peritonitis) or result in stenosis or atresia. Santulli and Blanc [61], Abrams, Koga et al, and Tovar et al, confirmed these findings in various experimental studies performed on foetal rabbits, sheep, dogs, and chick embryos [57]. In 2001, Sweeney and associates noted a higher incidence of associated anomalies in infants with jejunal atresia (42%) than ileal atresia (2%) and suggested that some cases of jejunal atresia may arise from a malformative process [64]. Glüer reported the occurrence of jejuno-ileal atresia in four sets of twins following intra-amniotic injection of dyes and theorised a teratogenic mechanism [65]. In a rat model using adriamycin, Gillick et al documented

that abnormal development of the notochord in the area of the developing midgut was associated with multiple intestinal atresias [57].

Frequent clinical instances of intestinal atresia as a result of late intra-uterine mesenteric vascular insults such as volvulus, intussusception, internal hernia, and constriction of the mesentery in a tight gastroschisis or omphalocoele defect have been observed [57]. The classification of atresias was revised in 1979 by Grosfeld et al, and this system has been used to describe these anomalies almost exclusively since that time [66].

De Lorimier et al [67] noted evidence of bowel infarction in 42% of 619 cases of jejuno-ileal atresia. Nixon and Tawes [68] observed macroscopic or microscopic intra-uterine peritonitis in 61 of 127 patients with atresia, with an obvious volvulus noted in 44. Murphy noted that 5% of atresias were related to foetal internal hernia [57]. Reports by Santulli and Blanc [61], Nixon and Tawes [68], and Okmian and Kovamees [57] document instances of atresia related to bowel incarceration in an omphalocoele. Iatrogenic post-partum ileal atresia as a result of umbilical clamping of an occult omphalocoele was reported by Vassy and Boles and by Landor et al [57]. Grosfeld and Clatworthy [57] observed the occurrence of jejunal atresia with infarction of the entire midgut in a tight gastroschisis defect. In an American Academy of Pediatrics survey, jejuno-ileal atresia associated with gastroschisis was observed in 2% of such patients [67]. Recently however, the incidence of gastroschisis complicated by bowel atresia is more common, being noted in 10% to 25% of cases [57, 69]. Intra-uterine intussusception is an infrequently reported cause of atresia. Evans' review [56] of 1498 cases recognised only nine examples of atresia associated with intussusception. In contrast, in a recent report, Komuro decribed intra-uterine intussusception as a cause of intestinal atresia in 12 of 48 (25%) cases commonly associated with a single mid-small bowel atresia [70]. Intussusception was not detected as a cause of atresia in instances of high jejunal, apple peel, or multiple atresias. Similar to intussusception after birth, the cause of intra-uterine intussusception is unknown. Most of these infants are full-term without associated malformations and have a cord or gap type of atresia unassociated with cystic fibrosis [57]. Postnatal intussusception as a cause of jejunal atresia in a premature infant has also been described [71]. In the author's own experience with 194 patients with jejuno-ileal atresia or stenosis treated at the Riley Children's Hospital, Indianapolis, volvulus was detected in 64, malrotation in 32, intussusception in five, internal hernia in two, gastroschisis in 28, and evidence of meconium peritonitis in 24 [57]. The late occurrence of such events accounts for the relatively low incidence (7%) of associated extra-intestinal anomalies [67]. In rare instances, jejuno-ileal atresia has been observed to coexist with biliary atresia, duodenal atresia, colon atresia, gastric atresia, Hirschsprung's disease, arthrogryposis, and to occur in identical twins [57]. Fortunately, most infants with jejuno-ileal atresia have only this single abnormality and are otherwise normal. Gross *et al* reported familial instances of combined duodenal and jejunal atresia [72]. Guttman *et al*, Aigrain *et al*, Kimble *et al*, Puri and Fujimoto, and Fourcade *et al*, described hereditary instances of multiple intestinal atresias without evidence of vascular insults or bile pigment, lanugo hairs, or squames distal to the atresia, indicating a malformative process possibly due to an autosomal recessive transmission [57]. Kilani and associates described a familial pattern of jejunal atresia with renal dysplasia that was most likely inherited as an autosomal dominant trait [73]. Walker *et al* [74] described a case of multiple atresias of the bowel associated with graft-versus-host disease and immunosuppression. Rothenberg and colleagues noted an instance of multiple atresias associated with severe immunodeficiency characterised by agammaglobulinaemia, B-cell deficiency and impaired T-cell function [75].

In their textbook *Abdominal Surgery of Infancy and Childhood* in 1941, Ladd and Gross noted a 36% survival for infants with intestinal atresia [76]. Since then, technical advances in the care of these infants have included recognising the importance of resecting the proximal atretic segment and performing an end-to-oblique anastomosis in instances with relatively normal bowel length [57, 62, 67, 68], using antimesenteric tapering [77] or imbricating techniques [57, 78] to taper the proximal atretic segment in instances that require preservation of bowel length, and using the longitudinal lengthening procedure of Bianchi [79] and the Step procedure designed by Kim [80] to enhance bowel length in instances of short bowel syndrome. With the advent of antibiotics, advances in paediatric anaesthesia, modern neonatal intensive care units (NICU), improved surgical techniques and the availability of total parenteral nutritional support, the current survival rate for jejuno-ileal atresia nears 90% [57]. Intestinal transplantation has been added as a new method to salvage infants with short bowel syndrome that fail to adapt to other measures.

Anomalies of rotation and fixation

In 1898, Mall described the process of bowel rotation and fixation following studies of reconstructed embryos [81]. In 1923, Norman Dott published the classic paper on this subject that was the first clear clinical correlation with embryologic observations based on the findings in five cases [82]. Most articles that followed described clinical cases of malrotation according to Dott's thesis. In 1928, Waugh described two cases of volvulus due to non-rotation [83]. In the early 1930s, other reports concerning anomalies of rotation and fixation by Haymond and Dragstedt, Gardner and Hart, Wakefield and Mayo and McIntosh and Donovan appeared in the literature [84]. In 1932, Ladd [85] described ten cases of malrotation with volvulus and standardised the treatment by counterclockwise detorsion. In 1936, Ladd [86] described dividing the caecal bands that passed over the duodenum and placed the caecum in the left upper quadrant. Ladd's method of releasing the duodenum and placing the caecum in the left upper quadrant remains the cornerstone of surgical treatment for non-rotation with midgut volvulus [84]. The operation is still called the Ladd procedure and the bands are referred to as Ladd's bands. In 1953, Gross [18] reported 156 cases in the first comprehensive review of the subject at the Boston Children's Hospital. In 1954, Snyder and Chaffin [87] published a clear and insightful description of rotation in which the embryology of malrotation was compared to twisting of a loop of rope around a central band that represented the superior mesenteric vessels. Estrada's comprehensive review further clarified the various abnormalities that are clinically seen due to anomalous rotation and fixation [88]. Early recognition of this condition is essential to obviate the risk of midgut volvulus and strangulation of the midgut [84].

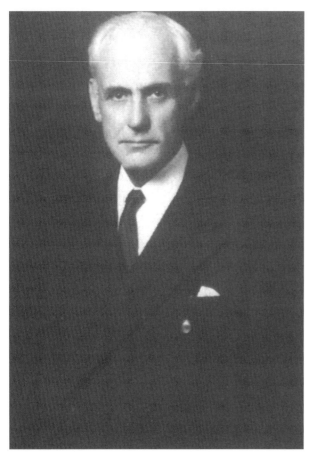

Figure 5. William E. Ladd (1880-1967). *Reproduced with permission from Springer Science and Business Media. Bill AH. William E. Ladd MD - Great Pioneer of North American Pediatric Surgery. Progr Pediatr Surg 1986; 20: 52-9.*

William E. Ladd (Figure 5) was born in the vicinity of Boston, Massachusetts in 1880. He attended both undergraduate school (1902) and medical school (1906) at Harvard University. He rowed in the crew for Harvard and maintained a life-long interest in the sport. Experience obtained in the care of children injured in the Halifax explosion, kindled his interest in limiting his surgical practice to the care of children. In addition to his pioneering work on anomalies of intestinal rotation and fixation, he was the first to describe the diagnostic findings on barium enema in instances of intussusception in 1913. Adopting Ramstedt's technique he was responsible for promoting the surgical cure of pyloric stenosis in the New England community and reported a mortality rate of 15% in 1918. He performed the first successful operation for a correctable case of biliary atresia in 1928 [38]. Dr. Ladd served as Surgeon-in-Chief of the Boston Children's Hospital from 1927-1947. He is

considered the 'father of American paediatric surgery' and was the mentor for many young men pursuing a career in children's surgery including Robert E. Gross, Orvar Swenson, Alexander Bill, and H. William Clatworthy. Thomas Lanman was his close associate for many years (1927-1945). He and Dr. Gross wrote the first modern paediatric surgical textbook in 1941. He was a founding member of the Section on Surgery at the American Academy of Pediatrics in 1948. Dr. Ladd retired in 1946 and died in 1967 at the age of 87 years. In his honour, the American Academy of Pediatrics developed the William E. Ladd Medal, the highest award given to paediatric surgeons of distinction in America in recognition of outstanding contributions in the field.

Colorectal conditions

Hirschsprung's disease (HD)

Hirschsprung's disease is a common cause of neonatal intestinal obstruction that occurs worldwide. The first observation concerning this condition is attributed to Frederick Ruysch (Figure 6), a Dutchman, in 1691 [89, 90].

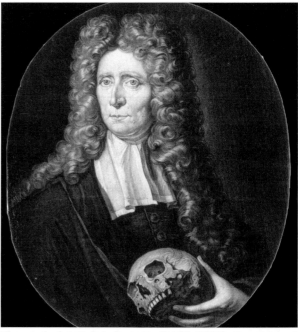

Figure 6. Frederick Ruysch (1638-1731). *Reproduced with permission from the Wellcome Library, London.*

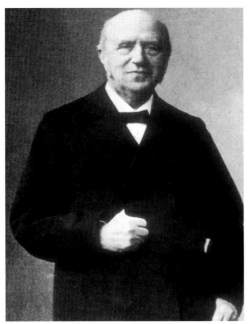

Figure 7. Harald Hirschsprung (1830-1916). *Reproduced with permission from Springer Science and Business Media. © 2006 Springer-Verlag, Heidelberg, 2006* [91].

In 1800, Battini (Italy) described an additional instance and Jacobi (New York) reported two infants that were likely to have had HD; one of them died following colostomy in 1869 [91]. In 1886 at a meeting of the Berlin Paediatric Society, Harald Hirschsprung (Figure 7), a Danish paediatrician from Copenhagen, presented a detailed description of severe constipation due to dilatation and hypertrophy of the colon in two infants who died at eight and 11 months respectively [92].

In 1898, Frederick Treves from London (Figure 13, Chapter 12) documented the presence of the narrow distal rectum in an affected child [93]. In 1899, Griffith reviewed 55 collected cases, and in 1900 Lennander from Sweden suggested a neurogenic origin for this condition [91]. In 1901, Tittel from Austria noted absence of the ganglia in the collapsed colon of a child with HD [94]. By 1904, Hirschsprung had accumulated ten personal cases; nine were boys [91, 95]. He focused on the dilated colon as the source of problems and considered this a congenital condition that was essentially lethal. He offered no specific recommendations for treatment. In 1923, Ishikawa from Kyushu, Japan [96], noted absence of

parasympathetic nerves in the pelvic colon and Dalle Valle [97] (1920) observed absent ganglion cells in the lower colon and ganglion cells present in the ileum in a baby with megacolon. Cameron confirmed these observations in 1928 [91]. In 1946, Ehrenpeiss from Stockholm focused on the narrow distal rectum as the cause of the obstruction, resulting in proximal colonic dilatation [91]. In 1948, Whitehouse and Kernohan described absence of ganglion cells in both Meissner's and Auerbach's plexeuses [98]. In 1949, Bodian and colleagues in London noted absence of ganglion cells in the narrow rectum in 11 babies with megacolon [99]. The mortality at the time was greater than 75%.

In the mid-1940s, Swenson (Figure 8) and Bill from Boston (Massachusetts) noted improvement in infants with congenital megacolon by performing a sigmoid colostomy. Attempts at colostomy closure resulted in recurrence of obstruction [100, 101]. In 1948, Swenson and Bill performed the first definitive

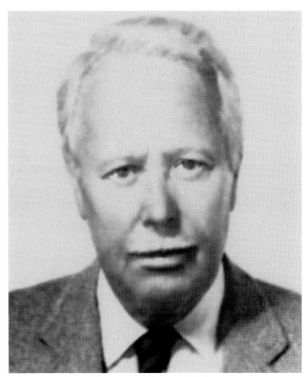

Figure 8. Orvar Swenson (born 1909). *Reproduced with permission from Springer Science and Business Media. © 2006 Springer-Verlag, Heidelberg, 2006* [91].

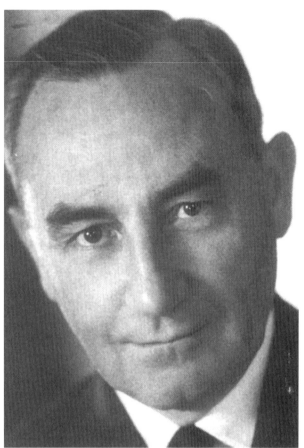

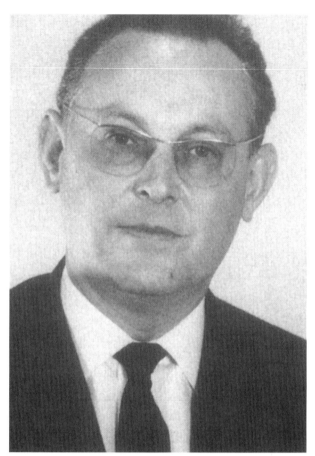

Figure 9. Fritz Rehbein. *Courtesy of Professor Alexander Holschneider, Cologne.*

Figure 10. Bernard Duhamel. *Reproduced with permission from Springer Science and Business Media. © 2006 Springer-Verlag, Heidelberg, 2006* [91].

corrective procedure for HD, namely rectosigmoidectomy and primary colo-anal anastomosis [102]. In 1955, they popularised the diagnostic full-thickness rectal biopsy [103]. State [104] and Rehbein [105] (Figure 9) described the use of variants of low anterior resection for HD patients. In 1956, Duhamel [106] (Figure 10) proposed the retrorectal pull-through procedure that was modified by Grob from Zurich, Martin from Cincinnati, Soper from Iowa, Ikeda from Fukuoka and Steichen and Ravitch from Pittsburgh [91, 103]. In 1960 Soave [107] from Genoa (Figure 11), described the endorectal pull-through operation that was further modified by Pellerin from Paris and Cutait from Brazil, using a delayed anastomosis and Boley from New York employing a primary anastomosis [91]. In 1965, Dobbins and Bill [108] described the submuscosal suction rectal biopsy for the diagnosis of HD and in 1967, Schnaufer *et al* [109]

reported on the anorectal manometric findings. The success rates observed for all the major procedures (Swenson, Duhamel and Soave) used for this condition are somewhat similar [92, 103]. Postoperative enterocolitis continues to be a significant problem and may be related to deficient mucus production [103]. Current trends include: primary transanal neonatal [110] and laparoscopic-assisted pull-through procedures [111] for patients with low segment disease; Soave or Duhamel operations for babies with total colonic aganglionosis with involvement of the mid to distal small bowel [103, 112]; and aganglionic patch enteroplasty [112, 113], myectomy-myotomy [114] and intestinal transplantation for extensive proximal small bowel aganglionosis [115]. So [116] and Carcassone [117] were early advocates of primary pull-through operations without a preliminary colostomy. Luis de la Torre [110] of Mexico City was the first to perform a primary transanal pull-through procedure and Keith Georgeson [111], from Birmingham, Alabama, has been a strong advocate of laparoscopic-assisted pull-through operations. The current mortality for this condition is now less than 2% [103].

Orvar Swenson was born on February 7th 1909 in Halsingborg, Sweden, a suburb of Malmo. His parents moved to America settling in Missouri. He attended undergraduate school at William Jewell College, Liberty, Missouri, graduating in 1933. He graduated from the Harvard Medical School in 1937. He was an intern at Ohio State University for one year and returned to Boston in 1938 as a resident in pathology at the Boston Children's Hospital and Peter Bent Brigham Hospital. He was a surgery resident at the Brigham (1939-1942) and Children's (1944-1945) Hospitals.

He joined the surgical staff at the Boston Children's Hospital under the direction of Drs. William E. Ladd and Robert E. Gross in 1945. Dr.

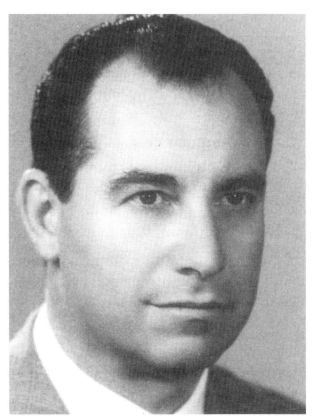

Figure 11. Franco Soave (1917-1984). *Reproduced with permission from Springer Science and Business Media. © 2006 Springer-Verlag, Heidelberg, 2006* [91].

Swenson became interested in the care of babies with severe constipation and congenital megacolon. He was an astute observer and performed colostomy as a life-saving measure in six babies with apparent colonic obstruction of unknown cause. Attempts at colostomy closure were followed by recurrent obstructive symptoms leading him to focus on the distal narrow rectum noted in these babies as the site of obstruction. Following dissections on puppies in the laboratory, Swenson and his colleague Alexander Bill developed the technique of sphincter-saving rectosigmoidectomy as the first operation to successfully treat congenital megacolon. At the time, there was considerable controversy surrounding the importance of the presence or absence of ganglion cells in this disorder. This played no role in the decision to proceed with the first pull-through operation in 1948 [102]. Reports concerning important histological findings by Whitehouse and Kernohan [98] and Bodian *et al* [99] were made regarding the absence of ganglion cells following this landmark surgical event in 1948 and 1949 respectively.

Swenson moved to the Boston Floating Hospital at Tuft's University in 1950 serving as the Surgeon-in-Chief. He was promoted to full Professor at Tufts in 1957. In 1960, he relocated to the Chicago Memorial Children's Hospital succeeding Dr. Willis Potts as Surgeon-in-Chief. He was appointed Professor of Surgery at Northwestern University and served as the Training Program Director in Children's Surgery. He was the mentor for numerous young paediatric surgeons. Dr. Swenson retired in 1974 at the age of 65 years. He maintained a faculty position at the University of Miami until 1980 when he fully retired from practice. He was an avid sailor and until recently, he and Melva, his wife of 65 years, would sail their boat in Maine during the summer and in Florida in the winter. Dr. Swenson was awarded the Ladd Medal from the American Academy of Pediatrics in 1959 and the Denis Browne Gold medal from the British Association of Paediatric Surgeons (BAPS) in 1979 for his seminal contribution. He was the 4th President of the American Pediatric Surgical Association from 1973-1974. Although retired he retained a keen interest in HD and continues to write about the subject more than 56 years later [118]. He is currently 97 years of age and lives with his wife in Charleston, SC.

Anorectal malformations

Soranus described dividing a thin anal membrane and dilating the opening in a baby in the 2nd century AD [119]. Paul of Aegina pierced an anal membrane and used a wedge-shaped tent dilator in the 7th century [120]. In 1676, Cooke treated a child by making a small incision over a blind anal membrane and dilated the aperture with an elder pith [121]. In 1693, Saviard was the first to attempt treatment of a high termination of the bowel by plunging a trocar through the perineum [120]. In 1787, Benjamin Bell [122] performed the first perineal dissection in two newborn infants finding the blind-ending rectum and inserting a trocar to evacuate meconium. Prolonged bouginage was required to preserve the open passage using a sponge tent. In 1792, Mantell published a report concerning a girl with a rectovaginal fistula in whom he had performed an incision in the perineum and carried it up to a probe placed through the vagina into the fistula to create an anal passage [123].

Following an autopsy in an infant with rectal atresia, Littré in 1710 proposed that the bowel be brought to the surface of the abdomen to function as an anus [124]. The first successful sigmoid colostomy for imperforate anus was performed by Duret in 1793 on a female infant who survived into adult life [125]. In 1798, Martin of Lyon suggested insertion of a sound in a colostomy and push it distally to identify the blind-ending rectum during a later perineal dissection [119]. In 1856, Chassignac reported successful use of this technique in two infants with a colostomy [119]. However, colostomy in the newborn was neither a popular procedure nor was it widely accepted at the time [120].

In 1834, J-N Roux tried to preserve external sphincter function and used a midline longitudinal incision extended towards the coccyx [126]. The incision continued through the elliptical sphincter ani muscle and levators and when the rectal atresia was palpated, a bistoury (trocar) was inserted into the bowel releasing meconium. Dressings and bouginage were required to prevent premature closure. In 1835, Jean Amussat (Figure 12) performed the first proctoplasty by suturing the opened rectal atresia to the perineal skin in the midline [127]. This operation was a landmark procedure at the time and gained wide acceptance and was used frequently for the rest of

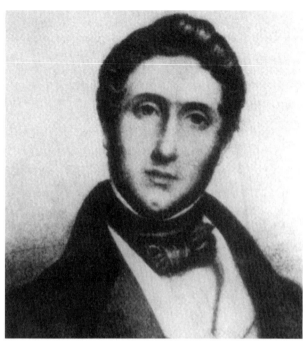

Figure 12. Jean Z. Amussat (1796-1856). *Reproduced with permission from the Wellcome Library, London.*

the 19th century. Amussat used an extensive T-shaped incision that basically destroyed the sphincter mechanism. In some instances he described removing the coccyx to aid exposure and mobilisation of the rectum [127].

In 1835, Amussat performed the first sutured proctoplasty for imperforate anus, and techniques to repair rectovaginal and rectovulvar fistulae were described by Dieffenbach in 1845 and Rizzoli in 1854 and again in 1869 [119, 120]. By 1860, Bodenhamer noted that in some instances of high rectal atresia, the sphincter muscles were detected, but not in all cases [128]. Despite this observation he shunned colostomy and recommended that an artificial anus should always be established in the perineum. He championed the midsagittal incision first described by Roux [126] 27 years earlier. In 1879, McLoed described an abdominoperineal (AP) procedure for instances in which the blind rectal atretic end was not found below [119]. By 1882, Amussat's procedure gained favour in the US [127]. Before the acceptance of Listerian principles, the operative mortality for both proctoplasty and colostomy was greater than 60% [120]. In 1886, McCormac was one of the few to suggest a two-stage procedure: preliminary colostomy and subsequent proctoplasty [129]. In 1897, Matas combined a sacral approach to rectal atresia with sacrotomy to aid exposure in instances of high-lying anomalies and predicted this would be the route of choice for these procedures in the future [130]. Matas was not a proponent of colostomy and favoured a one-stage procedure in the neonatal period [130]. His bias influenced the care of babies with anorectal malformations for the next four decades.

Textbooks of surgery in 1908 recommended colostomy only as a life-saving measure, otherwise the perineal approach was employed for all other cases [119]. In 1908, Mastin noted that the AP procedure had little to attract surgeons and scarcely could be viewed as a rational procedure [119]. By 1922, it was recognised that the perineal approach was often futile in instances of high rectal atresia [119]. Despite these observations, by 1926, laparotomy with or without a colostomy was considered a procedure of last resort and was associated with a high mortality [119].

In 1930, Wangensteen and Rice described the radiographic invertogram as a method to determine the level of termination of the rectal atresia and decide whether a perineal approach was rational [131]. In 1934, Drs. Ladd and Gross at the Boston Children's Hospital proposed a classification for anorectal malformations (Types 1-4) that closely resembled Bodenhamer's work published 74 years earlier [128, 132]. Only one of their 162 cases was managed by a one-stage AP approach and proctoplasty [132]. At the time the success rate for cases of rectovaginal fistula was 50%, recto-urethral fistula 20%, and the mortality was in excess of 50%. In 1936, Stone described transplantation of a low rectovaginal fistula to the anal site without splitting the rectum sagittally. He termed the condition imperforate anus with rectovaginal cloaca [119]. Before 1940, an early perineal operation was still considered the method of choice by many surgeons [119].

Following World War II, the availability of antibiotics and improvements in anaesthesia had a positive influence on reducing the septic complications associated with bowel surgery. In 1948, Rhoads and colleagues rekindled interest in a combined AP approach for cases of imperforate anus and high rectal

atresia [133]. In 1950, Denis Browne (Figure 13) of Great Ormond Street in London reclassified defects associated with rectal agenesis using a thesis originally described by Wood-Jones in 1904 and 1915 [119, 134]. The term 'covered anus' became popular and initial colostomy and subsequent AP pull-through through a hole stretched (not cut) in the pelvic floor was advocated for high lesions. Browne also popularised the 'cutback' anoplasty for instances of perineal fistula [134].

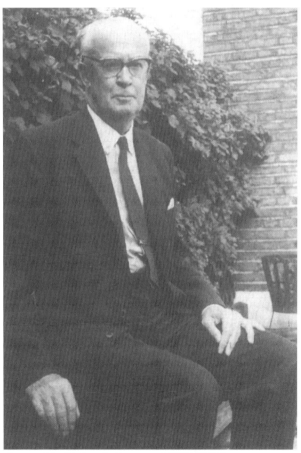

Figure 13. Sir Denis Browne (1892-1967). *Reproduced with permission from Springer Science and Business Media. Rickham PP. Denis Browne: Surgeon. Progr Pediatr Surg 1986; 20: 69-75.*

Denis Browne was born on April 28th, 1892 in Toorak, a suburb of Melbourne, Australia, and was raised on a sheep farm near Singleton in the Hunter Valley, New South Wales. He attended The King's School in Sydney at age 13 taking up tennis. At 18 he won a scholarship to St. Paul's University College,

Sydney University, to study medicine and excelled at tennis and shooting. Following graduation in 1915, he enlisted in the Australian forces in World War I, served in Gallipoli, Turkey, acquired typhoid fever and was sent home. He finished the war in Europe (in France) at the rank of Major in 1919 and stayed in England for surgical training, obtaining his FRCS in 1922. He confined his practice to children, becoming a Consultant Surgeon in 1926 and was the dominant figure in children's surgery at Great Ormond Street (GOS), London. He was a tall (6ft 4 inches), strapping, athletic man, who was somewhat controversial. He was rather intimidating to his junior staff, had a combative approach to his colleagues and an aggressive surgical technique [135]. In addition to his work in anorectal malformations, Browne made major contributions to the care of enlarged tonsils, club-foot, cleft palate, congenital dislocation of the hip, and hypospadias, and constructed innovative splints, instruments and other devices [136]. He was viewed as the father of paediatric surgery in the UK and taught many youthful enthusiasts to pursue this work as registrars (residents) at GOS. He continued his passion for tennis, played once at Wimbledon and practised strokes against a wall in a room in the hospital between cases! He welcomed students from abroad, especially those from Australia. He was founding President of the British Association of Paediatric Surgeons (BAPS) in 1953. He was awarded the Ladd Medal from the American Academy of Pediatrics, knighted by the English Queen Elizabeth in 1961 and in the same year he was awarded Chevalier Légion d'Honneur in France. He died in 1967 at the age of 74 years. He was survived by his second wife, Lady Moyra. The BAPS developed the Denis Browne Gold medal to recognise distinguished leaders in the field for outstanding contributions to paediatric surgery.

In 1953, Douglas Stephens (Figure 14) while working with Denis Browne in London, made the important contribution of sacroperineal rectoplasty, and emphasised the role of the levator ani muscle in the pelvic floor, but played down the importance of the internal and external anal sphincters [137]. Two of his four patients who had this procedure achieved continence.

F. Douglas Stephens was born in Australia in 1913. He attended medical school at the University of Melbourne, graduating in 1936. He served in the Australian Medical Corps in World War II. At the end of his duty he studied children's surgery under Sir Denis Browne at Great Ormond Street, London. He returned to Melbourne as a research surgeon at the Royal Children's Hospital in 1952, and was Director of Research from 1957-1975. He was an expert patho-embryologist with a special emphasis on the study of foetal abnormalities of the developing hindgut and genito-urinary tract. In 1975, he was appointed Professor of Urology and Surgery at Northwestern University in Chicago, Illinois and Research Director at the Children's Memorial Hospital. His fertile brain and academic approach led him to advance hypotheses of causation about diverse conditions, many of which were never published, and to interrupt his operating by making notes with sterile pencil and paper.

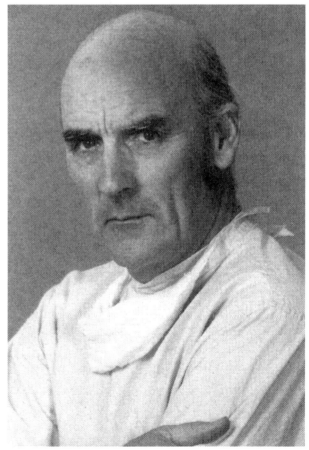

Figure 14. Douglas Stephens (born 1913). *Reproduced from the author's private collection.*

He retired in 1986 and returned to Melbourne as Honorary Research Fellow, Department of Surgery at the Royal Children's Hospital. He has continued to publish numerous textbooks and pursue his interest in anorectal malformations. At the age of 93 he remains an active tennis player and an artist with a passion for water colours.

In 1959, Fritz Rehbein of Bremen reintroduced the endorectal pull-through combined with an AP approach for boys with recto-urethral fistula [138]. The endorectal concept was initially described by Hochenegg in Austria in 1889 [139]. Rehbein divided the bowel at laparotomy, stripped the mucosa from the distal rectal atretic end and brought the proximal bowel through the resultant muscular sleeve to the anal dimple to perform an anoplasty [138]. He missed the puborectalis sling in performing this procedure. In 1960, Romauldi of Italy used the same approach for girls with a rectovestibular fistula [140]. In 1961, after extensive dissections, Stephens proposed the importance of the puborectalis muscle as the main muscle of continence but recognised that soiling accidents continued to occur because of mucus leakage from the anal canal due to total or functional absence of the external sphincter [119].

In 1963, Kiesewetter of Pittsburgh modified Stephens' operation by performing an abdomino-sacroperineal procedure [141]. He used the abdominal approach to isolate the recto-urethral fistula and the sacral route to enter the supralevator space by splitting the pubococcygeus and ileococcygeus in the midline. Unlike Stephens, Kiesewetter believed the external sphincter muscle was present and worth saving. Kiesewetter later met with Rehbein and adopted Rehbein's mucosal stripping and endorectal concept, while Rehbein added Stephens' inclusion of the puborectalis sling to his procedure [120]. In 1963, Stephens published the first modern major textbook on the subject [142]. In 1967, Kiesewetter and Nixon found the external sphincter muscle present in all nine cases of imperforate anus studied at autopsy but, found a gap between the sphincter and the puborectalis muscle [119]. In 1969, Justin Kelly of Australia reported the innovative use of cineradiographic defaecography in an attempt to evaluate function (of the puborectalis) following procedures for anorectal malformations [143]. In 1973,

a prone cross-table radiograph was recommended as an alternative to the classic invertogram in diagnosing the level of rectal atresia [119].

In 1970, a workshop was held in Melbourne, Australia, to reclassify anorectal malformations. A rather complex, male/female low, intermediate and high classification was developed. The contents of the workshop were published by Stephens and Smith in 1971 [144]. Stephens and Smith noted that the functional results of the AP procedure and sacroperineal operation were similar. However, they cited problems with the Kiesewetter/Rehbein operation, including mucosal prolapse at the anoplasty site, incomplete use of striated muscle, and loss of rectal storage capacity by using the atretic rectal segment for the muscle sleeve. Yet, they agreed that this procedure was more acceptable than an AP approach alone. The controversy continued, and in 1971, Stephens and Smith recommended the sacro-perineal approach for re-operative procedures after an initially inadequate rectoplasty [119]. Dissatisfied with the outcomes of other procedures, Mollard recommended in 1978 an anterior perineal approach bringing the atretic bowel down in front of the puborectalis sling [145].

Reports concerning the results of the procedures advocated by Stephens and Smith, Rehbein, and Kiesewetter suggested that different subjective criteria for grading and definitions used to assess function made it difficult to compare results [119]. Studies often focused on the area of specific interest to the surgeon that advocated the procedure. Comments like excellent, good, fair and poor characterised the studies, and continence was assessed according to whether one was evaluating puborectalis function or other sphincter activity [119]. Sphincter tone was frequently not mentioned. How motility was evaluated was often in question and terms like colonic inertia appeared to address failures and severe constipation that followed the procedure [144, 145]. In 1977, Kiesewetter noted an improvement over time from poor to good in low anomalies and from poor to fair in high anomalies, and that switching from an AP approach to abdominosacroperineal or sacroperineal approach did not improve function [120]. The same year, Nixon and Puri evaluated 47 children with high anomalies; only seven had a good outcome, 28 were fair, 11 poor and seven required a permanent colostomy [146]. The seven good outcome patients soiled to some degree for 6-17 years of follow-up. In 1979, Hecker and Holschneider presented a manometric and functional classification that evaluated external sphincter contraction, propulsive wave frequency and critical volume and noted that "an intelligent patient can effect social continence" [147].

Mucosal prolapse and stricture of the anoplasty site remained a problem and a variety of secondary plastic procedures were suggested to revise the anoplasty by Mollard and Rowe, Nixon, Becmeur *et al*, and Anderson *et al* [119]. Incontinence also continued to be a problem and free muscle transfer, reverse smooth muscle plasty, gracilis muscle flaps and artificial sphincters were used in an attempt to correct this problem with very marginal results [119, 120]. Re-operation for a missed puborectalis sling and failed previous procedures was also attempted [119].

The PSARP operation (posterior sagittal anorectoplasty) described by Peter de Vries and Alberto Peña (Figure 15) in 1982 was a new landmark event in the history of anorectal malformations [148]. It was just as influential as the contributions by Amussat and Stephens, and was rapidly adopted by many paediatric surgeons throughout the world [127, 136, 137, 148]. They resurrected the concept initially proposed by Roux [126] in 1834 and subsequently used by Bodenhamer in 1860 [128], and redefined the arrangement of the pelvic muscles and sphincters as a fused sphincter muscle complex. Peña completely divided all the muscles posteriorly in the midline from the anal dimple to the coccyx. He divided the recto-urethral fistula from within the atretic segment by separating the mucosa and smooth muscle to avoid urethral and neural damage. The distal atretic segment was tapered to fit within the muscle complex, and the divided muscles were sutured posteriorly around and to the neorectum before performing the anoplasty [149]. Slight tension was placed to the anoplasty site to draw the skin in and avoid prolapse. The popularity of the PSARP procedure was a reflection of discontent with the results obtained after other procedures. While the procedure allowed a precise anatomic reconstruction, it was not a panacea [150, 151]. Although the rate of continence improved, it became apparent that many

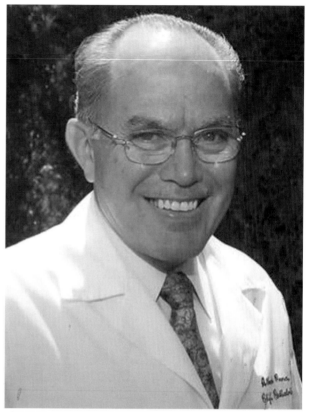

Figure 15. Dr. Alberto Peña (contemporary).
Reproduced from the author's private collection.

of the children had significant motility disorders and faecal retention was a major problem [152, 153]. Heightened awareness of this problem led to establishment of follow-up programmes to assure patient and parent compliance with postoperative anal dilatation and appropriate rectal washouts using enemas [119]. With the advent of the new procedure and continued controversy, an additional conference was held in 1984 at the Wingspread Conference Center in Wisconsin to re-evaluate anorectal malformations in regard to classification, embryology, anatomy and treatment. The Wingspread classification simplified the male/female low, intermediate and high variants decided upon in 1970 and transferred many female cloacal variants to separate subgroups and characterised the more uncommon anomalies as rare conditions [120]. Bladder and cloacal exstrophy and the various neuropathies were excluded. The presentations at the Wingspread Conference were edited by F. Douglas Stephens and E. Durham Smith and published in a Birth Defects monograph by the March of Dimes in 1988 [154]. The 1980s up to the early 1990s was a period that was also characterised by children's surgeons paying much closer attention to recognition and repair of cloacal anomalies. Dr. Raffensperger [155] of Chicago and especially Dr. Hendren [119, 156] of Boston were instrumental in developing methods of repair. Later, Peña and his associates employed the posterior sagittal approach to repair cloacal anomalies and developed considerable experience in the management of these patients [119, 157]. Peña also championed the concept of urogenital advancement in the repair of high cloacal defects with persistent urogenital sinus [158].

Alberto Peña (Figure 15) was born in Mexico and attended the Military Medical School in Mexico City. He served an internship and residency in surgery at the Central Military Hospital. He was an Assistant and Senior Resident in Paediatric Surgery at Boston Children's Hospital. He returned to Mexico and was appointed Surgeon-in-Chief, National Institute of Pediatrics and Professor of Pediatric Surgery at the University of Mexico. In 1980, along with Peter de Vries, he developed the posterior sagittal anorectoplasty for the treatment of anorectal malformations and advocated the urogenital advancement procedure for high urogenital sinus defects. From 1985-2005, Dr. Peña was Chief of Pediatric Surgery at the Schneider Children's Hospital, Long Island Jewish Medical Center and Professor of Pediatric Surgery at the Albert Einstein College of Medicine. He has organised annual hands-on courses to teach surgeons the nuances of caring for babies with anorectal malformations and has performed the PSARP operation in more than 2,000 cases around the world. He is currently Professor of Pediatric Surgery, University of Cincinnati College of Medicine and Director of the Colorectal Center, Children's Hospital Medical Center, Cincinnati, Ohio.

In 1992, Malone and associates described the antegrade colonic enema concept using an appendicostomy on the anterior abdominal wall or hidden within the umbilicus to flush the colon (MACE procedure) [159]. This was viewed as an attractive alternative to traditional retrograde enema washouts from below in children with incontinence or significant faecal retention [159]. The Chait percutaneous caecostomy tube and Gauderer sigmoid button were suggested as alternatives [119]. Brent and Stephens had identified the problem of rectal ectasia in 1976 and this was reaffirmed by Cloutier et al, Cheu and Grosfeld, and Peña and associates [119]. Rectal ectasia occurs more commonly in children with low anomalies and may result from longstanding distension of the rectal segment in-utero. Some of these patients (including those with megasigmoid) respond favourably to resection of the abnormal bowel [119]. Despite the apparent popularity of the PSARP operation, in the 1990s a number of articles appeared in the literature recommending anterior sagittal anorectoplasty, anterior perineal anorectoplasty, and other modifications of the Mollard approach [119, 160].

In the 1990s, advances in technology were used in the assessment of patients with anorectal malformations [119]. Transperineal ultrasonography was employed to locate the infracoccygeal level of atresia and identify fistulae. Magnetic resonance imaging proved useful in evaluating the pelvic and perineal muscles and identifying tethered cord, vertebral anomalies and spinal dysraphic syndromes. Anal endosonography became available to assess postoperative sphincter muscle function and the position of the pulled-through segment within the sphincter complex [119].

The advent of minimally invasive surgical techniques also influenced treatment. Georgeson [161] and others employed a laparoscopically-assisted one-stage abdominoperineal pull-through procedure that provided excellent exposure deep in the pelvis. They divided the fistula using a harmonic scalpel or endoscopic clips, identified the sphincter complex and puborectalis muscle and passed the colon through an intact sphincter to the anal dimple where an anoplasty was constructed in the neonatal period. Laparotomy and trans-sacral incisions were avoided and postoperative pain was diminished. Iwanaka et al [162] and Yamataka et al [163] used a laparoscopic muscle stimulator to accurately locate the sphincter during laparoscopic-assisted repair. Albanese and colleagues advocated one-stage correction of high imperforate anus in the male neonate as a method of preserving the neural framework for normal bladder and bowel function that exist at the time of birth [164]. Results are not yet available to determine whether these modifications will remain enduring and result in favourable long-term outcomes.

The current mortality for these anomalies has for the most part been very low and is related to the presence of associated anomalies and unfavourable chromosomal and genetic syndromes, rather than the result of treatment of the anorectal malformation *per se*. In general, agreement has been reached regarding some embryologic and anatomic considerations, diagnostic evaluation and pre-operative assessment [165, 166]. Most investigators would agree that results are better following repair of low defects when compared with intermediate and high anomalies and those with cloacae. There remains a number of areas of controversy regarding choice and timing of procedure and methodology to assess results. Certain poor prognostic factors have been identified including, abnormal sacrum, deficient pelvic innervation, poor perineal musculature and disorders of colonic motility [119]. An international conference on anorectal malformations held at Krickenbeck Castle near Cologne, Germany, in 2005 developed new classification systems and methods to assess function and outcomes [167].

Conclusions

Space limitations prevent the inclusion of many others that have contributed to the history of alimentary tract surgery in infancy. As the field of children's surgery is relatively young we chose specific individuals that were pioneers and seminal events that helped the specialty get off the ground. Selection of topics spanned the various areas of the alimentary tract from the oesophagus to the anorectum and focused mainly on important conditions that affected the newborn baby. Paediatric surgery is a field that is still evolving and remarkable advances have been made in the management of congenital and acquired conditions affecting many other organ systems that are beyond the scope of this chapter.

References

1. Durston W. A narrative of a monstrous birth in Plymouth October 22, 1670 with anatomical observations. *Philosophical Transactions of the Royal Society,* 1670; 2096.
2. Gibson T. *The anatomy of humane bodies epitomized,* 5th Ed. London: Thomas Warren for Awnsham and Churchill, 1697.
3. Ashcraft KW, Holder TM. The story of esophageal atresia and tracheoesophageal fistula. *Surgery* 1969; 65: 332-40.
4. Harmon CM, Coran AG. Congenital anomalies of the esophagus. In: *Pediatric Surgery,* 6th ed. Grosfeld JL, O'Neill JA, Jr, Fonkalsrud EW, *et al,* Eds. Philadelphia: Mosby, 2006.
5. Plass E. Congenital atresia of the esophagus with tracheo-esophageal fistula: associated with fused kidney. A case report and a survey of the literature on congenital anomalies of the esophagus. *Johns Hopkins Hospital Reports* 1919; 18: 259.
6. Steele C. Case of deficient oesophagus. *Lancet* 1888; 2: 764.
7. Hoffman W. Atresia oesophogi congenital et communicato inter oesapgaiu et tracheon. *Griefswald,* 1899.
8. Richter HM. Congenital atresia of the esophagus: an operation designed for its cure. *Surg Gynecol Obstet* 1913; 17: 397.
9. Lilienthal H. *Imperforate esophagus. Thoracic Surgery.* Philadelphia: WB Saunders, 1925: 12.
10. Gage M, Ochsner AO. The surgical treatment of congenital tracheo-esophageal fistula in the newborn. *Ann Surg* 1936; 103: 725.
11. Shaw R. Surgical correction of congenital atresia of the esophagus with tracheo-esophageal fistula. *J Thorac Surg* 1939; 9: 213.
12. Lanman TH. Congenital atresia of the esophagus: a study of thirty-two cases. *Arch Surg* 1940; 7: 1060-83.
13. Humphreys GH II, Ferrer JJ. Management of esophageal atresia. *Am J Surg* 1964; 107: 406-11.
14. Leven NL. Congenital atresia of the esophagus with tracheo-esophageal fistula. A report of successful extrapleural ligation of the fistulous communication and cervical esophagostomy. *J Thorac Surg* 1941; 10: 648-57.
15. Ladd W. The surgical treatment of esophageal atresia and tracheo-esophageal fistulas. *N Engl J Med* 1944; 230: 625-37.
16. Bae J-O, Widmann WD, Hardy MA. Cameron Haight: pioneer in the treatment of esophageal atresia. *Curr Surg* 2005; 62: 327-9.
17. Haight C, Towsley HA. Congenital atresia of the esophagus with tracheo-esophageal fistula. Extrapleural ligation of fistula and end-to-end anastomosis of esophageal segments. *Surg Gynecol Obstet* 1943; 76: 672-88.
18. Gross RE. *The surgery of infancy and childhood.* Philadelphia: WB Saunders, 1953.
19. Waterston DJ, Carter RB, Aberdeen E. Esophageal atresia: tracheo-oesophageal fistula. A study of survival in 218 infants. *Lancet* 1962; 1: 819-22.
20. Spitz L, Kiely EM, Morecroft GA, *et al.* Esophageal atresia: at-risk groups for the 1990s. *J Pediatr Surg* 1994; 29: 723-5.

21. Engum SA, Grosfeld JL, West KW, *et al.* Analysis of morbidity and mortality in 227 cases of esophageal atresia and/or tracheoesophageal fistula over two decades. *Arch Surg* 1995; 130: 502-8.

22. Livaditis A, Radberg L, Odensjo G. Esophageal end-to-end anastomosis. Reduction of anastomotic tension by circular myotomy. *Scand J Thorac Cardiovasc Surg* 1972; 6: 206-14.

23. Spitz L. Esophageal Replacement. In: *Pediatric Surgery,* 6th Ed. Grosfeld JL, O'Neill JA, Jr, Fonkalsrud EW, *et al.* Philadelphia: Mosby, 2006.

24. Bax KMA, Van der Zee DC. Feasibility of thoracoscopic repair of esophageal atresia with distal fistula. *J Pediatr Surg* 2002; 37: 192-6.

25. Little DC, Rescorla FJ, Grosfeld JL, *et al.* Long-term analysis of children with esophageal atresia and tracheoesophageal fistula. *J Pediatr Surg* 2003; 38: 852-6.

26. Mack H. A history of pyloric stenosis and its treatment. *Bull Hist Med* 1942; 12: 465-8.

27. Blair P. On the dissection of a child much emaciated. *Philosophical Transactions* 1717; 30: 631.

28. Ravitch MM. The story of pyloric stenosis. *Surgery* 1960; 48: 1117-43.

29. Hirschsprung H. Falle von angeborener pylorus-stenose, beobachtet bei saulingfen. *Jahrb der Kinderh* 1888; 27: 61-8.

30. Hernanz-Schulman M. Infantile pyloric stenosis. *Radiology* 2003; 227: 319-31.

31. Nicoll JH. Congenital hypertrophic pyloric stenosis. *Br Med J* 1900; 2: 571-3.

32. Dufour H, Fredet P. La Stenose hypertrophique du pylore chez le nourisson et son traitement chirurgical. *Rev Chir* 1908; 37: 208.

33. Ramstedt C. Zur operation der angeborenen pylorusstenose. *Med Klin* 1912; 8: 1702-5.

34. Schwartz MZ. Hypertrophic pyloric stenosis. In: *Pediatric Surgery,* 6th Edition. Grosfeld, JL, O'Neill JA, Jr Fonkalsrud EW, *et al*, Eds. Philadelphia: Mosby, 2006.

35. Thomson J. On congenital obliteration of the bile ducts. *Edinb Med J* 1892; 37: 724.

36. Mowat AP. Biliary atresia into the 21st century: a historical perspective. *Hepatology* 1996: 23: 1693-5.

37. Holmes JB. Congenital obliteration of the bile ducts: diagnosis and suggestions for treatment. *Am J Dis Child* 1916; 11: 405-31.

38. Ladd WE. Congenital atresia and stenosis of the bile ducts. *JAMA* 1928; 91: 1082-5.

39. Altman RP, Buchmiller TC. The jaundiced infant: biliary atresia. In: *Pediatric Surgery,* 6th edition, Grosfeld JL, O'Neill JA, Jr, Fonkalsrud EW, *et al*, Eds. Philadelphia: Mosby, 2006.

40. Kasai M, Suzuki S. A new operation for 'non-correctable' biliary atresia: hepatic portoenterostomy. *Shujyutsu* 1959; 13: 733-9.

41. Kasai M, Kimura S, Asakura Y. Surgical treatment of biliary atresia. *J Pediatr Surg* 1968; 3: 665-75.

42. Altman RP, *et al.* A multivariable risk factor analysis of the porto-enterostomy (Kasai) procedure for biliary atresia: twenty-five years of experience from two centers. *Ann Surg* 1997; 226: 348-53.

43. Grosfeld JL, *et al.* The efficacy of hepatoportoenterostomy in biliary atresia. *Surgery* 1989; 106: 692-700.

44. Ando H, Ito T, Nagaya M. Use of external conduit impairs liver function in patients with biliary atresia. *J Pediatr Surg* 1996; 31: 1509-11.

45. Meyers RL, *et al.* High-dose steroids, ursodeoxycholic acid, and chronic intravenous antibiotics improve bile flow after Kasai procedure in infants with biliary atresia. *J Pediatr Surg* 2003; 38: 406-11.

46. Escobar MA, Jay CL, Brooks RM, *et al.* Effect of corticosteroid therapy on outcomes in biliary atresia after Kasai portoenterostomy. *J Pediatr Surg* 2006; 41: 99-103.

47. Endo M, *et al.* Extended dissection of the portahepatis and creation of an intussuscepted ileocolic conduit for biliary atresia. *J Pediatr Surg* 1983; 18: 784-93.

48. Ogasawara Y, *et al.* The intussusception antireflux valve is ineffective for preventing cholangitis in biliary atresia: a prospective study. *J Pediatr Surg* 2003; 38: 1826-9.

49. Bismuth H, Houssin D. Reduced-sized orthotopic liver graft in hepatic transplantation in children. *Surgery* 1984; 95: 367-70.

50. Broelsch CE, *et al.* Liver transplantation in children from living related donors - surgical techniques and results. *Ann Surg* 1991; 214: 428-37.

51. Otte JB, de Ville de Goyet J, Reding R, *et al.* Sequential treatment of biliary atresia with Kasai portoenterostomy and liver transplantation: a review. *Hepatology* 1994; 20 (Suppl): 41S-48S.

52. Martinez-Ferro M, Esteves E, Laje P. Laparoscopic treatment of biliary atresia and choledochal cyst. *Semin Pediatr Surg* 2005; 14: 206-15.

53. Karrer, FM, *et al.* Biliary atresia registry, 1976 to 1989. *J Pediatr Surg* 1990; 25: 1076-80.

54. Society JBA. Nationwide Registry of Biliary Atresia, 1998. *J Pediatr Surg* 2000; 36: 311-4.

55. Professor Ryoji Ohi, Sendai, Japan. Personal communication, 2006.

56. Evans CH. Atresias of the gastrointestinal tract. *Surg Gynecol Obstet* 1951; 92: 1-8.

57. Grosfeld JL. Jejunoileal atresia and stenosis. In: *Pediatric Surgery,* 6th Ed. Grosfeld JL, O'Neill JA, Jr, Fonkalsrud EW, *et al*, Eds. Philadelphia: Mosby, 2006.

58. Tandler J. Zur Entwicklungsgeschichte des menschlichen Duodenum in fruhen Embryonalstadien. *Morphol Jahrb* 1900; 29: 187.

59. Fockens P. Ein operativ geheilter Fall von Kongenitaler Duenndarm Atresie. *Zentrlbl Chir* 1911; 38: 532.

60. Louw JH, Barnard CN. Congenital intestinal atresia: observations on its origin. *Lancet* 1955; 2: 1065-7.

61. Santulli TV, Blanc WA. Congenital atresia of the intestine: pathogenesis and treatment. *Ann Surg* 1961; 154: 939-48.

62. Nixon HH. An experimental study of propulsion in isolated small intestine and applications to surgery in the newborn, *Ann R Coll Surg Engl* 1960; 24: 105-24.

63. Cywes S, Millar A, Rode H. From a Louw beginning - paediatric surgery in South Africa. *J Pediatr Surg* 2003; 38 (Suppl): 44-7.

64. Sweeney B, Surana R, Puri P. Jejunoileal atresia and associated malformations: correlation with timing of in-utero insult. *J Pediatr Surg* 2001; 36: 774-6.

65. Glüer S. Intestinal atresia following intraamniotic use of dyes. *Eur J Paediatr Surg* 1995; 5: 240-2.

66. Grosfeld, JL, Ballantine TVN, Shoemaker RS. Operative management of intestinal atresia and stenosis based on pathologic findings. *J Pediatr Surg* 1979; 14: 368-75.

67. de Lorimier AA, Fonkalsrud EW, Hays DM. Congenital atresia and stenosis of the jejunum and ileum. Surgery 1969; 65: 819-27.

68. Nixon HH, Tawes R. Etiology and treatment of small intestinal atresia: analysis of a series of 127 jejunoileal atresias and comparison with 62 duodenal atresias. *Surgery* 1971; 69: 41-51.

69. Snyder CL, Miller KA, Sharp RJ, et al. Management of intestinal atresia in patients with gastroschisis. *J Pediatr Surg* 2001; 36: 1542-4.

70. Komuro H, Hori T, Amagai T, et al. The etiologic role of intrauterine volvulus and intussusception in jejunoileal atresia. *J Pediatr Surg* 2004; 39: 1812-4.

71. Puvabandisin S, Garrow E, Sanransamraujkit R, Lopez LA. Postnatal intussusception in a premature infant causing intestinal atresia. *J Pediatr Surg* 1996; 31: 711-2.

72. Gross E, Armon Y, Abu-Dalu K, et al. Familial combined duodenal and jejunal atresia. *J Pediatr Surg* 1996; 31: 1573.

73. Kilani RA, Hmiel P, Garver MK, et al. Familial jejunal atresia with renal dysplasia. *J Pediatr Surg* 1996; 31: 1427-9.

74. Walker MW, Lovell MA, Kelly TC, et al. Multiple areas of intestinal atresia associated with immunodeficiency and post-transfusion graft-versus-host disease. *J Pediatr* 1993; 123: 93-5.

75. Rothenberg ME, White FV, Chilmonczyk B, Chatila T. A syndrome involving immunodeficiency and multiple intestinal atresias. *Immunodeficiency* 1995; 5: 171-8.

76. Ladd WE, Gross RE. *Abdominal surgery of infancy and childhood.* Philadelphia: WB Saunders, 1941.

77. Weber TR, Vane DW, Grosfeld JL. Tapering enteroplasty in infants with bowel atresia and short gut. *Arch Surg* 1982; 117: 684-8.

78. de Lorimier AA, Harrison MR. Intestinal imbrication in the treatment of atresia. *J Pediatr Surg* 1983; 18: 734-7.

79. Bianchi A. Experience with intestinal lengthening and tailoring. *Eur J Pediatr Surg* 1999; 9: 256-9.

80. Kim HB, Fauza D, Garza J, et al. Serial transverse enteroplasty (STEP): a novel bowel lengthening procedure. *J Pediatr Surg* 2003; 38: 425-9.

81. Mall FP. Development of the human intestine and its position in the adult. *Bull Johns Hopkins Hosp* 1898; 9: 197

82. Dott NM. Anomalies of intestinal rotation: their embryology and surgical aspects with report of five cases. *Br J Surg* 1923; 11: 251.

83. Waugh GE. Congenital malformation of the mesentery: a clinical entity. *Br J Surg* 1928; 15: 438.

84. Smith S. Anomalies of rotation and fixation. In: *Pediatric Surgery*, 6th Ed, Grosfeld JL, O'Neill JA, Jr. Fonkalsrud EW et al, Eds. Philadelphia: Mosby, 2006.

85. Ladd WE. Congenital obstruction of the duodenum in children. *N Engl J Med* 1932; 206: 277.

86. Ladd WE. Surgical diseases of the alimentary tract in infants. *N Engl J Med* 1936; 215: 705.

87. Snyder WH, Chaffin L. Embryology and pathology of the intestinal tract: presentation of 48 cases of malrotation. *Ann Surg* 1954; 140: 368.

88. Estrada RL. Anomalies of intestinal rotation and fixation. Springfield, Ill: Charles C Thomas, 1958.

89. Leenders E, Sieber WK. Congenital megacolon, observation by Frederici Ruysch 1691. *J Pediatr Surg* 1970; 5: 1-3.

90. Ruysch F. *Observationum anatomico-chirurgicarum centuria.* Amstelodami, 1691.

91. Grosfeld JL. Hirschsprung's disease: an historical review 1691-2005. In: *Hirschsprung's disease and allied disorders,* 3rd Ed. Holschneider AH, Puri P, Eds. Heidelberg: Springer-Verlag, 2006.

92. Hirschsprung H. Struhltragheit Neugeborener in folge von Dilatation and Hypertrophie des colons. *Jahrbuch fur Kinderheilkunde* 1888; 27: 1-7.

93. Treves F. Idiopathic dilatation of the colon. *Lancet* 1898; 1: 276-9.

94. Tittel K. Uber eine angeborene Missbildung des Dickdarmes. *Wien Klin Wschr* 1901; 14: 903-7.

95. Cass D. Hirschsprung's disease: an historical review. *Prog Pediatr Surg* 1986; 20: 199-214.

96. Ishikawa N. Experimentelle und klinische Untersuchungen uber die Pathogenese und das Wesen des megacolons. *Mitt Medfak kaiserl, Kyushu Univ* 1923; 7: 339.

97. Dalle Valle A. Richerche istologiche su di un caso di megacolon congenito. *Pediatria* 1920; 28: 740-52.

98. Whitehouse FR, Kernohan JW. Myenteric plexus in congenital megacolon. *Arch Int Med* 1948; 82: 75-111.

99. Bodian M, et al. Hirschsprung's disease and idiopathic megacolon. *Lancet* 1949; 1: 6-11.

100. Swenson O. My early experience with Hirschsprung's disease. *J Pediatr Surg* 1989; 24: 839-44.

101. Swenson O. How the cause and cure of Hirschsprung's disease were discovered. *J Pediatr Surg* 1999; 34: 1580-1.

102. Swenson O, Bill AH. Resection of rectum and rectosigmoid with preservation of the sphincter for benign spastic lesions producing megacolon: an experimental study. *Surgery* 1948; 24: 212-20.

103. Teitelbaum D, Coran AG. Hirschsprung disease and related conditions. In: *Pediatric Surgery,* 6th edition. Grosfeld JL, O'Neill JA, Jr, Fonkalsrud EW, et al, Eds. Philadelphia: Elsevier, 2006.

104. State D. Surgical treatment for idiopathic congenital megacolon (Hirschsprung's disease). *Surg Gynecol Obstet* 1952; 95: 201-12.

105. Rehbein F. Intraabdominalle Resektion oder rectosigmoidektomie (Swenson) bei der Hirschsprungschen Krankheit? *Chirurg* 1958; 29: 366-9.

106. Duhamel B. Une novelle operation pan le megacolon congenital l'abaisement retrorectal et transanal du colon of san application posible au traitement de quelques autros malformation. *Presse Méd* 1956; 64: 2249-50.

107. Soave F. A new surgical technique for treatment of Hirschsprung's disease. *Surgery* 1964; 56: 1007-14.

108. Dobbins WO, Bill AH. Diagnosis of Hirschsprung's disease excluded by rectal suction biopsy. *New Engl J Med* 1965; 272: 990-3.

109. Schnaufer L, *et al*. Differential sphincteric studies in the diagnosis of ano-rectal disorders of childhood. *J Pediatr Surg* 1967; 2: 538-43.

110. de la Torre-Mondregon L, Ortega-Salgado JA. Transanal endorectal pull-through for Hirschsprung's disease. *J Pediatr Surg* 1998; 33: 1283-6.

111. Georgeson KE, *et al*. Primary laparoscopic-assisted pull-through for Hirschsprung's disease in infants and children. *J Pediatr Surg* 1995; 30: 1017-22.

112. Escobar MA, Grosfeld JL, West KW, Rescorla FJ, Scherer LR, Rouse TM, Engum SA. Long-term outcomes in total colonic aganglionosis: a 32-year experience. *J Pediatr Surg* 2005; 40: 955-61.

113. Kimura K. A new surgical approach to extensive aganglionosis. *J Pediatr Surg* 1981; 16: 840-9.

114. Ziegler MM, *et al*. Extended myotomy-myectomy: a therapeutic alternative for total intestinal aganglionosis. *Ann Surg* 1993; 218: 504-9.

115. Revillion Y, *et al*. Improved quality of life by combined transplantation in Hirschsprung's disease with a very long aganglionic segment. *J Pediatr Surg* 2003; 38: 422-4.

116. So H, *et al*. Endorectal pullthrough without preliminary colostomy in neonates with Hirschsprung's disease. *J Pediatr Surg* 1980; 15: 470-1.

117. Carcassone M, *et al*. Primary corrective operation without decompression in infants less than three months of age with Hirschsprung's disease. *J Pediatr Surg* 1982; 17: 241-3.

118. Swenson O. Hirschsprung's disease - a complicated therapeutic problem: some thoughts and solutions based on data and personal experience over 56 years. *J Pediatr Surg* 2004; 39: 1449-53.

119. Grosfeld JL. Anorectal malformations: an historical review. In: *Anorectal Malformations in Children: Embryology, Diagnosis, Surgical Treatment, Follow-up*. Holshneider AH, Hutson J, Eds. Heidelberg: Springer-Verlag, 2006.

120. de Vries PA. The surgery of anorectal anomalies: its evolution, with evaluation of procedures. *Curr Probl Surg* 1984; 21: 1-75.

121. Cooke J. *Mellificium Chirurgiae: or the marrow of Chirurgery much enlarged*. London: Marshall, 1685: 669 and 4th Ed: 158.

122. Bell B. *A system of surgery*, 3rd Edition. Edinburgh, 1787; 2: 275-82

123. Mantell T. Case of imperforate anus successfully treated. *Med Soc London Mem* 1792; 3: 389.

124. Littré A. Diverses observations Anatomatiques. *Paris Histoire de l'Academie Royale de Science* 1710: 36-7.

125. Duret C. Observation sur enfant un. ne sans anus, et auguel it a ete fait une ouverture pour y suppléer. *Receuil de la Societé de Médicine de Paris* 1793: 4: 45-50.

126. Roux J-N. Observation d'imperforation de l'anus et de l'uretre. *Memoires de l'Academie Royale de Medicine* 1835; 4: 183-90.

127. Amussat JZ. Histoire d'une operation d'anus practique avec success par un nouveau procede. *Gaz Med Paris* 1835; 3: 753-8.

128. Bodenhamer W. *Aetiology, pathology and treatment of the congenital malformations of the rectum and anus*. New York: Samuel and William Wood, 1860.

129. McCormac W. On a case of impeforate anus. *Lancet* 1886; 2: 12.

130. Matas R. The surgical treatment of anorectal imperforation considered in the light of modern operative procedures. *Transactions of the American Surgical Association* 1897; 15: 45.

131. Wangensteen OH, Rice CO. Imperforate anus. *Ann Surg* 1930; 92: 77.

132. Ladd WE, Gross RE. Congenital malformations of the anus and rectum. *Am J Surg* 1934; 23: 167.

133. Rhoads JE, *et al*. A simultaneous abdominal and perineal approach in operations for imperforate anus with atresia of the rectum and rectosigmoid. *Ann Surg* 1948; 127: 552.

134. Browne D. Some congenital deformities of the rectum, anus, vagina and urethra. *Ann R Coll Surg Engl* 1951; 8: 173-92.

135. Smith ED. Denis Browne: Maverick or master surgeon? *ANZ J Surg* 2000; 11: 770-7.

136. Smith ED. Close to and far from the origins. *J Pediatr Surg* 2003; 38 (Suppl): 27-32.

137. Stephens FD. Congenital imperforate rectum, recto-urethral and recto-vaginal fistulae. *ANZ J Surg* 1953; 22: 161-72.

138. Rehbein F. Opeartions der anal-und Rectumatresie mit Recto-Urethralfistal. *Chirurg* 1959; 30: 417-8.

139. Hochenegg J. Beitrage zur chirurgie des rectum und der Beckenorgane. *Wien Klin Woschr* 1889; 2: 55.

140. Romauldi P. A new technic for surgical treatment of some rectal malformations. *Langenbecks Arch Klin Chir Ver Dtsch Z Chir* 1960; 296: 371-7.

141. Kiesewetter WB, Turner CR. Continence after surgery for imperforate anus: a critical analysis and preliminary experience with the sacro-perineal pull-through. *Ann Surg* 1963; 158: 498-512.

142. Stephens FD. *Congenital malformations of the rectum, anus and genitourinary tracts*. Edinburgh and London: E and S Livingston, 1963.

143. Kelly JH. Cineradiography in anorectal malformations. *J Pediatr Surg* 1969; 4: 538-46.

144. Stephens FD, Smith ED. *Anorectal malformations in children*. Chicago: Year Book Medical Publishers, 1971.

145. Mollard P, *et al*. Surgical treatment of high imperforate anus with definition of the puborectalis sling by an anterior perineal approach. *J Pediatr Surg* 1978; 13: 499-504.

146. Nixon HH, Puri P. The results of treatment of anorectal anomalies: a thirteen to twenty-year follow-up. *J Pediatr Surg* 1977; 12: 27-37.

147. Hecker WCh, Holschneider AM. Complications, lethality and long-term results after surgery of anorectal defects. In: *Long term Follow-up in Congenital Anomalies*. Kiesewetter WB, Ed. Pittsburgh: Pediatric Surgical Symposium, 1970.

148. de Vries PA, Peña A. Posterior sagittal anorectoplasty. *J Pediatr Surg* 1982; 17: 638-43.

149. Peña A, de Vries PA. Posterior sagittal anorectoplasty: important technical considerations and new applications. *J Pediatr Surg* 1982; 17: 796-811.

150. Hedlund H, *et al*. Long-term anorectal function in imperforate anus treated by posterior sagittal anorectoplasty: manometric investigation. *J Pediatr Surg* 1992; 27: 906-9.

151. Smith ED. The bath water needs changing, but don't throw away the baby: an overview of anorectal anomalies. *J Pediatr Surg* 1988; 22: 335-48.

152. Peña A, el Behery M. Megasigmoid: a source of pseudoincontinence in children with repaired anorectal maformations. *J Pediatr Surg* 1993; 28: 199-203.

153. Peña A, Levitt MA. Colonic inertia disorders in pediatrics. *Curr Probl Surg* 2002; 39: 666-730.

154. Stephens FD, Smith ED. *Anorectal malformations in children.* Update 1988. March of Dimes Birth Defects Foundation Series; Hendren WH: Urogenital 24: (4). New York: Alan R Liss, Inc., 1988.

155. Raffensperger JG, Ramenofsky M. The management of a cloaca. *J Pediatr Surg* 1980; 8: 647.

156. Hendren WH. Cloacal malformations: experience with 105 cases. *J Pediatr Surg* 1992; 27: 890-901.

157. Peña A, *et al.* Surgical management of cloacal malformations: a review of 339 patients. *J Pediatr Surg* 2004; 39: 470-9.

158. Peña A. Total urogenital mobilization - an easier way to repair cloacas. *J Pediatr Surg* 1997; 32: 263-7.

159. Malone PS, *et al.* Preliminary report: the antegrade continence enema. *Lancet* 1990; 336: 1217-8.

160. Okada A, *et al.* Anterior sagittal anorectoplasty for rectovestibular and anovestibular fistula. *J Pediatr Surg* 1992; 27: 85-8.

161. Georgeson KE, *et al.* Laparoscopic-assisted anorectal pull-through for high imperforate anus - a new technique. *J Pediatr Surg* 2000; 35: 927-31.

162. Iwanaka T, *et al.* Findings of pelvic musculature and efficacy of laparoscopic muscle stimulator in laparoscopy-assisted anorectal pull-through for high imperforate anus. *Surg Endosc* 2003; 17: 278-81.

163. Yamataka A, *et al.* Laparoscopic muscle electrostimulation during laparoscopy-assisted anorectal pull-through for high imperforate anus. *J Pediatr Surg* 2001; 36: 1659-61.

164. Albanese CT, *et al.* One-stage correction of high imperforate anus in the male neonate. *J Pediatr Surg* 1999; 34: 834-6.

165. Stephens FD, Smith ED. Classification and assessment of surgical treatment of anorectal anomalies. *Pediatr Surg Int* 1986; 1: 200.

166. Peña A. Anorectal anomalies. *Semin Pediatr Surg* 1995; 4: 35-47.

167. Holschneider A, Hutson J, Peña A, *et al.* Preliminary report on the International Conference for the development of standards for the treatment of anorectal malformations. *J Pediatr Surg* 2005; 40: 1521-6.

Appendix

Biographical notes

By all chapter authors

The main pioneers listed here are in alphabetical order, but many others are found amongst the chapters within this book. For each selected pioneer, the name, date of birth and demise, where relevant, the main institution where they worked and the contribution or contributions that they gave to surgical posterity is recorded. It is hoped this will serve as a useful rapid source of information to all readers. Far from all the pioneers are listed, but those selected are mostly chosen for their contribution made to surgical gastroenterology, and some admittedly for their additional colourful lives.

We have not included all the possible references; many of the details have been gleaned from historical sources met in our research, which include principally: *An Introduction to the History of Medicine*, by Fielding Garrison in his third expanded edition. WB Saunders Company, 1924; and *Classic Descriptions of Disease. With Biographical Sketches of the Authors.* Third Edition, 5th printing. Ralph H. Major (Professor of Medicine, University of Kansas School of Medicine). Charles C. Thomas, Publisher. Springfield Illinois, USA, August 1959.

More unusual references are appended at the bottom of the corresponding biographical note. We apologise for the abbreviated style of writing; minimum wording has allowed us to include more pioneers.

ABBE, Robert (1851-1928).

Main institution: Surgeon, St. Luke's Hospital, New York, USA.

A contemporary and friend of Charles McBurney. In 1892, he devised a safe method of anastomosing intestine using catgut plates in a similar way to the bone plates described by Senn in 1889. However, he later found a double layer of continuous silk sutures by the Lembert principle in 1892 superior, as the lumina did not contract as much as the bone and catgut ring techniques (Chapter 10). He preceded Courvoisier with a successful choledochotomy for obstructive jaundice due to stones (Chapter 7). He also devised a retrograde method of dilating hard oesophageal strictures between the mouth and a gastrostomy by the 'string saw' technique (Chapter 4).

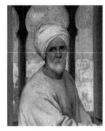

ABU AL-QASIM (approximately 936-1013 AD). Portrait in Chapter 14.

Also spelled ABUL KASIM, in full ABU AL-QASIM KHALAF IBN 'ABBAS AZ-ZAHRAWI, Latin, ALBUCASIS

Main institution: Chief Physician, Baghdad, Iraq.

Born near Cordoba in Spain, he was considered to be Islam's greatest physician and surgeon in Arab medicine. He was appointed a chief physician at the age of 18! His comprehensive medical text, combining Middle Eastern with Greco-Roman classical teachings shaped European surgical procedures until the Renaissance. Abu al-Qasim was Court Physician to the Spanish caliph, Abd ar-Rahman III an-Nasir, and wrote *At-Tasrif liman ajaz an at-Ta`alif*, or *At-Tasrif* ('The Method'), a medical work in 30 parts. The last chapter, with its drawings of more than 200 instruments, constitutes the first illustrated, independent work on surgery. He noted tumours of the oesophagus as a cause of dysphagia and wrote five books or canons, some of which were in standard use at the University of Montpelier up to the mid-17th century. Although he was largely ignored by physicians of the eastern Caliphate, the surgical treatise had tremendous influence in Christian Europe. His work was translated into Latin in the 12th century by the scholar, Gerard of Cremona, and it stood for nearly 500 years as the leading textbook on surgery in Europe. It was preferred for its concise lucidity to the works of Galen.

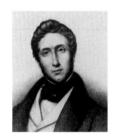

AMUSSAT, Jean Zuléma (1796-1856). Portrait in Chapters 9 and 16.

Main institution: Charité Hopital, Paris, France.

Amussat suffered from poor health most of his professional life. A brilliant medical student rewarded by membership in the Académie de Médecine before graduation, he was a fine surgeon with an international reputation as a teacher, despite his poor financial background. He was an expert on lithotomy for bladder stones, as well as his famous operation of lumbar colostomy for obstruction.

AMYAND, Claudius (1681-1740).

Main institution: Founder of, and principal surgeon, St. George's Hospital, London, UK.

First recorded appendicectomy in 1736, which is described in Chapter 12. This book's authors strongly support the belief that a groin hernia containing the appendix should eponymously be called an 'Amyand hernia'. Honours included appointment of Sergeant-Surgeon to King George II, and Master of the Company of Barber Surgeons (an old Guild in the City of London). An alleged pioneer for vaccination against smallpox, he vaccinated the whole Royal Family before Jenner's cowpox vaccine. He was a senior surgeon to the Westminster Hospital and was made a Fellow of the prestigious Royal Society.

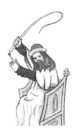

ARDERNE, John (1307-1390). Cartoon style portrait in Chapter 15.

Main institution: Norwich and London.

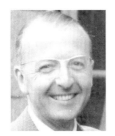

Self-taught surgeon in Norwich and London, who gained much experience in the 100-year war under the Duke of Lancaster and said to be an "excellent scholar, gentleman and trained surgeon, possessing a wide experience and excellent surgical judgement". He is described as the first English proctologist. He was one of the earliest to lay open anal fistulas. He also knew ischiorectal abscesses frequently preceded fistula as mentioned in Chapter 15. He published several treatises in Latin, which gained him an international reputation. His work on fistulas was re-published by Sir D'Arcy Power into English. In addition, he gave a good description of rectal cancer. He wrote (in Latin): "An abscess bred in any place of the body, if it be not healed by three or four months turns into a fistula or cancer". Hobbies included astrology, botany and charms!

ARNOUS, Jean (1908-1981). Portrait in Chapter 15.

Main institution: Hôpital Léopold Bellan, Paris, France.

Born in Angers, he graduated as an intern from Hôpitaux de Paris in 1934. He soon created a renowned Department of Proctology in Hôpital Bichat and later in Hôpital Saint-Antoine in Paris. In 1950, he was appointed Head of the Service of Gastroenterology in Hôpital Léopold Bellan; he transformed it into the first French Service of Proctology in 1961, and led it until 1979. Introduced in France Milligan's and Morgan's haemorrhoidectomy (Figure 11, Chapter 15). His attention was especially drawn to anorectal fistulae and abscesses, for which he established an original classification and precise surgical techniques. In 1954, he wrote with Ernest Parnaud a modestly entitled book called *La Petite Chirurgie des Fistules Anales.* Léopold Bellan Hospital became a famous proctological school, where French and international gastroenterologists and surgeons came for conferences or training. He became the co-founder and later Chairman of the French National Society of Proctology, and of the European and Mediterranean Society of ColoProctology. He died in Paris in 1981.

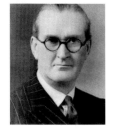

BARRETT, Norman Rupert (1903-1979).

Main institution: Surgeon, St. Thomas's Hospital, and Brompton Chest Hospitals, London, UK.

A fine teacher and kind to staff and patients. Between 1935-1936, he gained a Rockefeller Fellowship under Evarts Graham. An authority on hydatid disease of the lung, he pioneered cytological examination of sputum for malignant disease of the bronchus. He achieved the first recorded survival after surgery for spontaneous ruptured oesophagus, and was eponymously associated with 'columnar-lined oesophagus' (Chapter 4). He was the first surgical editor of *Thorax* journal and remained on the editorial staff for 25 years. He served as Vice-President of the Royal College of Surgeons of England before retirement.

1.   Lord RVN. Norman Barrett and the Esophagus. In: *Barrett's Esophagus.* Tilanus HW, Attwood SEA. Kluwer Academic Publishers, 2001: 1-15.

Image reproduced with permission from The Royal College of Surgeons of England.

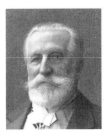

BERGMANN, Ernst von (1837-1907). Portrait in Chapter 3.

Main institution: Succeeded Langenbeck in Berlin, Germany, after Billroth declined the position.

Born in Riga in 1837, then part of Germany, and graduated in Dorpal in 1860. In 1878, he was appointed Chairman of Surgery in Würzburg, and in military surgery took a much more conservative line in treating gunshot wounds than his contemporaries. In 1882, he accepted the post of Chairman of Surgery in Berlin when it was declined by Billroth, who preferred Vienna. In 1886, he organised steam sterilisation, after adopting the Listerian method of antisepsis. He was fortunate to have Schimmelbusch on his staff, who introduced new theatre furniture (Figure 6, Chapter 3). He died after an operation for appendicitis on March 25th 1907.

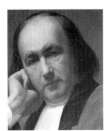

BERNARD, Claude (1813-1878). Portrait in Chapter 7.

Main institution: University of Paris, France.

He was a brilliant physiologist initially working under François Magendie who he eventually succeeded in his laboratory in the Hôtel Dieu de Paris. He was later Professor of Physiology at the Collège de France and then at the Natural History Museum. He graduated in 1843, and in 1853 was awarded Doctor in Natural Sciences. In 1854, he became a Member of the Academy of Sciences. In 1865, he wrote the famous *Introduction à l'étude de la Médecine Expérimentale* (introduction to the study of experimental medicine) and was one of the first to use chemistry in his experiments and to establish the main principles of experiment in physiological research. In 1868, he became a Member of the French Academy. In the following year he was nominated as Senator of the Second French Empire. He discovered glycogen and its importance in carbohydrate metabolism, discussed in Chapter 7. He reported the importance of the cell in relation to its environment ('milieu intérieur'). He also established the importance of vasomotor reflexes.

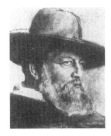

BILLROTH, Christian Albert Theodor (1829-1894). Portraits in Chapter 6.

Main institution: Second and later first Chair of Surgery, Vienna, Austria.

See the biography in Chapter 6.

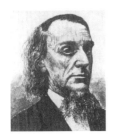

BOBBS, John Stough (1809-1870). Portrait in Chapter 7.

Main institution: Surgeon, Indianapolis, Indiana, USA.

He was born in Greenville, Pennsylvania on December 28th 1809. He studied medicine by apprenticeship in Harrisburg, Pennsylvania, followed by a degree course in Jefferson Medical College for a further two years. When he graduated in 1836, he went to practice in Indianapolis. He performed the first cholecystotomy on 15th June 1867, which is described briefly in Chapter 7. It took place in a woman of 32 who had a large mucocoele of the gallbladder initially thought to be a large ovarian cyst. The patient outlived her surgeon and lived for another 45 more years and died of arteriosclerosis. In 1869, Bobbs became Professor of Surgery in the new University of Indiana and founded the still famous Bobbs Library.

1. Bobbs JS. A case of lithotomy of the gallbladder. *Trans Ind State Med Soc* 1868; 18: 68.

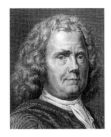

BOERHAAVE, Hermann (1668-1738). Portrait in Chapter 4.

Main institution: Professor of Botany, Clinical Medicine, and Chemistry, University of Leyden, The Netherlands.

Founded a postgraduate medical institution in Leyden long before Edinburgh and London were recognised. He was mentor to numerous famous pioneers in medicine and surgery, including Lorenz Heister, William Cullen and many others. He gave a famous description of a ruptured oesophagus in Baron de Wassenaer, Grand Admiral of the Dutch Fleet in 1723. The whole account, including the clinical features and autopsy results, were meticulously recorded in Latin a year later; the details are found in Chapter 4 (Boerhaave's syndrome; so-called spontaneous rupture of the oesophagus). His works in medicine and chemistry were translated into many European languages; also in Arabic.

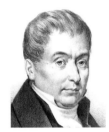

BOYER, Alexis (1757-1833). Portrait in Chapter 15.

Main institution: Chief Surgeon, Charité Hospital, Paris, France.

He was born in Corrèze, France, in poor circumstances, but was apprenticed to a local barber surgeon. He survived a severe attack of typhoid fever. He was apointed Professor of Pathology in the Faculty of Medicine in Paris, and later Professor of Surgery at the Hôpital de Charité. In 1805, he was posted as First Imperial Surgeon to Napoleon and followed the Grande Armée during the campaigns of 1806 and 1807. In 1825, he became a Member of the Academy of Sciences in Paris and laid open or excised fistulas and invented a radical sphincterotomy for anal fissure (Chapter 15). After Waterloo he said: "Today I lost my endowment of 25,000 francs and my post of Imperial Surgeon. I have got five horses, I shall sell three of them. I shall keep my carriage which does not cost me a penny. I shall read this evening a chapter from Séneque and will not think about it afterwards." In fact, he was later reinstated as Surgeon to the Court three kings afterwards.

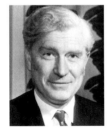

BROOKE, Bryan Nicholas (1915-1998). Portrait in Chapter 13.

Main institutions: Consultant Surgeon, Queen Elizabeth Hospital, Birmingham, and later, Professor of Surgery, St. George's Hospital, London, UK.

He had a lifelong interest in the study of inflammatory bowel disease. He designed a much improved everted ileostomy giving at least 3cm clearance into a suitable bag. The edges of the ileum were anastomosed to the dermis of the circular skin incision, whose site was decided on by a stoma nurse before the operation.

1.   Brooke BN. The management of an ileostomy including its complications. *Lancet* 1952; 2: 102.

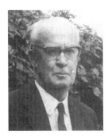

BROWNE, (Sir) Denis John Wolko (1892-1967). Portrait in Chapter 16.

Main institution: Great Ormond Street Hospital, London, UK.

See the biography in Chapter 16.

1.   Smith ED. Denis Browne: Maverick or master surgeon? *ANZ J Surg* 2000; 11: 770-7.
2.   Smith ED. Close to and far from the origins. *J Pediatr Surg* 2003; 38(Suppl): 27-32.

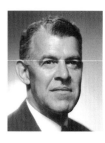

CATTELL, Richard (1900-1964). Portrait in Chapter 13.

Main institution: Lahey Clinic, Boston, Massachusetts, USA.

Cattell had a huge reputation in life-saving results from surgery for severe ulcerative colitis, described in Chapter 13. He had a fine reputation also in biliary surgery for complications after cholecystectomy. He operated on Anthony Eden, Prime Minister of the UK, for biliary stricture after cholecystectomy in 1956, mentioned in Chapter 7.

CHEEVER, David William (1831-1915).

Main institutions: Professor of Surgery, Harvard Medical School, and Attending Surgeon, Boston City Hospital, Boston, USA.

Born in Portsmouth, New Hampshire, USA, he pursued general studies in Harvard 1848-1852 before travelling to Europe for a year. In 1854, he studied medicine at Harvard Medical School until 1859 and worked under Oliver Wendell Holmes in 1859, who found him to be a gifted anatomy teacher. He soon became Editor of the *Boston Medical and Surgical Journal*. His surgical achievements included: expertise at tonsillectomy, including the removal of a large malignant tonsil by a cervical approach; oesophagotomy for impacted foreign bodies; knowledge of nasopharyngeal tumours; pharyngotomy; and a radical cure of hernias. In 1886, he became Professor of Surgery at Harvard. Cheever was early to exploit steam tents to alleviate airway oedema and frequently avoided the need for tracheostomy. Quote: "I never thought I excelled as an operator, but rather as a pains-taker!"

1.   Childs WA, Phillips RB. Experience with intestinal plication and a proposed modification. *Ann Surg* 1960; 152: 258-65.

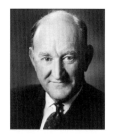

COLLIS, Jack Leigh (1911-2003).

Main institution: Queen Elizabeth Hospital, Birmingham, UK.

Graduate of Birmingham University and started his career in surgery there, before working under famous pioneer thoracic surgeons in the Brompton Hospital in London. He is remembered for his painstaking work on the anatomy of the diaphragm and for his work on complicated and uncomplicated gastro-oesophageal reflux. He emulated Billroth by conducting an honest audit on all his results on oesophageal cancer. His mortality before retirement for this severe disease was as low as that of many top-ranked contemporaries. A meticulous surgeon, he expected 'the right thing' from his students, juniors, peers and mostly from himself. His gastroplasty for oesophageal stricture is now combined with a fundoplication and much exploited by thoracic surgeons.

1.   Orringer MB. Combined Collis gastroplasty-Nissen fundoplication operation for reflux oesophagitis. *Surgical Rounds* 1978; 1: 10-9.

Image reproduced with permission from the editor's private collection.

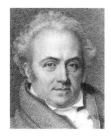

COOPER, Sir Astley Paston (1768-1841). Portrait in Chapter 9.

Main institution: Guy's Hospital, London, UK.

He was born in Norwich and became a student at St. Thomas's Hospital under Henry Cline. He attended John Hunter's demonstrations and was appointed Lecturer in Anatomy at St. Thomas's at the early age of 21, and at the Royal College of Surgeons two years later. Like Hunter, he acquired bodies from illegal sources to teach students. In 1800, he was appointed Surgeon at Guy's Hospital. He resigned the lectureship at St. Thomas's in 1825. When he was replaced by a Mr. South, rather than by his nephew Bransby Cooper, he persuaded the Treasurer of Guy's to found a separate medical school, with Bransby as Lecturer in Anatomy. He claimed successful ligations of carotid and femoral aneurysms; he also ligated the aorta (but the patient died hours later) and performed an early successful amputation through the hip. In 1820, he removed a sebaceous cyst from the scalp of King George IV and was rewarded with a baronetcy. He became twice President of the Royal College of Surgeons. He wrote: "Sir Astley Cooper was a good anatomist, but never was a good operator where delicacy was required."

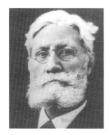

COURVOISIER, Ludwig (1843-1918). Portrait in Chapter 8.

Main institution: Professor of Surgery, Basle, Switzerland.

He graduated from Basel and studied in London under William Fergusson and Spencer Wells. He later spent time in Vienna with Billroth and Czerny. He is known for his eponymous law on obstructive jaundice, described in Chapters 7 and 8. One of the first to successfully extract gallstones from the common bile duct. He was a world expert on butterflies.

CRILE, George (1864-1943).

Main institution: Chief of Surgery, Lakeside Hospital, Columbus, Ohio, USA (later known as the Cleveland Clinic).

The death of a close friend from crush injury to the legs after an accident made a profound impression on Crile's career. He studied and treated shock and other metabolic disorders long before his peers. In 1892, he travelled abroad as many Americans did at that time, attending Billroth, where he saw radical thyroidectomies for malignant disease; also, von Eiselsberg and Trotter in the UK. In 1903, he wrote *Blood Pressure in Surgery*. He is reported to have performed the first human to human blood transfusion in America. He also invented the pressurised rubber suits for pilots in warplanes. As Cleveland was the 'goitre belt', he performed over 25,000 thyroidectomies in his lifetime. He pioneered radical neck dissections for cancer. In 1912, with Finney, he co-founded the American College of Surgeons and in the following year was elected to the Royal College of Surgeons of England with Harvey Cushing, William Mayo and John B. Murphy. He was the joint organiser of the Hospital Services of the American Expeditionary Forces in World War I in France. He founded The Cleveland Clinic with a group of physicians and pathologists. He served as the second President of the ACS.

1. Hermann RE. George Washington Crile (1864-1943). *J Med Biog* 1994; 2: 78-83.

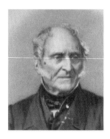

CRUVEILHIER, Jean (1791-1874). Portrait in Chapter 6.

Main institution: Professor of Surgery and Anatomy and later in Pathology, Paris, France.

He was born in Limoges, France, a son of an army surgeon. He was a student disciple of Morgagni, and achieved his MD in Paris in 1816. In 1823, he was appointed Professor of Surgery in Montpellier (thanks to the influence of Dupuytren) and returned to Paris as Professor of Descriptive Anatomy in 1825. In 1830, his description of simple gastric ulceration earned him the eponym for gastric ulcer as 'Maladie de Cruveilhier'. He was a co-founder with Dupuytren, Boyle and Laennec of the Grande École Française d'Anatomie Pathologique. In 1836, he became Professor of Surgical Pathology in Paris, appointed by Dupuytren's dying wish. He wrote a biography called *Life of Duypuytren* in 1840, and was the author of a beautifully illustrated book, *Anatomie pathologique du corps humain*.

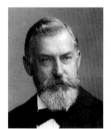

CZERNY, Vincenz von (1842-1916). Portrait in Chapter 4.

Main institutions: Professor of Surgery, Freiburg and later Heidelberg, Germany.

He was born in Trautenau in Bohemia (Czech Republic), the son of a pharmacist. He was certainly one of Billroth's brightest assistants, a fine teacher and in 1873, he assisted Billroth in total laryngectomy. He was later son-in-law to internist Adolf Kussmaul. In 1877, he performed the first successful oesophagectomy for cancer situated in the cervical oesophagus. Other surgical feats included: vaginal hysterectomy (1879); first pyelolithotomy in Germany (1880); alleged first removal of uterine fibroids (1881); first excision of benign gastric ulcer (1883); preliminarily sutured the gallbladder to the abdominal wall before cholecystostomy to remove gallstones (1888). In 1887, he accepted the Chair of Surgery in Heidelberg. Soon after, he removed a tumour of the large bowel. For himself he invented a style of intestinal suture invaginating and avoiding the mucosal layer described in Chapter 10. He declined Billroth's Chair in 1894, because he had dedicated his life to cancer research, and in fact he founded the Cancer Institute of Germany and the Heidelberg Samariterhaus in 1906. He wrote 160 scientific papers; most about carcinoma and gastrointestinal surgery. In addition, he wrote about thyroid disease, bone, tuberculosis and fat-embolism. An Honorary Member of the American Surgical Association, he was President of the Deutsche Gesellschaft für Chirurgie (German Surgical Society) in 1901, and died in 1916 of chronic leukaemia.

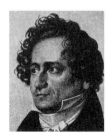

DIEFFENBACH, Johann Friedrich (1792-1847).

Main institution: Charité Hospital, Berlin, Germany.

He succeeded von Graef as Professor in Berlin. He had a great interest in experimental and clinical plastic surgery, including urethrotomy for stricture. He was the first to succeed in intestinal anastomosis using Lembert's method (see Chapter 10).

1.   Dieffenbach JF. *Die Operative Chirurgie*. Leipzig, 1845-1848.

Image reproduced with permission from the Académie de Médecine, Paris, France.

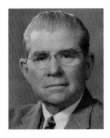

DIXON, Claude F (1893-1968). Portrait in Chapter 14.

Main institution: Mayo Clinic, Rochester, Minnesota, USA.

Dixon was a practising surgeon at the Mayo Clinic, Rochester, Minnesota. He was the father of modern anterior resection, an operation Dixon performed entirely from the abdomen. He used a double-layered, hand-sewn, end-to-end anastomosis to connect the colon to the rectal stump. This operation was initially developed for carcinomas of the rectosigmoid and upper third of the rectum, provided there was 5cm of normal mucosa below the tumour; hence the 5cm rule. However, with Wangensteen he questioned the alleged length of downward spread of cancer being more than a short distance. This philosophy reduced the number of abdominoperineal resections in those times (see Parks and elsewhere).

1. Dixon C. Surgical removal of lesions occurring in the sigmoid colon and the rectosigmoid. *Am J Surg* 1939; 46: 12-7.

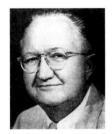

DRAGSTEDT, Lester Reynold (1893-1975). Portrait in Chapter 6.

Main institution: University of Illinois, Chicago, USA.

Born in Anaconda, Montana, USA, his parents were Swedish immigrants; his father was a blacksmith. Initially, he was a pure physiologist, and achieved professorial status in the Department of Physiology in 1921. Later he was encouraged by Phemister to get surgical training. Besides training locally, he visited European centres including Ernst Polya's unit in Budapest. He underwent nephrectomy for tuberculosis on his return to America. He always had a great interest in gastric acid secretion and the neural and hormonal influences. On 18th January 1943, he performed the first truncal vagotomy through the chest; when this often produced gastric stasis, he switched to the abdomen, in order to add gastroenterostomy. With colleague Weinberg, he standardised gastric drainage as a one-layered pyloroplasty. To reduce ulcer recurrence, he added a 40-50% gastrectomy to the vagotomy, called 'vagotomy and antrectomy'. At one time it was the most effective and frequently used ulcer operation in the US.

DUKES, Cuthbert (1890-1977).

Main institution: St. Mark's Hospital, London, UK.

An English pathologist with research interests in proctology and colorectal cancer. He was appointed the first full-time pathologist of the St. Mark's Hospital for Diseases of the Rectum and Colon in London, and working with Lockhart-Mummery, developed the pathological staging system for colorectal cancer that bears his name. He also founded the Ileostomy Association of Great Britain, and devoted considerable research to improving the quality of life for ileostomy patients.

1. Shampo M. Dukes and Broders: pathologic classifications of cancer of the rectum. *Journal of Pelvic Surgery* 2001; 7(1): 5-7.

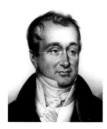

DUPUYTREN, Guillaume (1777-1835). Portrait in Chapter 12.

Main institution: Head of Surgery, Hotel Dieu Hospital, Paris, France (appointed in 1815).

Dupuytren trained during the hard times of the French Revolution. Whilst a medical student, he led an austere life surviving on bread and cheese for months on end. His talents as a teacher and skills as a surgeon seem to have been above reproach, and so wealth and honours were heaped upon him. He was a cold, tough, arrogant man, quarrelsome with his colleagues and rough with patients. Known by Lisfranc as "The brigand of the Hotel Dieu"; by others as "The first of surgeons and the least of men!" Despite being a son of the Revolution he adorned himself with many of the unpleasant characteristics of the Royalist 'ancien regime'. He even failed to appear at his arranged wedding, when due to marry the daughter of his old chief, Alexis Boyer. According to Lindskog, he was reputed, at one time to have had over 200 assistants in his entourage. He founded the Société Anatomique de Paris in 1803, and was elected as a Member of the prestigious Académie des Sciences in 1825. Louis XVIII awarded him his baronetcy, despite his failed management of the politically powerful Duke de Berry, who was stabbed in the chest by an assassin. Besides being very talented, his was the right face in the right place at the right time. He was Chief Surgeon to King Charles X. A brilliant teacher and operator, combined with a very cold personality gained him few friends. In his time he was one of the wealthiest men in France, and was in a position to lend the King of France one million francs. He established a Chair in Pathological Anatomy, while being described by a contemporary as the "Dictator of Surgery in Paris from 1815 to 1835", clearly a man who though gifted, had little modesty and sensitivity. He is quoted as saying: "I have been mistaken, but I have been mistaken less than others!" He suffered a severe stroke in November 1833 and died in 1835. His other surgical exploits were: in 1812, the first excision of the mandible, in a young man for osteomyelitis; in 1815 and 1819, he was one of the first to ligate the external iliac and subclavian arteries for an aneurysm; in 1822, he instigated the subcutaneous division of the sternomastoid muscle for torticollis; in 1832, he described and performed an operation for excision of palmar fascia due to his eponymous contracture. His name is associated with fractures, dislocations and bilocular hydrocoeles.

1. Dupuytren G. Mémoire sur une méthode nouvelle pour traiter les anus accidentels, par Monsieur le baron Dupuytren. *Mémoires de l'Académie Royale de Médecine* 1828; 1: 259-316.

EISELSBERG, Anton von (1860-1939).

Main institutions: Utrecht, The Netherlands; Königsberg, Germany; and Vienna, Austria.

He was born in Austria, and studied medicine in Würzburg, Zurich, Paris and Vienna. When he qualified in 1884, he assisted Billroth until 1887. He left Vienna for Utrecht and learnt fluent Dutch in three months. He achieved an excellent low mortality for his gastric surgery and alleged no anastomotic leaks. He was famous for research in sarcoma in rats, and thyroid cancer in patients. He was an early operator for acromegaly by performing hypophysectomy. He was honoured worldwide before retirement at 75. He did much work on abdominal surgery, plastic surgery, trauma, thyroid, and neurosurgery, and devised an antrum-exclusion operation for irresectable carcinoma. He served as President of the German Surgical Society and Honorary doctor of: Athens, Budapest, Debreczin, Edinburgh, Geneva, Leyden, Vienna, Paris. He also became an Honorary Member of the American Surgical Association and was befriended by William Halsted at Johns Hopkins. He reluctantly performed exploratory laparotomy on Mikulicz who self-diagnosed inoperable stomach carcinoma. In 1927, he was awarded an Honorary Fellowship of the Royal College of Surgeons. Nineteen of his pupils became heads or chairmen of various surgical departments. In 1939, he died in a train accident, attributed to war-time blackout precautions.

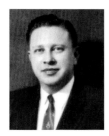

ELLISON, Edwin Homer (1918-1970). Portrait in Chapter 8.

Main institution: Marquette School of Medicine, Milwaukee, Wisconsin, USA.

See the biography in Chapter 8.

FABRY, Wilhelm (1560-1634).

Main institution: Hilden, Düsseldorf, Germany.

Alias Wilhelm Fabricius von Hilden. Born in Hilden near Düsseldorf, and was often described as the father of German surgery. He invented a tourniquet for limb amputation and was said to be among the first to have a survival following amputation of the thigh. He described gallstones after autopsy, and designed an instrument for extracting foreign bodies from the oesophagus, usually employing thin waxed tapers. He removed metal splinters from the eye with magnets.

1. Wilhelm F. *Opera quae extant omnia. Observationum Centuria IV.* Frankfurt: Dufour, 1682: 320. (Translated by or for RH Major, qv. p640-2.)

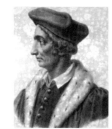

FERNEL, Jean (1497-1558).

Main institution: Physician to the Dauphin (Crown Prince) of France, later Henry II and also Diane of Poitiers.

Born in Montdidier near Clermont in France, he was also known as a philosopher, mathematician, astronomer and very celebrated physician during the Renaissance. In Paris, he calculated the exact dimensions of one-degree meridian latitude. He studied medicine later and graduated aged 38. He was so successful and popular in a short time that he soon became personal physician to the Dauphin of France. Medically he gave an early clinical description of gonorrhoea, and described physical properties of gallstones. He was incorrectly alleged to have made the first description of perforated appendicitis, but on careful scrutiny, he described peritonitis from perforation of the distal ileum near the appendix, by a hard fruit called a quince of 5cm diameter. His final words of wisdom were: "The history will be of value to those who in excessive flow of abundant and toxic fluid from whatsoever cause, hasten intemperately to stop and subdue it to the greatest misfortune to the patient."

1. Fernel J. *Universa Medicina. De partium morbis et symptomis.* Liber VI. Frankfort: Wechlus, 1581: 592.
Image reproduced with permission from the Musée de L'Histoire de la Médecine, Paris, France.

FINSTERER, Hans (1877-1955).

Main institutions: Königsberg, Germany; Innsbruck and Vienna, Austria.

Born in Weng, Austria, he started his medical studies in Vienna, graduating in 1902. He completed surgical training under Hochenegg and von Hacker in 1887 and became assistant to Billroth before returning to von Hacker in Innsbruck. During his surgical training in Billroth's clinic, he visited Charcot and Péan in Paris, Robert Koch and Joseph Lister. He is eponymously associated with Hofmeister for the modified gastrectomy like that devised by Polya, illustrated in Chapter 6. He was a strong promoter of gastric resection and in his lifetime he performed 5000 resections (only 23 gastrojejunostomies), most of them under local anaesthesia. He also devised an operation for recurrent dislocated shoulder. In 1896, he was appointed Professor of Surgery in Königsberg. In 1901, at 58 years, he became the Chief of the Department of Surgery of Allgemeine Krankenhaus and Professor at the University of Vienna.

FINNEY, John Miller Turpin (1863-1942).

Main institution: Surgeon, Johns Hopkins, Baltimore, USA.

His mother died at five months, so he was brought up by an Afro-Caribbean nurse. Graduated in Princetown and Harvard before working under Halsted in Baltimore. In 1903, he invented the inverted U-shaped pyloroplasty (described and illustrated in Chapter 6), which is very applicable for the control of bleeding duodenal ulcers in the second part of the duodenum. The same principle is exactly that which is still being used for the relief of obstruction of long small bowel strictures due to Crohn's disease described in Chapter 9. In Baltimore, he founded the Provident Hospital for black patients, which was a new concept. Finney was the co-founder, with George Crile, and first President, of the American College of Surgeons.

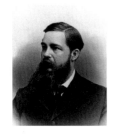

FOWLER, George Ryerson (1848-1906). Portrait in Chapter 12.

Main institution: Surgeon, Brooklyn Hospital, New York, USA (appointed in 1895).

In 1890, he was founder of the Brooklyn Red Cross and lecturer in First Aid to the National Guard. In 1893, he performed his first thoracoplasty for tuberculosis. In 1900, he published an important aid to the management of advanced peritonitis of any cause including perforated appendicitis before the advent of antibiotics, called the 'Fowler Position', allowing dependent drainage via the rectum described in Chapter 12. In 1901, he described the value of de-cortication of the lung after empyema. In 1906, despite his added pioneering for the safe management of appendicitis by early intervention, it was ironic that he himself succumbed to postoperative ileus secondary to acute gangrenous appendicitis.

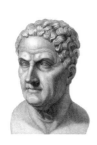

GALEN, Claudius Galenicus (approximately 130-200 AD). Portrait in Chapter 1.

Main institution: Imperial Court, Rome, Italy.

Physician and writer, born in Pergamum, of Greek parents. After studying in Greece, Asia Minor and Alexandria, he returned to Pergamum, where he served as Physician to the Gladiatorial School. He resided chiefly in Rome from c.162. He was noted for his lectures and writings, and established a large practice and eventually became Court Physician to Emperor Marcus Aurelius. He is credited with some 500 treatises, most of them on medicine and philosophy; at least 83 of his medical works are extant. He correlated earlier medical knowledge in all fields with his own discoveries (based in part on experimentation and on dissection of animals) and systematised medicine in accordance with his theories, which emphasised purposive creation. His work in anatomy and physiology are especially notable. He demonstrated that arteries carry blood instead of air and added greatly to knowledge of the brain, nerves, spinal cord, and pulse. Until the 16th century, his authority was virtually undisputed, thus discouraging original investigation and hampering medical progress.

1. *Chambers Biographical Dictionary*. Magnus Magnusson, Ed. W & R Chambers Ltd., 43-45 Annandale Street, Edinburgh, EH7 4AZ. Reprinted 1996.

GERSUNY, Robert (1844-1924).

Main institution: Vienna, Austria.

He was born in Bohemia (Czech Republic) and qualified in Prague. He achieved much of his surgical training under Billroth, and was particularly interested in the formation of adhesions. He performed the first of several cholecystogastrostomies, which is described in Chapter 7. Outside gastroenterological surgery he invented a colporrhaphy for uterine prolapse, and demonstrated before Kocher that Dupuytren's contracture could be cured by fasciectomy.

GOLIGHER, John (1912-1998).

Main institution: Leeds General Infirmary, Leeds, UK.

He was born in Londonderry, Northern Ireland in 1912, and received his medical degree from the University of Edinburgh in 1934. He trained at the Royal Infirmary, Edinburgh, St. Mark's Hospital and St. Mary's Hospital in London before accepting the Chair at the Department of Surgery at the University of Leeds and at the Leeds General Infirmary in 1955. His operating technique resembled serial pages in a textbook of operative surgery. Goligher was one of the pioneers of gastrointestinal stapling and an eminent clinical researcher. His most appreciated contribution was, perhaps, his textbook of colorectal surgery: *Surgery of the Anus, Rectum and Colon*. This book has been widely read by surgeons and has been published in five editions. He introduced randomised clinical trials in surgery and is remembered for surgical progress in colitis, Crohn's disease and rectal cancer.

GROSS, Samuel David (1805-1884).

Main institution: Jefferson Medical College, Philadelphia, USA.

He was born in Easton, Pennsylvania, and graduated in Louisville, Kentucky, USA. He was appointed to the Chair in Surgery, Louisville, from 1840-1856, and conducted a huge amount of work on pathological anatomy, for example, in 1843, he studied intestinal wounds and suturing in laboratory animals. In 1851, he was an acknowledged expert on gastric ulceration, and in 1854, an expert on foreign bodies in the oesophagus and air passages. Afterwards, in 1859, he wrote two textbooks of surgery. He was a staunch advocate of early operation for rupture of the bladder. In 1873, he wrote a masterpiece of sternomastoid myotomy for 'wryneck' (torticollis), 51 years after the original publication by Dupuytren. In his spare time he wrote biographies on Francis Drake, Ephraim McDowell, John Hunter, Johann Paul Richter and Ambroise Paré.

GUSSENBAUER, Carl von (1842-1903).

Main institutions: Liege, Brussels; Prague, Czech Republic; and finally, Vienna, Austria.

Born in Obervallach, Austria, he obtained his medical degree in Vienna in 1866. He is remembered for the anatomy of the atrioventricular valves in the human endocardium. He also devised an internal metal splint for ununited fractures. With Alexander Winiwarter he showed a method for safe excision of the pylorus in dogs. This gave impetus to Billroth to perform the first successful pylorectomy in man in 1881, described in Chapter 6. He described the first excision of a tumour of the bladder performed by Billroth in 1875 and was the first to marsupialise pancreatic cysts. He succeeded Billroth at the Second Surgical Clinic in Vienna, and in 1894, he became President of the German Surgical Society.

HACKER, Victor von (1852-1933).

Main institutions: Sophia Hospital, Vienna, Innsbrück and Graz, Austria.

He was born in Vienna and qualified there in 1878. In 1880, he received his surgical training under Billroth and became successor to Mikulicz. He was an assistant to Billroth in the historic first pylorectomy on Thérèse Heller. In 1885, he performed a first retrocolic posterior gastroenterostomy. After Billroth's death in 1894 he was appointed interim Head of Second Surgical Clinic for nine months. As this was not made permanent, he was appointed, in 1895, the Head of the Surgical Department in Innsbrück. In 1889, he performed the first extraction of a foreign body by means of an endoscope, mentioned in Chapter 4. In 1902, he succeeded Nicoladani in Graz in Austria as Chief Professor of Surgery. Von Hacker was acclaimed to be a leading expert after Mikulicz, on oesophageal surgery, particularly including gastroscopy, and the management of impacted foreign bodies and stricture; he was also an expert in plastic surgery. In 1908, he excised a carcinoma of the cervical oesophagus and larynx in which the patient survived. In 1913, he performed an oesophagoplasty using the transverse colon. In 1930, he was made an Honorary Member of the German Surgical Society.

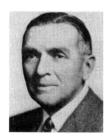

HAIGHT, Cameron (1901-1970). Portrait in Chapter 16.

Main institution: Faculty of Surgery, University of Michigan, Ann Arbor, USA (1932).

See the biography in Chapter 16.

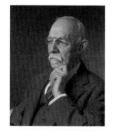

HALSTED, William Stewart (1852-1922). Portrait in Chapter 10.

Main institution: Johns Hopkins Hospital, Baltimore, USA.

Halsted graduated from Yale University in 1874, and after internships he visited Vienna, Leipzig and Würzburg. He returned to surgical practice in New York in 1881. While experimenting with cocaine as a local anaesthetic, he became addicted and for a time had to withdraw from practice. In 1887, his friend Claude Welch provided him with a job in the laboratory at Johns Hopkins, Baltimore, where he was appointed Surgeon in Chief two years later. He organised a system of postgraduate surgical training and his department produced a stream of distinguished surgeons including Finney and Harvey Cushing. He studied wound healing, and was an originator of careful operating technique, to minimise blood loss. He introduced radical mastectomy, a method of inguinal herniorrhaphy and also instituted gutta percha drains and silver foil dressings. When his theatre nurse developed contact dermatitis (from the antiseptic mercury bichloride (not phenolic spray), he devised rubber gloves in 1890. He subsequently married her (see Chapters 9 and 10).

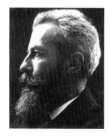

HARTMANN, Henri Albert Charles Antoine (1860-1952).

Main institution: Professor of Surgery, Paris, France.

In 1891, he described the pouching of the gallbladder usually encountered in gallstone disease, which is now thought to be a pathological deformity rather than an anatomical one. In 1909, he described the removal of the upper rectum and / or sigmoid colon initially for inoperable cancer (see Chapter 14), closing the rectal stump, and leaving above an end colostomy in the left iliac fossa (this operation nowadays is more often performed as an emergency operation for complicated diverticular disease).

Image reproduced with permission from The Royal College of Surgeons of England.

HEINECKE, Walther Hermann (1834-1901).

Main institution: University of Ehrlangen, Germany.

In 1886, he performed the first successful pyloroplasty for stenosis, due to scarring of the duodenum by ulceration [1]. It is now known as the 'Heinecke-Mikulicz' pyloroplasty described in Chapter 6. Exactly the same procedure was being used wrongly for achalasia by Wendel as described in Chapter 4 but rightly used as a strictureplasty in Crohn's disease [2].

1. Fronmuller F. *Operation der pylorusstenose.* Erlangen dissertation. Furth: Schroder, 1886.
2. Greenstein AJ. The Surgery of Crohn's disease. In: *Gastroenterology,* 4th edition. Berk JE, *et al*, Eds. Volume 4. Philadelphia: WB Saunders, 1985: 2332.

HEISTER, Lorenz (1683-1758).

Main institutions: Professor of Surgery, Altdorf and Helmstedt, Germany.

Born in Frankfurt-am-Main, at school he excelled in the arts, including poetry and music. He studied medicine first in Giessen, then Leyden and Amsterdam to study under Ruysch and Rau. Lectured by Boerhaave in Leyden, and served in the Dutch Army for several years. He described one of the first reports of peritonitis due to appendicitis in a criminal at post mortem when Professor of Pathology in Altdorf (Chapter 12). He also saved the life of a cavalryman with a strangulated hernia, which did not require resection of the intestine, during the battle of Oudenard. He is also alleged to have given the first description of direct inguinal hernia.

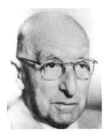

HELLER, Ernst (1877-1964). Portrait in Chapter 4.

Main institution: Professor of Surgery, Leipzig, Germany.

In 1913, he performed the first myotomy for achalasia described in Chapter 4. This procedure did not catch on for many years until support from Barrett and Franklin in 1949. He described the double myotomy of the lower oesophagus, found to be reproducible across the world, replacing the multiple bypasses and cardioplasties of the time, which had high complication rates.

1. Barrett NR, Franklin RH. Concerning the unfavourable late results of certain operations performed in the treatment of cardiospasm. *Br J Surg* 1949; 37: 194-202.

HILL, Lucius D (born 1921).

Main institution: Department of Surgery, University of Washington, Seattle, Washington, USA.

Dr. Hill graduated from the University of Virginia in 1944 with much initial experience in military surgery. His postgraduate training was at the University of Virginia and the Lahey Clinic, before his appointment as Assistant Professor of Surgery in Seattle in Washington State in 1964. He became full Professor there in 1976. He described a partial posterior fundoplication for reflux oesophagitis, which included a gastropexy accentuating the cardio-oesophageal angle mentioned in Chapter 4. He achieved much expertise in highly selective vagotomy, both in animal and clinical studies before the advent of ulcer-healing drugs, described in Chapter 6, were available.

HIPPOCRATES (ca 460-450 BC to 377-370 BC).

Widely regarded as the founder of medicine; although his dates and life are largely uncertain, his existence is historical. Born on the Island of Cos in the Greek Dodecanese in the Aegean Sea, the legend implies he was a descendant of the half-God, Aesculapius. He was much travelled in the Greek world and in Egypt and Scythia. He embraced all the fields of medicine and surgery, and created a School containing many disciples, including his two sons. His written works were numerous, some of which he was probably not the sole author. Some experts suspect there was more than one physician writing under the name of Hippocrates. Most famous are his aphorisms, a series of clear and short sentences with a pedagogical objective. Some of these were required to be learnt by heart until the 19th century by generations of young European physicians. The Hippocratic Oath is still quite up-to-date with our deontological standards. His main contribution will undoubtedly remain to have stressed the importance of writing down medical history and clinical observations methodically. He took care over anatomical and physiological studies, and so allowed the emancipation of medicine from magic, religious rites and philosophical theories. His death according to tradition is recorded between 377 and 370 BC, making him more than one hundred years old.

HUTCHINSON, Jonathan (1828-1913). Portrait in Chapter 9.

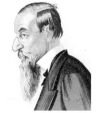

Main institution: Consultant Surgeon, London Hospital, UK.

He was born in Selby in Yorkshire, UK, but studied medicine in the City of York in the UK at first before going to London at St. Bartholomew's Hospital, Moorfields Eye Hospital and The London Hospital. He had a strong interest in ophthalmology and a notable expertise on syphilis, prophesying that a microbe would prove to be the cause. In 1858, the notched incisors of congenital syphilis were named after him, and he described the triad of interstitial keratitis, labyrinthine disease and the cusped teeth. The 'Hutchinson's facies' in ophthalmoplegia and the 'Hutchinson's mask' in tabes dorsalis were also named after him. He also described unequal pupils in meningeal haemorrhages. In 1871, he was the first surgeon to reduce an intussusception in a two-year-old infant by operation with a successful outcome, mentioned in Chapter 9. He was at first opposed to antiseptic surgery and to women entering the medical profession!

JURASZ, Antoni Aleksander Tomasz (1882-1961).

Main institution: Professor and Director of the Poznan Clinic, Poznan, Poland.

He was the first instigator of internal drainage of a pancreatic pseudocyst by a large posterior gastrostomy, mentioned in Chapter 8. This principle is still used today by endoscopists and radiologists, so that now it is an outpatient procedure.

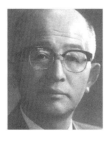

KASAI, Morio (born 1922). Portrait in Chapter 16.

Main institution: Chairman of the Department of Surgery, Tohoku University, Japan.

See the biography in Chapter 16 (personal communication to Professor Jay Grosfeld from Professor Ryoji Ohi, Sendai, Japan, in 2006).

KIRSCHNER, Martin (1879-1942).

Main institutions: Königsberg and Heidelberg, Germany.

He was famed for stabilisation of bone fragments and joints with wire in limb problems, and he achieved the first successful pulmonary embolectomy by his mentor's 'Trendelenburg operation' in 1924. He was probably the first to prove that the fundus of the stomach could reach the neck after mobilisation in the abdomen, by preserving the branches of the right gastric vessels as described and illustrated in Chapter 4. He described synchronous combined excision of the rectum in 1934, after seeing that posterior excision had a lower mortality but a higher local recurrence rate than abdominoperineal excision. His procedure was published in Germany well before Morgan and Lloyd-Davies in 1936 but was not accepted for political reasons during this period when Germany was isolated.

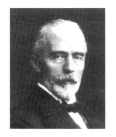

KOCHER, Theodor (1841-1917). Portrait in Chapter 12.

Main institution: Professor of Surgery, University of Berne, Switzerland.

This surgical giant was a fine technician and an inspiration to his assistants and his visitors, such as Harvey Cushing from the US. His sensible approach for patients suspected to have appendicitis is referred to in Chapter 12. In addition, he devised his own forceps in gallbladder and gastroenterological surgery, as well as his incision for cholecystectomy, which gave good exposure before good relaxant anaesthesia was available. It is known that the 8th or 9th intercostal nerves are in jeopardy by this approach, yet in his own textbook of surgery he stressed that these nerves should be preserved to prevent an incisional hernia. He is known for his duodenal-mobilising manoeuvres described in 1903, mostly for gastric operations (for the record the manoeuvre was described by Jourdan in 1895 and performed in biliary surgery by Vautrin in 1886). He invented closed reduction (by manipulation) for shoulder dislocation. He was the first surgeon to win the Nobel Prize, mainly for his exemplary work on the physiology and surgery of the thyroid gland. He performed over 2000 thyroidectomies with a 4% mortality rate, remarkable at that time. Kocher's rule: "A surgeon is a doctor who can operate and who knows when not to."

KUSSMAUL, Adolf (1822-1902).

Main institution: Professor of Surgery, Strasburg, Germany.

This physician was born in Graben near Karlsruhe, and became Professor of Medicine, first at Heidelberg in 1857, next to Erlangen in 1859, then Freiburg in 1863 and finally, Strasburg in 1876. He gave the first description of mesenteric thrombosis in a living subject in 1864. He attempted oesophagoscopy in 1869, thwarted by lack of good light and suction. He described peri-arteritis nodosa in 1866, progressive bulbar paralysis in 1873 and acetonaemia and air hunger in 1874. He also performed a series of intubations and irrigation of the stomach in acute gastric dilatation in 1867-1869. He stressed to the surgical fraternity the need for surgical relief of pyloric obstruction, perhaps via his son-in-law, Vincenz Czerny. In 1868, he demonstrated a gastric ulcer with bismuth, and performed a thoracocentesis.

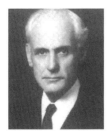

LADD, William E (1880-1967). Portrait in Chapter 16.

Main institution: Professor of Paediatric Surgery, Harvard University, and Boston City Hospital, Boston, USA.

See the biography in Chapter 16.

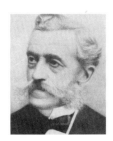

LANGENBECK, Bernhard von (1810-1887). Portrait in Chapter 6.

Main institution: Berlin, Germany.

His uncle, Konrad Langenbeck, was Professor of Surgery in Göttingen, so Bernard started his surgical career there from 1830-1834. He was said to be one of the greatest clinical teachers of his time. Initially, he worked in Kiel, then succeeded Dieffenbach at the Charité Hospital in Berlin. Pupils under him included Billroth, von Bergmann, Krönlein, Trendelenburg, Witzel and Esmarch. He was the founder of *Archive fur Klinische Chirurgie* (initially called *Langenbeck's Archives*), and also founded the German Surgical Society. There are said to be 21 eponymous operations, mostly bone and joint operations.

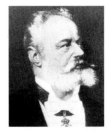

LANGENBUCH, Carl Johann August (1846-1901). Portrait in Chapter 7.

Main institution: Director of the Lazarus Hospital, Berlin, Germany (from 1873).

Carl Langenbuch was born in Kiel in 1846 and graduated in 1869. The very next year he served as a surgeon in the Franco-Prussian war, and on demobilisation was an Assistant Surgeon to Max Wilms for three years, which gave him tremendous surgical experience. A remarkable surgeon, he carried out procedures in human cadavers in the local mortuary, before applying new techniques on live patients. In 1877, he performed the first nephrectomy for malignant disease, and in 1879 he performed a duodenostomy. He practised Listerian principles in abdominal surgery. On July 15th 1882, he performed the first cholecystectomy on a man of 43 who was a morphine addict because of repeated attacks of biliary colic. The patient was out of bed on the 12th day and fit to go home after six weeks. He became Director of the new hospital in Berlin, the Lazaruskrankenhauss, where he worked until his death in 1901.

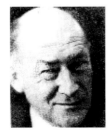

LATARJET, André (1877-1947). Portrait in Chapter 6.

Main institution: University of Lyon, France.

A French surgeon and Professor of Anatomy, he became famous for his description of the eponymous anterior and posterior vagus nerves entering the lesser curvature. He performed several operations described by him as 'enervation gastrique', now called selective vagotomy, for various dyspepsias, some he called 'gastropathie vago-sympathique' and some for duodenal ulcers. His last published scientific article appeared in 1923.

LEMBERT, Antoine (1802-1851).

Main institution: Hotel Dieu Hospital, Paris, France.

Born in Nancy in 1802. He was assistant to Dupuytren in Paris and applied the new principles of suturing described by Travers, ensuring that only the serous surfaces are apposed to each other. He warned the surgical world against creating too large a phlange by excessive inversion of the suture line. This became the foundation of all modern gastric and intestinal surgery (Chapter 10). He was named laureate of the Académie des Sciences for his research of 'la methode iatraleptique'. He died of carcinoma of the stomach aged 49.

1. Lembert A. Memoire sur l'enteropathie avec la description d'un procede nouveau pour practiquer cette operation chirurgicale. *Rep Gen Anat Physiol Pathol* 1826; 2: 100.
2. Bogardus GM. Antoine Lembert and his method of intestinal anastomosis. *West J Surg Obstet Gynec* 1962; 70: 286-8.

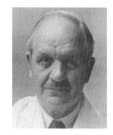

LEWIS, Ivor (1895-1982). Portrait in Chapter 4.

Main institution: Consultant Surgeon, North Middlesex Hospital, London, UK. Later, Royal Alexandra Hospital, Rhyll, North Wales.

Trained at University College, Cardiff and also at University College Hospital, London. In 1933, he was appointed to the North Middlesex Hospital in London. He pioneered daily visiting to patients by relatives. He achieved the first successful pulmonary embolectomy (Trendelenburg procedure) in the UK in 1939 (see Kirschner, Martin). His patient lived for 12 years, and there was no lung disease at autopsy. In 1946, he devised the two-stage approach for carcinoma of the middle third of the oesophagus, which is the most used approach in the UK (Chapter 4). This right-sided approach was much criticised by several peers for many years. Lewis was a fine poet, musician, classical scholar and ardent Welshman.

1. Morris-Stiff G, Hughes LE. Ivor Lewis (1895-1982). Welsh pioneer of the right-sided approach to the oesophagus. *Dig Surg* 2003; 20: 546-58.

LISFRANC de SAINT-MARTIN, Jacques (1790-1847).

Main institution: L'Hôpital de la Pitié, Paris, France.

This French surgeon started his education in Lyon before studying under Dupuytren in Paris. Most of his interests lay in diagnosis and management of orthopaedic injuries. Renowned for his operative speed, he reportedly could perform a transmetatarsal amputation in less than one minute. Credited with the first successful resection of a rectal cancer by means of a perineal incision and amputation of the rectum proximal to the tumour. In 1826, he had his own Department of Surgery at L'Hôpital de la Pitié in Paris. He was a famous teacher, but had such an aggressive style that students and colleagues found co-operation very difficult.

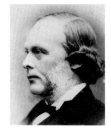

LISTER, Joseph (Baron Lister of Lyme Regis) (1827-1912). Portraits in Chapter 3.

Main institutions: Professorial Chairs at Glasgow, Edinburgh and King's College Hospital, London, UK.

See the biography in Chapter 3.

LITTRÉ, Alexis (1658-1726).

Main institution: Académie des Sciences, Paris, France.

As a famous anatomist and surgeon, he was known for his hernia containing a Meckel's diverticulum; also known for the glands around the male urethra and occlusion of part of the intestine in a strangulated hernia. He successfully performed a colostomy in neonatal obstruction in rectal atresia.

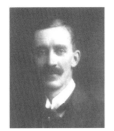

LOCKHART-MUMMERY, John Percy (1875-1957). Portrait in Chapter 13.

Main institution: Surgeon, St. Mark's Hospital, London, UK.

In 1899, he graduated from St. George's Hospital. Father of H.E. Lockhart-Mummery, Consultant Surgeon at St. Thomas's Hospital in London. He introduced the electrically illuminated sigmoidoscope in 1904, having used Strauss' lighted rectoscope in the early 1900s. He was first Secretary of the British Proctological Society in 1913 (this later became the Proctological section of the Royal Society of Medicine). Later, he became President of the Royal Society of Medicine. He devised a perineal excision of the rectum in 1925, modified from Kraske's pioneer perineal resection, first described in 1882. He described the early results of surgery for ulcerative colitis (Chapter 13). He started an audit with Dukes and Gabriel on the follow-up of colorectal cancer, which in those days was new. He started a familial polyposis register. He also founded the Imperial Cancer research fund that became Cancer Research UK (CRUK).

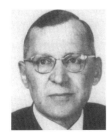

LOUW, Jan Hendrik (1915-1992). Portrait in Chapter 16.

Main institution: Director of Paediatric Surgery, University of Cape Town, South Africa.

See the biography in Chapter 16.

MACEWEN Sir William (1848-1924.)

Main institution: Professor of Surgery, Glasgow Royal Infirmary, Glasgow, UK (in 1892).

Born in Rothesay on the Isle of Bute. In 1865, he moved to Glasgow and graduated from the Royal Infirmary in 1869. He was a surgical dresser (student) to Joseph Lister, a major influence on his practice. In 1892, he became Regius Professor of Surgery at Glasgow Western Infirmary. He studied and described precisely the processes of wound healing, and the true function of the peritoneum. He was the first in the successful practice of laryngeal intubation and introduced both oral and nasal endotracheal tubes for general anaesthesia, following huge experience in the treatment of airway obstruction from diphtheria. As a result, he was an early pioneer in thoracic surgery. He declined the Chair of Surgery at Johns Hopkins, Baltimore, that later went to William Halsted. He was interested in the rehabilitation of amputees using primitive prosthetic limbs; he also was the first practitioner in bone grafting and osteotomy, and the surgery of transverse fractures of the patella. He was a pioneer in neurosurgery, and was famous for dramatic results from drainage of cerebral abscesses.

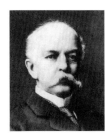

McBURNEY, Charles (1845-1913). Portrait in Chapter 12.

Main institution: Professor of Surgery, College of Physicians and Surgeons, New York, USA (Columbia Presbyterian).

Born in Roxbury, Massachusetts on the 17th February 1845, he undertook general and medical studies at Harvard University until 1869 and was a student in New York when Willard Parker drained an appendix abscess. He subsequently became a surgical intern at Bellevue Hospital, New York and conducted further postgraduate studies in Paris, Berlin, Vienna and London. In 1873, he returned from Europe to New York and was an anatomy demonstrator and lecturer until 1894. From 1894 to 1907, he was Professor of Surgery at the College of Physicians and Surgeons in New York (Columbia Presbyterian) and Staff Surgeon at the Roosevelt Hospital, New York. After enumerable cadaver examinations, he calculated the site of the base of the appendix, known as McBurney's point. With Murphy (q.v.) he advocated appendicectomy in the early stages of the disease. He independently described the gridiron approach for early appendicitis about the same time as McArthur, but gave the latter the credit. He instigated the transduodenal access for stone extraction from the lower end of the common bile duct (see Chapters 7 and 12).

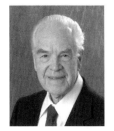

MASON, Edward E (born 1920). Portrait in Chapter 5.

Main institution: University of Iowa, Iowa, USA.

See the biography in Chapter 5.

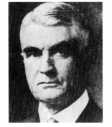

MAYO, William James (1861-1939). Portrait in Chapter 7.

Main institution: The Mayo Clinic, Rochester, Minnesota, USA, which was founded with his father William Worrall and brother Charles Horace in 1889.

Mayo served as President of the American Medical Association in 1906. In 1911, he founded The Society of Clinical Surgery and became a Member of the American Surgical Association in 1913. In 1917, he started with his brother, Charles Horace, the Foundation for Medicine and Research, parallel to the town hospitals. In 1925, he joined the American College of Surgeons. His name was attached to several surgical procedures and instruments, and he wrote innumerable scientific articles.

MAYO, William Worrall (1819-1911).

Main institution: Founder of the Mayo Clinic, Rochester, Minnesota, USA.

Born in Manchester, UK and emigrated to North America in 1845. He received his medical degree in Missouri University in 1853 and settled down as a surgeon in Rochester, Minnesota in 1863. In 1858, he founded the Minnesota State Medical Society. His two sons became surgeons: William James (1861-1939) described above, and Charles Horace (1865-1939). The three formed a surgical practice together and developed great productivity and prominence. They made the Mayo Clinic a world-famous centre for surgical care, training and research. Charles Horace was more modest, but the three built up an enormously successful and productive department, performing several thousands of operations per year. The Mayo Clinic became a role model in the US and the whole world. In 1915, they founded the Mayo Foundation for education and research.

1.   Rutkow IM. *Surgery, an illustrated history.* Mosby-Year Book Inc., 1993: 500.

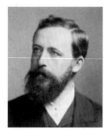

MIKULICZ-RADECKI, Johann (1850-1905) (later Germanised as Johann von Mikulicz.). Portrait in Chapter 4.

Main institutions: Krakow, Poland; Königsberg, Germany; and finally Breslau (Wroclaw), Poland.

Born at Czernowitz in Poland in 1850, the family soon moved to Austria. He disobeyed his father by studying medicine instead of law, so he maintained himself as a medical student by giving piano lessons. He trained in Vienna, and was awarded an MD in 1875. He worked for Billroth until 1878, becoming surgical assistant to Billroth until 1881, and was said to be Billroth's most brilliant pupil. Occasionally, he played in quartets including both Billroth and Brahms! In 1881, he became known as the 'father of oesophagoscopy and gastroscopy'. In 1882, he was appointed Professor of Surgery at Krakow. His name is associated with the syndrome of hypertrophy of the salivary glands and xerostomia, described the same year. He was an early advocate of antiseptic surgery and was one of the first to use (cotton) gloves and mask, moving on to rubber gloves later. In 1883, he excised a pharyngeal tumour via a lateral pharyngotomy. An early user of the multi-layered large gauze pad to retract abdominal viscera. In 1884, he performed a successful operation for a typhoid ulcer of the intestine. He advocated and practised partial thyroidectomy called 'wedge thyroidectomy'. In 1885, he performed the first, although an unsuccessful attempt, simple closure of a perforated peptic ulcer. The condition had been well known as a lethal cause of death since 1817. In 1886, he performed resection of the cervical oesophagus for tumour. He was appointed Professor of Surgery at Königsberg the following year. In the same year, he performed a successful pyloroplasty for duodenal stenosis a year after Heinecke; the commonest pyloroplasty with truncal vagotomy was since called the 'Heinecke-Mikulicz' pyloroplasty (Chapter 6). The same procedure is still used for relief of strictures in the intestine, due to Crohn's disease today. He subsequently devised an enterotome to anastomose adjacent loops of intestine by a delayed gradual crushing procedure. In 1890, he was appointed Professor of Surgery at Breslau (now Wroclaw). He was a mentor to Ferdinand Sauerbruch in Breslau and believed that surgeons should not marry until becoming a professor! (Philosophy also adopted by Sauerbruch). In 1892, he described the symmetrical inflammation of the lachrymal glands, named as Mikulicz syndrome, and the folowing year, the first two-stage resection of the colon; he also inserted a successful shunt for hydrocephalus.

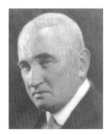

MILES, Sir William Ernest (1869-1947). Portrait in Chapter 14.

Main institution: Surgeon, The Royal Marsden Hospital and Gordon Hospitals, London, UK.

In 1908, he performed the first abdominoperineal resection of the rectum. The principle was that the regional lymphovascular pedicle and the levator ani muscles lateral to the rectal wall were removed en bloc with the rectum and distal sigmoid colon. Miles reasoned that the downward spread of the tumour necessitated the removal of the whole rectum and anal canal in all rectal cancers. He introduced the 'cylinder' of tissue removed with the rectum to achieve adequate removal. He championed rectosigmoidectomy for rectal prolapse, and his textbook ran into four editions.

1. Miles WE. The radical abdominoperineal operation for cancer of the rectum and of the pelvic colon. *Br Med J* 1910; 2: 941-3.

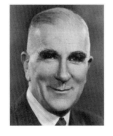

MILLIGAN, Edward Thomas Campbell (1886-1972). Portrait in Chapter 15.

Main institution: St. Mark's Hospital, London, UK.

An Olympic ski medallist for Australia before qualification as a doctor, he was associated with the anatomical landmark of the columns with Naunton Morgan. He pioneered debridement and delayed suture of shrapnel and bullet wounds in World War I, the principle decried by a senior surgeon in London who demanded his removal from the frontline battle stations because of his "wild colonial methods". Later, he was reinstated and decorated by King George Vth of Britain after the war. His philosophy of delayed suture of contaminated wounds has saved thousands of lives in major wars ever since. His haemorrhoidectomy operation has survived at least half a century. He was a devoutly religious man who always preceded his operating sessions with prayer.

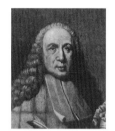

MORGAGNI, Giovanni Battista (1682-1771). Portrait in Chapter 15.

Main institution: Professor of Anatomy, Padua, Italy (in 1715).

A founder of pathological anatomy, he was born in Forli, Italy. A pupil of Valsalva, he published his work in his 79th year. He was an instigator of scientific medicine and according to Virchow, Morgagni was the first to introduce the anatomical and not the humoral reasoning into medical practice. Alleged to have said: "Signs and symptoms are the cry of the suffering organs within!" Numerous anatomical structures and conditions are named after him: posterior diaphragmatic hernia; cerebral gummata; aneurysms; diseased cardiac valves; yellow atrophy of the liver; and heart block, later described clinically as Stokes-Adams attacks. He attributed cerebral abscesses to middle ear infection, and was the first to note that a lesion of the cerebral cortex caused a paralysis on the contralateral side.

MORTON, William Thomas Green (1819-1868).

Main institution: Various, but including the Massachusetts General Hospital, Boston, USA.

Born in Charlton, Massachusetts, he studied dentistry in Baltimore, Maryland. Morton encountered a public demonstration of the soporific effects of nitrous oxide in 1844, and he noticed the subject felt no pain. This commenced a series of painless dental extractions, before he decided to study medicine. Despite the failed demonstration of painless tooth extraction by colleague Horace Wells, he was able to demonstrate the anaesthetic properties of sulphuric ether to senior surgeon, John Warren, thanks to the introduction by Henry Jacob Bigelow. He was able to repeat the effect during another operation three weeks later. His attempts to patent sulphuric ether mixed with air were rejected by Henry Bigelow, but Morton's legal battles with entrepreneur Charles Jackson led him into poverty and an early grave.

MOYNIHAN, Berkeley George Andrew (1865-1936).

Main institution: Surgeon, Leeds General Infirmary, Leeds, UK.

Born on the Island of Malta. In 1887, he graduated from London University and achieved an MS diploma from Leeds University. In 1890, he achieved the Fellowship Diploma at the Royal College of Surgeons in London and in 1896, was appointed surgeon to Leeds General Infirmary, UK. He was known as one of the finest abdominal surgeons in his time. Founder of the Association of Surgeons of Great Britain and Ireland, he also founded the *British Journal of Surgery* and became a sub-editor to *Surgery, Gynecology and Obstetrics*, requested by J.B. Murphy. He published his work on duodenal ulcer, establishing its clinical importance separate from gastric ulcerations; he also advocated that patients should 'earn' their operation for ulceration and gallstones. He apparently first described 'hunger pain' associated with duodenal ulceration. He was famous, too, for his aphorism "A gallstone is a tombstone to the memory of the germ which lies within it." He designed strong forceps still used by many for grasping the gallbladder during open cholecystectomy. According to Cushing, French surgeons

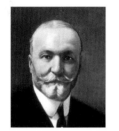
visiting Moynihan noticed his lack of spilling of blood during operations. They asked if "English blood is really as precious as all that?"

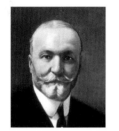

MURPHY, John B (1857-1916). Portrait in Chapter 10.

Main institutions: North Western and Rush Colleges of Surgery (now University of Illinois), Chicago, USA.

Born in Appleton, Wisconsin in 1857, he graduated from, and later became Professor of Surgery at Rush Medical College of Chicago and Professor of Surgery, North Western University, Chicago. He served as President of the AMA in 1911 and the American College of Surgeons in 1913. He was the first editor of *Surgery, Gynecology and Obstetrics* and was the first author of *Surgical Clinics of North America* (they were initially known as *Clinics of J.B. Murphy*). After graduation he spent 18 months visiting centres in Europe, such as Billroth in Vienna, and others in Berlin and Heidelberg. He was admired by Lord Moynihan of Leeds who said: "Murphy was without question the greatest clinical teacher of his day." To ensure uniform sharpness of his scalpels, he used new disposable razor blades fixed to a designated handle for each patient. An early advocate of Listerian antisepsis. He was also an early practitioner for artificial pneumothorax for tuberculosis. He attended President Theodore (Teddy) Roosevelt when an attempted assassination was made by a bullet fired into his right chest, successfully treating it conservatively. In 1887, he introduced end-to-end suturing of blood vessels. He successfully saved a patient's limb following embolectomy from the common iliac artery. In 1892, he invented his celebrated button (Chapter 10). Others used the button for suprapubic bladder drainage, for vascular anastomoses, after lower oesophageal resections, and for occluding oesophageal varices. He was subsequently conferred the order of Christian Knighthood and Apostolic Blessing by the current Pope of the day. In 1904, he advocated early as well as interval appendicectomy to prevent recurrent appendicitis. According to George Crile, although Murphy was then a sick man, he mobilised many medical and surgical resources for the American contribution to the Allied effort in World War I. He died on Mackinac Island on the 11th August 1916.

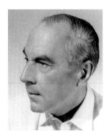

NISSEN, Rudolf (1896-1981). Portrait in Chapter 4.

Main institution: Professor of Surgery, Basle, Switzerland.

See the biography in Chapter 4.

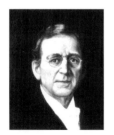

OCHSNER, Albert John (1858 1925). Portrait in Chapter 12.

Main institution: Augustana Hospital, Chicago, and University of Illinois, Chicago, USA.

Born in Baraboo in Wisconsin of German-Swiss origin, his family had emigrated to America. He achieved a BSc in 1884, followed by an MD at Rush University, Chicago in 1886. He learned the basic ABO blood types for major surgery and while visiting a European centre, he saved the life of a colleague who had a massive haemorrhage from a peptic ulcer, by setting up and cross-matching a blood transfusion. Known for the emergency treatment of incarcerated hernia in children, he was appointed Professor of Surgery at the University of Illinois between 1900-1925 and served as President of the American Surgical Association in 1923-1924. In 1902, he outlined the indications for the conservative treatment of appendicitis when over-enthusiasm for appendicectomy was rife (Chapter 12). James Sherren from London, independently advocated this approach three years later. The medical establishment agreed to call the conservative approach, the 'Ochsner-Sherren' regime.

OCHSNER, Edward William Alton (1896-1981). Portrait in Chapter 9.

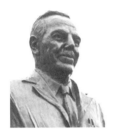

Main institutions: Tulane University and the Ochsner Clinic, New Orleans, Louisiana, USA.

Ochsner qualified from Washington University, St. Louis in 1920. He obtained a surgical residency under his older cousin, Albert Ochsner, in Chicago, who then arranged visits to Zurich and Frankfurt. (Alton generally referred to Albert as 'uncle' but he was his cousin.) After a year in private practice in Chicago, he accepted a reduction in income in moving to the University of Wisconsin Medical School to do research into bronchiectasis. In 1927, he succeeded Rudfolf Mattas as Chairman of Surgery at Tulane. In 1939, he published an article with Michael De Bakey suggesting a link between cigarette smoking and lung cancer. In 1942, he and others established a group practice clinic. The independent surgeons were jealous of its success, leading to his being dismissed from the Chairmanship at Tulane in 1946, although he retained his Professorship. He tried, unsuccessfully, to integrate the Ochsner Clinic with the medical school. He was President of, among other organisations, the American College of Surgeons, the Society of Vascular Surgery, The International Society of Surgery and the American Cancer Society.

PARÉ, Ambroise (1510-1590). Portrait in Chapter 1.

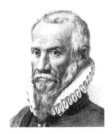

Main institution: Fellow of the prestigious Collège de St. Cômbe, Paris, France.

Paré was born near Laval in Northern France. After an apprenticeship in Paris, he became a military surgeon in various battlefields, and made some remarkable artificial limbs for the wounded. He published in French rather than Latin. A surgeon to five Kings of France, Premier Chirurgien et Conseiller du Roi, and famous for several especial advances: rejection of boiling oil in treatment of gunshot wounds; ligature instead of cautery for vessels; podalic version in difficult breech presentations in pregnancy; attempted implantation of teeth. His published work was translated into Latin, German and several other languages.

PARKS, Alan (1920-1982). Portrait in Chapter 13.

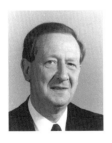

Main institution: St. Mark's Hospital, and The Royal London Hospital, London, UK.

See the biography in Chapter 13.

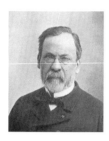

PASTEUR, Louis (1822-1894). Portrait in Chapter 3.

Main institution: Professor of Chemistry, the Sorbonne, Paris (1867).

Born in 1822 in Dôle in French Jura, he first worked on the polarisation of light and on crystals and so allowed the emergence of stereochemistry (1848). In 1849, he was appointed Professor of Chemistry in the Faculty of Strasbourg, and in 1854, became Dean of the Faculty of Lille, and Director of the prestigious Ecole Normale Supérieure in Paris in 1857. His main studies were devoted to the role of micro-organisms but were greeted by many with scepticism. Nevertheless, his discourses had many industrial applications, including preventing a disease of silk-worms, perfecting the making of vinegar, and protecting wines and beers by the invention of the process of pasteurisation. From the 1870s, he turned to medical applications, proving the importance of sterilising surgical instruments, studying carbuncles (1877) and chicken cholera (1878). In 1881, he was elected at the Académie Française; his fame evolved into the status of a national hero when he succeeded in saving a boy, aged nine, from rabies; it was the first attempt of curative vaccination. In 1888, the Institut Pasteur was founded in Paris. This institution was to be the home of many famous microbiologists and would give birth to many discoveries on infectious diseases and vaccinations. He died in 1894.

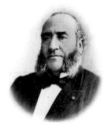

PÉAN, Jules (1830-1898).

Main institution: St. Louis Hospital, Paris, France (later his own Clinic).

Born in Chateaudun in France, he trained with Denonvilliers and under Nélaton. He was a sound technical surgeon who realised that most vessels needed to be tied or crushed, so he invented his own forceps (such haemostasis was called 'Par le pincement de Péan'). Actually, Charrière and Koeberle had invented haemostatic forceps before Péan. He instigated: pincement préventatif; pincement temporaire; and pincement définatif. He always operated in evening dress with a towel around his neck to protect his shirt front! Nélaton and he visited Lister, adopted his principles, but avoided the spray. In 1865, he was one of the first to remove a large ovarian cyst successfully, and in 1867, he first successfully performed splenectomy for an accidental injury during ovarian cystectomy! In 1879, he was the first surgeon recorded to resect a tumour of the stomach; however, the patient died after four or five days, despite transfusions of blood which had not been cross-matched. He never attempted gastrectomy again. He contributed much to urology and gynaecology and pioneered hysterectomy, but was heavily criticised by others who could not emulate his survivals. He was the first surgeon to excise a bladder diverticulum. A true 'workaholic', on his death bed he advised his juniors: "Je vous quitterai sur un mot qui résume tout; Travailler." ("I am leaving you with one word which says it all: Keep working!"). A press communication which described his 'gung-ho' approach to surgery quoted: "De l'audace, encore l'audace, toujours l'audace" ("of audacity, again audacity, and always audacity"). There is a portrait by Toulouse Lautrec in the Sterling and Francine Clark Institute in Williamstown, Massachusetts.

1.   Brochin A. L'œuvre de Péan. In: *La France médicale*, 1900: 126-9.
Image reproduced with permission from the Académie de Médicine, Paris, France.

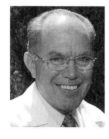

PEÑA Alberto. Portrait in Chapter 16.

Main institution: Professor of Pediatric Surgery, University of Cincinnati College of Medicine and Director of the Colorectal Center, Children's Hospital Medical Center, Cincinnati, Ohio.

See the biography in Chapter 16.

POLYA, Eugene ('Jeno') (1876-1944).

Main institution: Surgeon-in Chief, St. Stephens Hospital, Budapest, Hungary (1906).

Born in Budapest on the 30th April 1876, he graduated from Budapest in 1898. He modified the Billroth II operation with a retrocolic gastrojejunal anastomosis, shortening the afferent loop, and described an ingenious method of closing the duodenal stump (Chapter 6). He was a protagonist of conservative treatment of pancreatitis. An Honorary Fellow of the American College of Surgeons in 1938, he retired in 1941, after over 500 publications, especially in gastric and biliary surgery. He was a linguist, musician, chess and bridge player of renown. Politically, he was a Jew and a liberal. He was alleged to have been murdered by the Nazis in 1944 for being a Zionist, but according to more accurate information provided by R.M. Kirk, he was transported to Siberia by the order of Stalin (as was the famous Swedish philanthropist, Raoul Wallenburg), and never heard of since.

1.   Kirk RM. Contemporary. Personal communication.

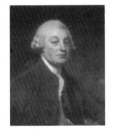

POTT, Percival (1714-1788). Portrait in Chapter 9.

Main institution: St. Bartholomew's Hospital, London, UK.

A well educated pupil of Edward Nourse and William Cheselden at St. Bartholomew's Hospital in London, he described paralysis from tuberculosis of the spine, later called 'Pott's paraplegia'. Eponymous fracture of the ankle, which he had sustained himself from falling off a horse. While recovering he wrote his *Treatise on Ruptures*. Pott, in his day, was an authority on head injuries, especially extradural haematoma and abscess. In addition, his name is associated with occupational diseases such as 'Chimney sweep's cancer of the scrotum', which was due to the carcinogenic properties in soot, and oedema of the scalp, due to underlying osteomyelitis of the skull, known as 'Pott's puffy tumour'. He appreciated the need for urgent surgery of strangulated hernias, but there is no record of results, described in Chapter 9.

1.   Sebastian A. *A Dictionary of the History of Medicine.* New York and London: Parthenon Publishing Group, 1999.

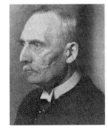

RAMSTEDT, Conrad Wilhelm (1867-1962). Portrait in Chapter 16.

Main institution: Surgeon, Rafael Clinic, Munster, Germany.

See the biography in Chapter 16.

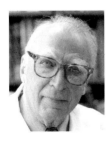

RAVITCH, Mark (1910-1989). Portrait in Chapter 11.

Main institution: Head of the Department of Surgery, University of Pittsburgh, Pittsburgh, USA.

See the biography in Chapter 11.

ROUX, César (1857-1934). Portrait in Chapter 4.

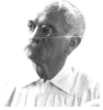

Main institution: Professor of Surgery, University of Lausanne, Switzerland.

Roux was the eighth child of a Protestant refugee from Catholic France. He was a favoured pupil of Kocher, (q.v.) at the University of Bern and Kocher's assistant 1876-80. He was Chief Surgeon at the Cantonal Hospital, Lausanne, in 1887 and co-founder of the new University Hospital in Lausanne in 1890. He disliked the fashion of surgical travels, but was consequently visited by distinguished peers. He was feared and respected by students, but was a great teacher and brilliant illustrator on blackboards in the operating theatre. According to Cushing, Roux was a "rough diamond, brilliant, showy and rapid in his work", until the advent of improved general anaesthesia when he became slower and more meticulous. He became famous for his retrocolic 'Ansa-en-Y' gastrojejunostomy and was the first surgeon to remove a phaeochromocytoma successfully. He resected and bypassed a caustic oesophageal stricture in a child of 12 in two stages over four years starting in 1906 (Chapter 4). He was an early protagonist for long-term nasogastric tubes to preserve the lumen in caustic strictures until all cicatrisation complete, before a programme of dilatations. In retirement, he embarked on social schemes including supporting women's suffrage. He retired in 1926 from the University. He continued operating for a while until his vision became impaired by bilateral cataracts. He died on the 21st December 1934 from myocardial insufficiency during a clinical consultation.

RYDYGIER, Ludwig (1850-1920). Portrait in Chapter 1.

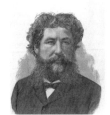

Main institutions: University Departments of Surgery, Krakow, Lvov and Poznan, Poland.

Born in Dusocin in Poland, he trained in Germany at Greifswald, also in Berlin and Strasbourg and spent a few years in private practice in his home town, Chelmno, Poland. He succeeded von Mikulicz as Professor of Surgery in Krakow in 1887. Subsequently, he was appointed Professor of Surgery in Lvov. An ardent Polish Nationalist, he founded the Polish Association of Surgeons. His MD thesis confirmed the antiseptic qualities of carbolic acid, but conversely, the toxic nature of concentrated solutions of the acid. He visited several European centres including Billroth in Vienna. He was the ambassador of Polish surgery in a very difficult time in Polish history when Poland, deprived of statehood, was split up into neighbouring states in the latter part of the 19th century. In 1880, he performed the second gastrectomy in history but it had a fatal outcome due to unrelenting haemorrhage. In the following year, he performed an identical gastrectomy as the 'Billroth I' for a benign gastric ulcer, which had bled intermittently for three years, but the procedure was eventually successful. The patient gave birth to five children and lived for another 25 years. Rydygier also performed subcapsular prostatectomy for benign hypertrophy preventing damage to the urethra; early successful resection of gangrenous loops of intestine for strangulated hernia and; he used a sacral approach for rectal cancer.

1.   Condensed from: Special comment by Rudowski Witold. In: *Surgery of the Esophagus, Stomach and Small Intestine*, 5th Ed. Nyhus LM, *et al.* Boston, New York, Toronto, London: Little, Brown and Company, 1995; 30: 382-5.

SALMON, Frederick (1796-1868). Portrait in Chapter 15.

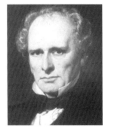

Main institution: Founder of St. Mark's Hospital, for Diseases of the Anus, Rectum and Colon, London, UK.

He succeeded in founding a specialist institution in the face of tremendous opposition from the surgical establishment. He felt problems such as fistula-in-ano were a neglected condition. His first inpatient institute was an eight-bedded ward in Aldersgate in the east end of London. He needed and found a larger site nearby in the parish of St. Mark's Church on the City Road. This became St. Mark's Hospital (Figure 3, Chapter 15). It became the centre for research and treatment of all colorectal disease. It moved to Northwick Park in Harrow in London in 1995.

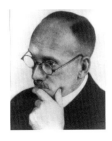

SAUERBRUCH, Ferdinand (1875-1951). Father of thoracic surgery.

Main institution: Professor of Surgery, Zurich and later, The Charité Hospital, Berlin, Germany.

He worked under Mikulicz, who he admired greatly; he was initially famous for developing a low-pressure chamber for both the patient and the surgeon, so that the lung would not collapse on opening the chest (before endotracheal intubation). He gained much experience in war wounds in World War I, and as Chief Surgeon to the German Army in World War II. He was also Hitler's surgeon in that war. Sauerbruch wrote an autobiography called *A surgeon's life (Das war mein leben)*, first published in 1953 by Andre Deutsch Ltd., 12 Thayer Street, Manchester Square, London W1, and was later translated by Fernand G. Renier and Anne Cliff. This was read after World War II by Nissen who, though he admired his old chief, believed the book was "probably written by a ghost writer, it was sensational and full of inaccuracies". He was known to be a fine technician, but perhaps was more known for his skills as an administrator.

Image reproduced with permission from Professor Bernard Launois, Department of Surgery, Rennes, France.

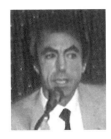

SCOPINARO, Nicola (born 1945). Portrait in Chapter 5.

Main institution: Professor of Surgery, University of Genoa Medical School, Genoa, Italy.

See the biography in Chapter 5.

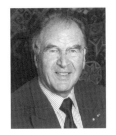

SEMM, Kurt (1927-2003). Portrait in Chapter 12.

Main institution: Gynaecological Surgeon, Director of the Department of Obstetrics and Gynaecology, and the Michaelis Midwifery School, Kiel, Germany.

Semm performed the first totally laparoscopic appendicectomy on September 13th 1980, and many other various gynaecological procedures. When he announced the operation at a meeting later, the President of the German Surgical Society demanded his suspension. His attempts to persuade the surgical establishment to use minimally invasive techniques for other operations such as cholecystectomy were likewise ignored. One colleague suggested that his mental state required a brain scan to exclude a tumour. He invented many instruments for minimally invasive surgery, including the first electronic carbon dioxide insufflator. He wrote many books on laparoscopic surgery, translated into several languages.

1.   Semm K. Endoscopic appendicectomy. *Endoscopy* 1983; 15: 59-64.

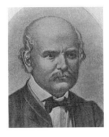

SEMMELWEISS, Ignaz Phillipp (1818-1865). Portrait in Chapter 3.

Main institution: University Hospital, Budapest, Hungary.

Born in Austria, Semmelweiss became a Hungarian nationalist when Hungary became part of the Austro-Hungarian Empire. He was an obstetrician and advocate for antisepsis in the prevention of puerperal sepsis by using soap, water and chlorine water. He reduced the mortality in his department from 10% to 1% by insisting on personnel washing their hands before attending patients.

After his friend died of an 'autopsy accident' from a penetrating wound, he noticed phlebitis, lymphangitis, peritonitis, pericarditis and meningitis as a result of the wound. He described this as 'corpse poison' and made his staff wash their hands with chloride of lime to destroy the poison. His theory was not believed and he was persecuted by his peers, including James Young Simpson, and eventually this led to insanity. Ironically, he died from septicaemia from an infection of his own finger.

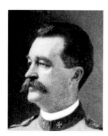

SENN, Nicholas (1844-1909). Portrait in Chapter 10.

Main institutions: Milwaukee and Rush University, Chicago, USA.

Born in Buchs in Switzerland, in 1852 he settled in Wisconsin. He studied at Rush Medical College, achieving an MD in Chicago in 1868. He investigated the action of digitalis, experimenting on himself and worked for three years in general practice in Wisconsin; then as an attending physician at Milwaukee Hospital, while doing experimental surgery in the basement at home. In 1886, he was appointed Foundation Professor of Surgery at the College of Physicians and Surgeons in Chicago; for the next seven years he commuted 80 miles on two or three days each week to lecture and conduct his clinics. In 1885, he described the clinical features of air embolism. In 1888, he became Professor of Surgery at Rush Medical College. He pioneered the use of X-rays in surgical diagnosis and invented the use of decalcified bone plates to approximate and suture divided intestine (Chapter 10). He had tremendous experience on active service and was in Cuba during the Spanish-American war. An expert on gunshot wounds of the abdomen and intestinal perforation, his career in Chicago paralleled that of Murphy, of whom he was a severe critic, until near to retirement. In 1891, he founded the Association of Military Surgeons (Brigadier General). In 1892, he served as President of the American Surgical Association, and in 1897, as President of the American Medical Association. In 1903, he treated leukaemia with radiotherapy. He made experimental work important in surgery and furthered both undergraduate and postgraduate medical education. He wrote several travel books (e.g. *Tahiti the island paradise*).

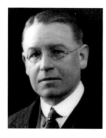

SHERREN, James (1872-1945). Portrait in Chapter 12.

Main institution: Surgeon, The London Hospital, London, UK.

Sherren went to sea aged 13. He obtained his Master's certificate aged 21 and became a medical student at the London Hospital in 1897, graduating in 1899; then made a Fellow of the Royal College of Surgeons in London in 1900. He conducted research on the nervous system, and demonstrated that apart from the oesophagus and rectum, all visceral sensations were referred. In 1905, he recommended removal of the appendix for early appendicitis, as delay and drainage of an appendix abscess was then the fashion (Chapter 12). He also advocated the conservative management of the appendix mass (the 'Ochsner-Sherren regime') for the late presentation of appendicitis. A renowned surgical technician, and at one particular time he was equated with Moynihan in Leeds, Finisterer in Vienna, and Balfour of the Mayo Clinic. However, most of his clinical research was in the nervous system. He did describe what is now known as 'Sherren's triangle', the area of hypersensitivity between the anterior superior iliac spine, the umbilicus and the pubic tubercle, when an obstructed or very badly inflamed appendix is present underneath. In 1911, he reported on the first excision of a double gallbladder. He suddenly retired without notice to colleagues and went back to sea.

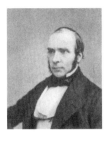

SNOW, John (1813-1858). Portrait in Chapter 2.

Main institution: St. George's Hospital, London, UK.

Snow was probably the first specialist anaesthetist in the UK. He started medical studies in Newcastle on Tyne but completed them when he moved down to London. He discovered that a water pump in Soho in London was contaminated by a sewer. He is renowned for ordering the removal of the handle of that Broad Street pump during a cholera epidemic, which halted the epidemic in days. His discovery of the waterborne transmission of cholera was not accepted for many years. He anaesthetised animals before moving to human patients, with a fine record of low mortality with chloroform on his patients. He silenced his critics by the successful use of chloroform when Prince Leopold was born to Queen Victoria in 1853.

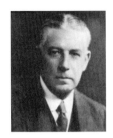

SOUTTAR, Sir Henry Sessions (1875-1964).

Main institution: Surgeon, The London Hospital, now The Royal London Hospital, London, UK.

He was an athlete and engineer before becoming a highly skilled endoscopist and surgeon at The London Hospital. He performed the first transauricular valvotomy in a young girl with mitral valve disease in 1925, despite the great Billroth's warning: "Let no man who wishes to maintain the respect of his medical brethren, dare to operate on the human heart!" Inventor of the first atraumatic needle, and the use of steam cautery for general haemostasis, he also pioneered the use of radon seed implants for tumours such as oesophageal cancers. Especially famous for his gold-plated spiral tube for palliation of dysphagia of oesophagogastric carcinoma illustrated in Chapter 4.

1.   Souttar HS. The surgical treatment of mitral stenosis. *Br Med J* 1925; 2: 603-6.
Image reproduced with permission from the Royal London Hospital Medical College Library.

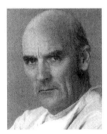

STEPHENS, F Douglas (born 1913). Portrait in Chapter 16.

Main institution: Royal Children's Hospital, Melbourne, Australia.

See the biography in Chapter 16.

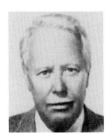

SWENSON, Orvar (born 1909). Portrait in Chapter 16.

Main institutions: Chicago Children's Memorial Hospital and North Western University, Chicago, USA.

See the biography in Chapter 16.

SYMONDS, Sir Charters James (1852-1932).

Main institution: Surgeon, Guy's Hospital, London, UK.

He was born in New Brunswick, Canada, and came to London with his widowed mother in 1859. His medical education was at University College and Guy's Hospital, London. In 1902, he was appointed full Surgeon to Guy's Hospital, London, where he had a reputation for being kind to his patients and the students under him. Later, he became a knight of the Realm. He removed a faecolith from an appendix at Guy's Hospital in 1883 with a good clinical result three years after Tait (vide infra). Like so many of his peers, he later advocated total appendicectomy. He founded the Royal Medical Benevolent Fund, and the Invalid Children's Aid Association. As a prototype ear, nose and throat surgeon, he had great experience in the intubation of malignant oesophageal disease starting in 1885 (Chapter 4). He once treated a rectal cancer successfully with pre-operative radiotherapy in 1913.

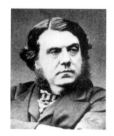

TAIT, Lawson Robert (1845-1899). Portrait in Chapter 12.

Main institution: Women's Hospital, Birmingham, UK.

Born in Edinburgh and trained in the Edinburgh Royal Infirmary until aged 22, Tait was a general surgeon and gynaecologist in Birmingham for most of his professional life. In 1870, he became a Fellow of the English and Edinburgh Colleges of Surgeons. He revived, reconstructed and presided over the Medical Defence Union. He was an ardent anti-vivisectionist, outwardly rejecting Listerian principles of antiseptic surgery, yet in reality practised aseptic surgery by careful cleansing of his hands, as well as the skin of the patient before operation. His many gynaecological achievements included: an ovariotomy in 1868; an ovariectomy in 1872; a hysterectomy for uterine fibroids employing silk ligatures instead of unreliable clamps in 1873; and finally, in 1879, he devised a perineal flap repair for posterior uterine prolapse and perfected cervical dilation for therapeutic and diagnostic purposes. In 1883, he achieved a successful outcome for ruptured tubal pregnancy. By this time, he established a dedicated hospital for women in Birmingham, UK. In hepatobiliary surgery in 1879, he performed his first cholecystostomy (Chapter 7), but believed cholecystectomy was too dangerous. In 1880, he performed the first hepatotomy for hydatid disease in nine patients and an abscess in one further patient. Otherwise, it was alleged he performed the first appendicectomy in the midst of an appendix abscess, although this case was not published until 9-10 years later. He wisely used two incisions due to the difficulty of the operation, reported in Chapter 12. In his final five years, he suffered from renal disease and stones.

1. Tait L. A case of perityphlitis successfully treated by abdominal section. *Br Med J* 1889; (Oct 5th): 763.
2. Tait RL. *Diseases of Women and Abdominal Surgery*. Leicester: Richardson, 1889.
3. Shepherd JA. Acute Appendicitis. A historical survey. *Lancet* 1954; 2: 298.
4. Shepherd JA. *Lawson Tait the Rebellious Surgeon (1845-1899)*. Kansas: Coronado Press, 1980.

TOREK, Franz (1872-1938).

Main institution: The German Hospital, New York, and New York Postgraduate Medical School, New York, USA.

He performed the first successful case of resection of the thoracic portion of the oesophagus for carcinoma, which led to the founding of the American Association for Thoracic Surgery. He employed the principle of restoring alimentary continuity outside the thorax and established a tube between the oesophagus in the neck and entering the stomach via a gastrostomy below (Chapter 4). In 1908, he perfected an orchidopexy operation which at the first stage held the mobilised previously undescended testis in the thigh.

1.　Torek F. The first successful resection of the thoracic portion of the oesophagus for carcinoma. *Surg Gynecol Obstet* 1913; 16: 614-7.

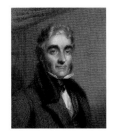

TRAVERS, Benjamin (1783-1858). Portrait in Chapter 10.

Main institution: Surgeon, St. Thomas's Hospital, London, UK.

Initially a pupil of Astley Cooper at Guy's Hospital, later, he became a surgeon to St. Thomas's Hospital. In 1809, he described the physical sign of an audible bruit through the skull due to a carotico-cavernous fistula. In 1811, he ligated the common carotid artery in an attempt to cure Berry aneurysm. In the following year, he demonstrated in animal studies that all layered sutures cut through to the lumen of intestine, but adhesions healed the bowel at the site of the sutures. This finding opened the floodgates for surgery of the intestines. He was the first demonstrator to show that provided there is mucosa-to-mucosa contact all round an anastomosis, an everting technique will work. He also became interested in ophthalmology at the London Infirmary for Diseases of the Eye. Quoted by Lembert in his classic paper 17 years later.

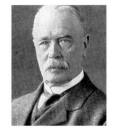

TRENDELENBURG, Friedrich (1844-1924).

Main institutions: Professor of Surgery, Bonn and Leipzig, Germany.

Born and later graduated in Berlin in 1866, his father sent him for a year to Scotland studying anatomy, embryology and physics. He attended some of Lord Lister's clinical surgery lectures. He returned to Berlin and was much influenced by Bernhard von Langenbeck. In 1875, he succeeded König at Rostock and from 1882-1895, he was appointed Professor of Surgery in Bonn. In 1895, he succeeded Thiersh at Leipzig. In 1872, as co-founder of the German Surgical Society, he was elected first President. He introduced elective tracheotomy for major surgery to the thorax, head and neck, to prevent aspiration during operations (Chapter 2) and invented an endotracheal tube with a surrounding tampon to prevent aspiration in 1877. In 1878, he was the first German to suture a ruptured patella after traumatic fracture and in 1881, he became known for the Trendelenburg position for a patient, although described by others long ago. Willy Meyer from New York publicised the head-down position as the 'Trendelenburg position'. He is also associated with the gluteal insufficiency test ('sound side sinks') in hip disease. In 1908, he devised a sternal split approach for the emergency operation of pulmonary embolectomy. At one attempt he nearly succeeded, but his pupil, Martin Kirschner, performed a successful pulmonary embolectomy 16 years later. In 1877, he was alleged to have performed the first gastrostomy to treat starvation due to oesophageal stricture. His name is also associated with a test for saphenofemoral insufficiency, although Benjamin Brodie had described the test earlier in 1846. He retired in 1911 and died in 1924, due to carcinoma of the lower jaw.

1.　Roger Maltby JR, Ed. *Notable names in Anaesthesia.* London: Royal Society of Medicine Press Ltd., 2002: 213-5.

Image courtesy of www.historiadelamedicina.org.

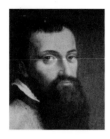

VESALIUS, Andreas (André Wesel) (1514-1564). Portrait in Chapter 1.

Main institution: Professor of Anatomy, Padua, Italy (at the age of 23).

See the biography in Chapter 1.

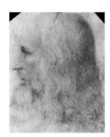

VINCI, Leonardo da (1452-1519). Portrait in Chapter 12.

Main institutions: Scientist and painter, Florence and later, Rome, Italy.

Founder of iconographic and physiological anatomy, he persuaded the Catholic Church to allow dissection of the human body in those not destined for Heaven, i.e. criminals. Although the Church was not officially against human dissection, many relatives of patients were against it. He became one of the earliest to dissent of 'Galenism'. He was an originator of cross-sectional anatomy, now part of CT scanning examinations. He discovered the A-V conducting fibres of the heart. He used a powerful exterior flame light source and a metal tube to examine the peritoneal cavity of animals as an early method of laparoscopy. He made the first illustration of the human appendix around 1515, although it was not published until later; about the same time as Vesalius' sketch in 1543. The portrait above was by his pupil, Francesco Melzi, and the drawing of the appendix is shown in Figure 2 in Chapter 12.

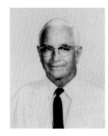

WANGENSTEEN, Owen Harding (1898-1981). Portrait in Chapter 9.

Main institution: Professor of Surgery, Minneapolis, Minnesota, USA.

See the biography in Chapter 9.

WARREN, John Collins (1778-1856).

Main institutions: Harvard University and Massachusetts General Hospital, Boston, USA.

Born in Boston, he was the eldest son of the founder of the Harvard Medical School. In 1799, he visited Astley Cooper in London, dissected at Guy's Medical School, London and later gained a MD degree at Edinburgh University. He subsequently visited Ribes, Sabatier, Chaussier, Cuvier and Dupuytren in Paris and in 1802, he returned to Boston later becoming Professor of Surgery in 1806. He founded the Massachusetts General Hospital and arranged the celebrated demonstration of ether anaesthesia in 1846. He is also one of the founders of the American Medical Association. He is alleged to be one of the first surgeons to operate on a strangulated hernia. He died aged 78.

WELLS, Thomas Spencer (1818-1897).

Main institution: St. Thomas's Hospital, London, UK.

Surgeon in the British Royal Navy and the Crimean War (1854-1856). In 1880, he had performed his 1,000th ovariotomy, with an operative mortality of 23%. He also removed uterine fibroids, performed hysterectomy, splenectomy, and nephrectomy before the establishment of full surgical asepsis. He performed his first hysterectomy for myoma in 1861 and first splenectomy in the UK in 1865, 39 years after Quittenbaum of Rostock in 1826, but the patient lived for only six days. He is noted for haemostasis by 'forci-pressure' by the crushing action of his designed forceps, rather than by tying or cauterising the pedicle nowadays. He introduced five different pedicle clamps before settling on his well-known unimanual pivoting haemostat, controlled by rack catches, and was first to measure the compression force exerted, at 22 pounds. He was known also for his bitter conflicts on surgical matters with Lawson Tait.

1. Wells TS. *Diagnosis and Surgical Treatment of Abdominal Tumours.* London: Churchill, 1885.
2. Shepherd JA. *Spencer Wells: the Life and Work of a Victorian Surgeon.* Edinburgh: Livingstone, 1965.

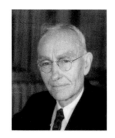

WHIPPLE, Allen Oldfather (1881-1963). Portrait in Chapter 8.

Main institution: Chief Surgeon, Presbyterian Hospital, New York, and Professor of Surgery, Columbia University, New York City, USA.

He is famous for the operation of pancreaticoduodenectomy for carcinoma of the head and ampulla of the pancreas. Although modified by recent surgeons, it still remains a standard operation for the attempted cure for carcinoma of the head and ampulla of the pancreas, and carcinoma of the proximal duodenum. He co-ordinated with the Radcliffe Infirmary, Oxford, UK, with the use of topical penicillin on burns in World War II. He was one of the earliest clinicians to co-ordinate physicians and surgeons to combine ward rounds on all gastroenterological patients. Also like Billroth, he instituted weekly audit meetings on mortality and morbidity in the US.

WÖLFLER, Anton (1850-1917).

Main institutions: University of Graz, Austria and Prague, Czech Republic.

A Bohemian, i.e. born in the current Czech Republic in Kopenzen on the 12th January 1850, Wölfler achieved his MD in 1874, and served under Billroth, and persuaded Billroth to 'Listerism'. He performed the first gastrojejunostomy in 1881 when he was 31. He became known as the 'father of gastrojejunostomy'. The hourglass sign due to mid-lesser curve gastric ulceration was known as 'Wölfler's sign'. He devised an 'inside to outside' suturing technique in intestinal surgery. In 1886, he was appointed as Professor of Surgery at Graz and became an expert in surgery of foreign bodies of the alimentary tract in his lifetime, and on surgery of the thyroid gland. In 1895, he was appointed as Professor of Surgery in Prague. He died in 1917 after a bout of depression ending in suicide.

ZAAYER, Johannes Henricus (1876-1932).

Main institution: Professor of Surgery, University of Leyden, The Netherlands.

Trained under Czerny in Heidelberg, he found Sauerbruch's negative pressure chamber costly and cumbersome. He developed positive pressure tracheal insufflation. He doubted von Mikulicz's dictum that achalasia was due to 'cardiospasm'. In 1913, he performed: two transpleural resections for carcinoma of the cardia, with success; and a two-staged procedure for carcinoma of the oesophagus, using the Sauerbruch chamber for the second stage. He also performed two Torek-style oesophageal resections.

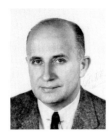

ZOLLINGER, Robert M (1903-1992). Portrait in Chapter 8.

Main institution: Professor of Surgery, Columbus, Ohio, USA.

See the biography in Chapter 8.